The Jossey-Bass Health Series brings together the most current information and ideas in health care from the leaders in the field. Titles from the Jossey-Bass Health Series include these essential health care resources:

E-Health, Telehealth, and Telemedicine

E-Health, Telehealth, and Telemedicine

A Guide to Start-Up and Success

MARLENE M. MAHEU

PAMELA WHITTEN

ACE ALLEN

Foreword by Evan Melrose, M.D.

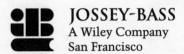

JOSSEY-BASS
A Wiley Company
San Francisco

Jossey-Bass books and products are available through most bookstores. To contact Jossey-Bass directly, call (888) 378-2537, fax to (800) 605-2665, or visit our website at www.josseybass.com.

Substantial discounts on bulk quantities of Jossey-Bass books are available to corporations, professional associations, and other organizations. For details and discount information, contact the special sales department at Jossey-Bass.

Manufactured in the United States of America on Lyons Falls Turin Book. This paper is acid-free and 100 percent totally chlorine-free.

Library of Congress Cataloging-in-Publication Data

E-health, telehealth, and telemedicine: A guide to start-up and success ; Marlene M. Maheu, Pamela Whitten, Ace Allen.
    p. cm.—(Jossey-Bass health series)
    Includes bibliographical references and index.
    ISBN 0-7879-4420-3
    1. Telecommunication in medicine. 2. Medical information. 3. Medicine—Communication systems. 4. Telemedicine—organization & administration. I. Maheu, Marlene M. II. Whitten, Pamela. III. Allen, Ace. IV. Series.
    R119.95.M334 2000
    362.1'028'21—dc20   00-59093

HB Printing   10 9 8 7 6 5 4 3 2 1   FIRST EDITION

CONTENTS

FOREWORD

I f you are involved in health care, telecommunication technologies, or
the study of either field, you owe it to yourself to read this book. This is
the first book I have seen in the telemedicine genre that was not dated by
the time it went to press. It is the optimal book to provide you with an in-
depth look at a wide range of issues in the field of health care and telecommunication technologies. I recommend this book for a variety of readers,
including health administrators, health practitioners, telecommunication
and technology specialists, and academics and their students.

I am highly impressed with this publication for three reasons. First, it
acknowledges that the use of telecommunication technologies in health
care has evolved far beyond traditional notions of telemedicine. The authors had the courage to tackle traditional telemedicine and telehealth issues, as well as the vast frontier of e-health. Readers are getting two books
for the price of one—and an overview of how technology and health are
evolving together.

Second, the range of topics covered in this book is quite impressive.
Telehealth and e-health are complex phenomena that span technological, organizational, regulatory, and clinical issues. This book tackles each of these
issues in depth and then some. For example, the authors address the development, management, and research-related aspects of telehealth and
e-health. However, they do not simply graze through a vast array of content.
Instead, each chapter is well researched and thorough. I invite you to examine the References section; this book is perhaps the most thoroughly researched publication in this field to date. The authors also include pragmatic

information from professionals with real experiences in this field. I was especially impressed with the testimonies presented in several of the chapters and in Appendix A. The Resources section is also quite extensive.

Finally, this book is well written and easy to read. Although there is a great deal of information, the writers have written the book in basic business English to allow readers from any field to easily grasp the underlying principles and apply them to their particular situations. In addition, each chapter is so well organized that readers can readily find specific topics and see how they fit into the overall schema.

It would be remiss of me to conclude these comments without acknowledging the scope of expertise and experience among the three authors of this book. Marlene Maheu, Ph.D., is a licensed psychologist with years of experience in Internet-based health care delivery and consultation with dot-com companies. Pamela Whitten, Ph.D., possesses practical experience gained through running a wide variety of telehealth and e-health projects; she is also one of the most active academic researchers in this field. Ace Allen, M.D., is truly a pioneer in the field of telemedicine as a provider and as the editor and publisher of the most respected trade publication in this field.

I encourage you to dive into this book. I think you will find much of the information both practical and thought provoking.

Philadelphia   Evan Melrose
November 2000

Evan Melrose, M.D., is a founder and managing director of eHealth Capital Network, a global network of incubator-investment hubs and strategic partners dedicated to developing the e-health market space. He is on the family medicine faculty at the University of Pennsylvania School of Medicine and is finishing his M.B.A. studies at the Wharton School.

PREFACE

Technological development is accelerating in two areas that will influence health care dramatically: the fields of medicine and communication. This book is primarily about the influence of communication technologies on health care. It will only secondarily mention various developments in medical technology as they complete the discussion of communication technology. However, it must be kept in mind that as this decade advances, the boundary between medical and communication technologies will increasingly blur.

Unprecedented change in health care is upon us. The use of telecommunication technology (including the Internet) in health care is indispensable from a competitive standpoint, as well as transformative from a global standpoint. Many federally funded pilot programs have proved and disproved the feasibility of various approaches to improving on bricks-and-mortar health services. The best of these services face the true test as they begin to share a common platform and migrate to the Internet.

Lessons learned in pilot programs will streamline services. Marketplace forces are now forging a new health care system offering increasingly less invasive strategies that are deliverable around the globe in a matter of minutes. Legislative and technological advances will make the use of technology increasingly appealing. Professional groups of all types are already forming strategic planning committees to assess opportunities and entry points for staking a claim in this new territory. Workshops and seminars related to e-health, telehealth, and telemedicine are already popular at national and international conferences.

Many professionals and their organizations are awakening to the enormous potential for service delivery through technology. Most have been slow to adopt change, however. Although they are curious about offering immediate, high-quality care to their patients and having easier access to continuing professional education, they have not found it easy to integrate technology into their traditional work flows.

In the midst of this changing landscape, a definitive work is needed to point the way to the practicalities of design, implementation, and management of successful start-ups. Professionals still lack a basic text describing what is currently available to them and where to begin. This book aims to fill that gap by guiding you through the steps to building successful e-health, telehealth, and telemedicine services and products.

This book is written for the health care executive, administrator, practitioner, and student. It has captured the successful components of telecommunication technology's influence on health care and presented an integrated review of the existing literature to offer you practical information about getting started. It serves as a general resource guide for accessing nuts-and-bolts information for those interested in developing or improving health care in government, military, and hospital systems, as well as in the private sector. It shows how health care professionals can bring innovative communication tools to the full range of health care settings, including private or group practice. It reviews essential elements of program development, ethics, laws, and technical options, all while providing examples of e-health, telehealth, and telemedicine models that are already established and flourishing.

The overarching goal of the book is to provide a well-researched yet practical guide to setting up remote health care services using a variety of technologies. Our primary attempt has been to outline general principles that work for many people who have developed successful programs and companies. We provide useful information to inspire your creativity. This book, then, is a guide for making sense of what has been learned, combining this information with solid business principles, and creating flexible blueprints for developing and managing a successful start-up in the new and exciting health care marketplace.

OVERVIEW OF THE CONTENTS

The book begins by setting the historical stage and introducing the benefits of and challenges to telecommunication technology. Chapter One also gives a brief overview of the major issues to be discussed in greater detail throughout the book. Chapter Two is an overview of current and emerging opportunities provided by e-health technologies. Chapter Three focuses on how to choose the best equipment to meet specific programmatic needs and how to optimize the use of this equipment. Chapter Four outlines specific clinical applications to various medical specialties, such as radiology, home care, and behavioral health. Chapter Five describes telemedicine and telehealth applications in military, correctional, school, and other specialized settings. Chapter Six reviews the trend toward computerization of medical records both through private programs and e-health. It also discusses changes in the laws regulating this movement. Chapter Seven examines in detail the issues of privacy, confidentiality, security, and data integrity, giving tips and suggesting practical approaches to organizations and professionals for protecting themselves and their patients in the electronic health care environment. Chapter Eight discusses legal developments on both the state and federal levels, along with ethical and credentialing information. It covers confidentiality and other informed consent issues, proper documentation, staff training, and vendor selection. Chapter Nine highlights malpractice issues, and offers a number of points to consider when developing risk management policies. Because people need to understand how to develop their own programs and companies, Chapter Ten offers a blueprint for building a successful business plan, obtaining funding, maximizing referral networks, and managing other critical aspects of getting started. Chapter Eleven details approaches to research and to outcome assessment. The last chapter discusses what to expect in the next decade and examines national and international trends.

Throughout the book, vignettes highlight information we have gleaned through our direct contact with many of the key companies and organizations that are involved in e-health, telehealth, and telemedicine. These vignettes describe challenges, successful strategies, and experiences with start-up, vendors, and management. Specific Web site names will be mentioned throughout this book. Given the wide variety of Web sites available, selection of those mentioned was based on two factors: Web site owners' responses to our direct inquiries for interviews and the authors' opinions of exemplary Web sites in operation at the time of this writing.

We have also included a glossary of telehealth terms (boldfaced at their first appearance in the book), and the Resources section lists Web sites, e-mail addresses, and publications related to e-health, telehealth, and telemedicine. Appendix A presents a collection of lessons learned from some of the leading professionals across the country. Appendix B discusses issues related to vendor agreements and offers a checklist for vendor agreements, and suggests a sampling of teleconferencing and videoconferencing vendors. Finally, Appendix C provides tips for videoconference room layout and videoconferencing etiquette.

Business leaders as well as practitioners at every level need to have a comprehensive text explaining the practical, ethical, legal, technical, and future applications of telecommunication technology in health care. The overall intent of this book, then, is to serve as a how-to guide for the business owner, professional, administrator, and vendor. It is written for those interested in getting started in the delivery and processing of e-health, telehealth, and telemedicine. This book is more than an anecdotal text of our opinions, however. We have rigorously researched and documented the experiences of dozens of health care providers, administrators, vendors, and business executives who are experienced in the use of telecommunication technology.

ACKNOWLEDGMENTS

Special appreciation is given to Tim Mount for his precision and dedication in the monumental task of compiling information and preparing this manuscript for publication. Ryan Thurman also deserves mention for his work in researching much of the literature and assisting with the manuscript. Laura Struhl deserves acknowledgment for her unfailing support throughout the research and writing process.

In addition, this project has benefited from the collaboration of our many students and colleagues. They have generously donated their time and talent to brainstorm and research, and to distill their experiences. Some have even rewritten portions of the manuscript for us. We are grateful to them all for making this a better guide for those who seek the wisdom of the pioneers in telemedicine, telehealth, and e-health: David Adams, George Alexander, Robert Ax, Ofir Baharav, Bruce Bennett, Marshall Brackbill, John Bringenberg, Cathy Britain, Heather Brytan, Craig Buchholz, Tom Caffrey, Jeanne Callan, Dan Carnicom, Bonnie Cassidy, Suresh Challa, David Chazin, Nancy Cobble, Linda Cole, Ted Cooper, Susan Cossette, Robert Cox, Sally Davis, Susan Day, Gary Doolittle, Richard Dorsey, John Economos, Hans Ehrnrooth, Wendy Everett, Tom Ferguson, Richard Flanagan, Tom Friar, Daniel Frieling, Michelle Gailiun, Ann Garnier, Victoria Garshnek, Robert Glueckauf, Mitchell Gold, Barry L. Gordon, William Grigsby, Robin Hawkins, Robert Higginson, J. Gil Hill, Jeff Hitton, Jerry Hodges, Michael Hurst, John Ingram, Leigh Jerome, Kent Johnson, Warren Karp, Janice Kennedy, Jennifer Kohn, Gerald Koocher, Tracy Kormylo, Shannah Koss, G. Ed Kriese, Vince Kuraitis, Kristine Kurth, Robert Levine, Debi Lewinski, John Mack, Phil Magaletta, Don McBeath, Joe McMenamin, Evan Melrose, John Miller, Carolyn Moeller, Lynn Morris, Thomas Nagy, Konjit Page, John-Ashley Paul, Tony Pavel, Myron Pulier, Dena Puskin, Robert Pyke, Karen Rau, James Reid, Harry Rhodes, Sheila Richards, Holly Russo, Elizabeth Saindon, Jay Sanders, Steven Schelhammer, Loretta Schlachta, Paul Schneider, Jenny Schweiters, Nancy Sharpe, Amit Sheth, Joey Skroski, Michael

Smith, Scott St. Clair, B. Hudnall Stamm, Steven Strode, Rosa Ana Tang, Carol Tomlinson-Keasey, Tom Trabin, Carl Tsukahara, Glen Tullman, Emily Van Ness, Star Vega, Michael Weiss, Jeremy Wyant, Peter Yellowlees, Laura Young, Charles Zaylor, and Thomas Zeffiro.

San Diego, California   Marlene M. Maheu

East Lansing, Michigan   Pamela Whitten

Overland Park, Kansas   Ace Allen

November 2000

THE AUTHORS

Marlene M. Maheu, Ph.D., is the CEO and president of E-Health Interactive, an e-health company devoted to developing informational services for professionals and consumers. She is the founder and editor in chief of SelfhelpMagazine.com, an online community and informational ethics demonstration project. Established in 1994, this award-winning site was the first, and remains one of the largest, mental health portals on the Internet. Maheu has also developed Telehealth.net, a Web site for professionals who want to keep abreast of news and research related to telehealth and e-health. She also administers several e-mail discussion groups and two newsletters for online professionals and consumers.

Maheu holds a Ph.D. degree (1985) in clinical psychology from the California School of Professional Psychology and a B.A. degree (summa cum laude, 1977) from the University of Hartford. She is currently the director of telehealth for the Alliant University, where she oversees a postgraduate professional training program in telehealth and e-health. She also serves the American Psychological Association as a member of the Committee on Professional Practice Standards and as the APA Division 46 cochair for the Task Force for Media and Telehealth. In working with the California Psychological Association, she serves as the chair for the Presidential Task Force for Telehealth, as a member of the Committee for Continuing Education, and as a member of the Innovations in Psychology Task Force.

An internationally recognized speaker, Maheu organizes as well as participates in numerous e-health and telehealth symposia. Maheu is a licensed psychologist in San Diego, California, and offers consultation to organizations interested in developing ethical and secure e-health services.

Pamela Whitten, Ph.D., is currently an assistant professor in the Department of Telecommunication at Michigan State University. She has been actively involved in telehealth throughout the last decade from an administrative as well as evaluative perspective. Prior to her recent move to Michigan, Whitten was the director of telemedicine services at the University of Kansas Medical Center. In this role, she was initially responsible for developing a sustainable telemedicine organizational and economic infrastructure, and subsequently managed all telemedicine operations at the University of Kansas Medical Center. Under her administration, the telemedicine program evolved into a system that made dozens of medical services available to clients located at rural hospitals, mental health centers, patients' homes, elementary schools, and a jail. In addition, she was responsible for implementing a wide range of health education programs for health providers as well as for the general population.

To shift the focus of her professional life to research and evaluation, Whitten joined the faculty at Michigan State University in fall 1998. In her current position, she conducts technology- and health-related research as well as teaches graduate and undergraduate telecommunications courses. Whitten has published numerous studies in academic journals; her research focuses on the use of technology in health care, with a specific interest in telehealth and its impact on the delivery of health care services and education.

Whitten holds a Ph.D. degree in organizational communication from the University of Kansas, an M.A. degree in communication from the University of Kentucky, and a B.S. degree in management from Tulane University.

Ace Allen, M.D., is a board-certified medical oncologist and associate professor in the Department of Medicine at the University of Kansas Medical Center. His interest in telemedicine began in 1991, when he became aware of the Kansas telemedicine pilot project begun in 1990. Allen staffed several oncology fly-in outreach clinics in rural Kansas, many of which would be periodically cancelled because of poor flying conditions. Frustration with the inefficiency and expense of the fly-in clinics prompted him to apply for a National Cancer Institute Career Development Award (KO-7 Grant) to allow him to pursue implementation and evaluation of a teleoncology outreach clinic. With award of the grant in 1993, he set up a series of teleoncology clinics between the University of Kansas Medical School in Kansas City and rural Hays, Kansas. These clinics have been carefully evaluated for patient and physician satisfaction. He is involved in research of satisfaction, efficacy, and cost-benefit considerations of other aspects of the Kansas Telemedicine Project, including home telehealth as well as teleoncology.

Allen is a founding member of the American Telemedicine Association, the International Society for Telemedicine, the Telemedicine Research Center, and the Association of Telemedicine Service Providers. He is also the editor in chief and publisher of *Telemedicine Today,* a bimonthly e-health magazine published since 1992, with an international circulation.

Allen is also CEO of Today Communications, an Internet health (e-health) company that matches consumers and professionals to the Internet-based information, products, and services that best meet their individual needs and requirements.

CHAPTER 1

History, Definitions, and Current Applications

Hector's earache flared up in the middle of the school day. Rather than call a parent to leave work and try to get a quick appointment with Hector's doctor, the teacher sent Hector to the school nurse, who obtained faxed permission from Hector's mother. She then set up a video link with an available consulting pediatrician located across town and got Hector's regular pediatrician's office to fax that doctor a copy of Hector's medical record. With the school nurse's help and hands, the consulting physician was able to examine Hector adequately. The nurse listened to Hector's heart and breathing sounds with an electronic stethoscope, checked his ears with an electronic otoscope, and looked down his throat. She talked with Hector to assess his mood and level of pain. From his medical record, she noted his history of chronic ear and throat infections and his allergy to penicillin. Through this teleconsult, the pediatrician diagnosed a recurrent ear infection, coordinated with Hector's regular physician, and had the nurse send a throat swab to the lab. Hector's classmates were not judged at risk of infection from Hector. When he took the school bus home, Hector had a set of printed instructions and a slip for a follow-up appointment with his regular pediatrician. The antibiotic prescription that the consulting physician had faxed to the pharmacy was delivered before dinner.

Telecommunication technologies are being used to change the health care industry in unprecedented and irreversible ways. At their best, these technologies are enabling delivery of health care to remote patients and facilitating information exchange between generalists and specialists. At their worst, they leave decision makers with far too many choices about the best use of technology, too little technical training with which to make those choices, and too many unanswered questions about efficacy, costs, **security,** privacy, ethics, risk management, return on investment, and other important matters.

This book focuses on the telecommunication technology–based service delivery systems that will reshape the standard of health care. Telemedicine, telehealth, and e-health are a progression in an inexorable transformation in health care. The question is no longer, Will these new technologies work in health care? but rather, How will we make them work best? This chapter introduces the subject matter by defining terms, looking at the underlying movements, and acknowledging the potential benefits and challenges.

DEFINITIONS

The following sections define three overlapping categories of electronic health care: telemedicine, telehealth, and e-health. Because the similarities between telemedicine and telehealth are greater than the differences, we define them in one section, e-health in another.

Telemedicine and Telehealth

As in any technological area, health care and telecommunication definitions change to adjust to the vagaries of language use and developing concepts. An example of this phenomenon is the distinction—or lack of distinction—between *telemedicine* and *telehealth*. Telemedicine—the provision of health care services, clinical information, and education over a distance using telecommunication technology—existed long before the **Internet.** Some authors note that telemedicine was broadly conceived even when the term was first coined nearly thirty years ago (Willemain & Mark, 1971). Some of the first telemedicine reports were of group therapy (Wittson, Affect, & Johnson, 1961), nursing interactions (Cunningham, Marshall, & Glazer, 1978), education and training (Menolascino & Osborne, 1970), **telemetry** (Fuchs, 1979), televisits to community health workers (Straker, Mostyn, & Marshall, 1972), medical image transmission (Jutras & Duckett, 1957), home care (Mark, 1974), and other applications. In many cases, no physician was involved, and interactivity was not a necessary part of the transaction.

Telehealth is seen by some authors as being a more encompassing term than telemedicine, which they define as restricted to interactive patient-physician teleconsultations. Other dimensions have been used to draw distinctions between the terms. For example, "telehealth is understood to mean the integration of telecommunication systems into the practice of protecting and promoting health, while telemedicine is the incorporation of these systems into curative medicine" (World Health Organization, 1997). It is of note that toward the end of the 1990s, the term telehealth grew in popularity and is now used by many as a synonym for the older term, telemedicine. A number of other terms, such as *health informatics, health telematics,* and *telecare* have been proposed for this newly forming field. Because of their slow acceptance and controversial definitions, we are omitting them from this book. The large and ever-changing number of terms reflects the field's dynamic nature and continual evolution (Bashshur, 2000).

E-Health

In 1999, e-health surfaced as a popular term that refers to Internet-based health care delivery (McLendon, 2000). The term is reflective of a sea change: the movement from innovative health care delivery through independent telemedicine and telehealth projects to the worldwide distribution **network** known as the Internet. Given the significance of this movement, a major portion of this text will be devoted to e-health.

E-health refers to all forms of electronic health care delivered over the Internet, ranging from informational, educational, and commercial "products" to direct services offered by professionals, nonprofessionals, businesses, or consumers themselves. E-health services encompass the "five C's": *content, connectivity, commerce, community,* and *clinical care* (Lee, Conley, & Preikschat, 2000), to which some would add a sixth: *computer applications* in the form of application service providers, or ASPs (Savas, Parekh, & Fisher, 1999). (Chapter Five discusses ASPs in more detail.)

E-health draws on the unique capabilities of the Internet while enabling delivery of the clinical services that have characterized telehealth and telemedicine. As a result, e-health is making health care more efficient, allowing patients and professionals to do the previously impossible through the efficiencies of the Internet.

E-health differs from telehealth and telemedicine by not being "professional-centric." In fact, there is no doubt that the e-health groundswell is being led by people who are not health professionals. Consumers are driving the bus and are demanding and using the services and tools that the Internet can provide. This is an unstoppable force and is what will impel distance health care into our general lives, especially as bandwidth availability soars and prices plummet. Another difference is that most e-health services are motivated by financial gain, whereas telehealth and telemedicine are not (Bashshur, 2000). (Please note, however, that many in the industry feel that the term *e-health* will eventually be used universally for telemedicine and telehealth applications as well as for the current conception of this term.)

THE HISTORY OF TELECOMMUNICATION TECHNOLOGY IN HEALTH CARE

Although e-health has captured the mind and heart of the global economy, we begin by reviewing the roots of telecommunication technology in health care: telemedicine. We will then look at the shift to telehealth and then the strong movement toward e-health.

The Birth of Telemedicine

Telemedicine technologies can be traced to the pretelevision era. In the early 1900s, radio communications were used for providing medical services to Antarctica (Sullivan & Lugg, 1995). The first transtelephonic "electrical stethoscope" was demonstrated in England in 1910 (Brown, 1910). As early as 1924, researchers were describing the potential of a remote "radio doctor" who could both see and be seen by the patient (Institute of Medicine [IOM], 1996). In 1950, radiological images were transmitted for the first time, between West Chester and Philadelphia, Pennsylvania (Gershon-Cohen & Cooley, 1950).

The first use of interactive video communications in health care occurred in the late 1950s, when the Nebraska Psychiatric Institute used a two-way interactive television system for telepsychiatry consultations with Norfolk State Hospital, 112 miles away. This link was developed for education, specialized treatment, and consultation between specialists and general practitioners (Wittson et al., 1961). Another experimental project became active in 1959, when a Canadian radiologist used images transmitted by coaxial cable for a diagnostic consult (Jutras, 1959). In the late 1960s, a teledermatology demonstration project linked a polyclinic from Logan International Airport in Boston to Massachusetts General Hospital. Using an interactive audio-video system, physicians were able to deliver services by using gray-scale screens (no color) to communicate relative degrees of erythema (Murphy & Bird, 1974).

The National Aeronautics and Space Administration (NASA) was also central in the early development of telemedicine. Concerned about the effects of zero gravity on the physical condition of astronauts, NASA had an early need to monitor vital signs during space missions (Bashshur & Lovett, 1997). Fueled by its successes, NASA supported the establishment of a comprehensive test bed system. Known as STARPAHC (Space Technology Applied to Rural Papago Health Care), this program was incubated on the Tohono Odham (formerly Papago) reservation in Arizona. Spanning approximately twenty years, the program tested **satellite**-based communications designed to provide both the reservation and astronauts with a wide range of medical services (Fuchs, 1979).

NASA was also a pioneer in distributing advanced telemedicine technology following the devastating earthquake that struck Mexico City in

1985 (Garshnek & Burkle, 1999a, 1999b). NASA furnished the Advanced Technology-3 communications satellite (ATS-3), enabling the American Red Cross and the Pan American Health Organization to communicate and coordinate disaster rescue operations within twenty-four hours after virtually all land-based communications were disrupted ("NASA Satellite," 1985).

NASA maintained its interest in disaster assistance through telehealth technology. In 1988, NASA conducted the first international telehealth program, known as Space Bridge (now called Space Bridge to Russia), to provide medical consultation to earthquake victims in Armenia. This program was based on technology originally developed for astronauts (Garshnek, 1991; Llewellyn, 1995). Consultants used satellite-based communication to deliver one-way video, voice, and facsimile medical care from four medical centers in the United States to a health center in Yerevan, Armenia, in the areas of psychiatry orthopedics, neurology, infectious disease, and general surgery (Garshnek & Burkle, 1999a, 1999b; Nicogossian, 1989).

In 1985, the SatelLife/HealthNet program began to provide health communication information and services in developing countries. It linked urban medical centers to remote clinics and practitioners in nine African nations, the Philippines, and three countries in the Americas (Ferguson, Doarn, & Scott, 1995). The system provided e-mail communications and CD-ROM availability via the HealthSat satellites (**LEO** satellites), for a fraction of the cost of **geostationary** satellites (Garshnek & Hassell, 1997).

These various programs demonstrated that telemedicine could overcome cultural, social, political, and economic barriers, and they set the stage for many similar experiments in subsequent years. Dozens of similar projects have since surfaced throughout the world, assimilating these basic concepts into many other applications. However, despite their many successes, most of these projects have folded. Their demise was not the result of a lack of efficacy or patient satisfaction. The main reason for their failure was their inability to sustain themselves financially upon withdrawal of external (often federal) funding. Although these early attempts were not ultimately accepted as a cost-effective alternative to the then-standard modes of health care delivery, they provided rich evidence for the clinical effectiveness of (and satisfaction with) remote consultation, education, and training.

Rebirth of Telemedicine, 1990–1995

By 1985, only one of the early North American telemedicine programs remained (House & Roberts, 1977). Founded in the 1970s by Dr. A. M. (Max) House and headquartered at Memorial University of Newfoundland, this relatively low-tech program continues to operate to the present day. It uses low-**bandwidth** telephone links to transmit two-way audio and one-way still images for medical education, and to transmit tele-EEGs for remote diagnosis. (In the mid-1990s, this program began to expand its services using higher-bandwidth interactive video technologies.)

The beginning of the 1990s saw the rebirth of telemedicine. The telemedicine renaissance in the United States was spawned by changes in the health care environment, with recognition that there was inequitable access to medical care in rural areas. As a political consequence, there was a significant increase in federal funding of rural telemedicine projects. For instance, in 1991, Dr. Jay Sanders was asked by the governor of Georgia and the president of the Medical College of Georgia to develop a statewide telemedicine program. This program became the first statewide program in the United States, and it generated much enthusiasm. It received site visits from more than thirty interested parties and inspired the development of numerous other telemedicine programs (J. Sanders, personal communication, May 29, 2000). The 1990s also brought advances in image **digitization** and **data compression** technology, which enabled interactive **videoconferencing** over lower-bandwidth lines. This meant that programs could function without having to use high-cost satellites or other options.

By 1993, there were ten telemedicine programs using interactive videoconferencing technology in the United States (Allen, 1993). Since then, the number of programs has approximately doubled each year, with a pari passu increase in the number of clinician-patient interactions. Figure 1.1 shows this growth of the two most common types of technologies used in telemedicine between 1993 and 1999: interactive televideoconferencing and **store-and-forward** technologies. Both are discussed in greater detail in Chapter Three.

Early funding between 1993 and 1995 led to increased awareness of and interest in telemedicine projects and set the stage for further funding of broader applications to be developed in the years that followed.

Figure 1.1. Clinical Telemedicine Activity in the United States, 1993–1999

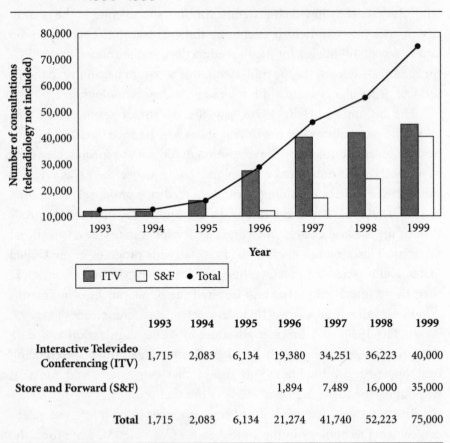

	1993	1994	1995	1996	1997	1998	1999
Interactive Televideo Conferencing (ITV)	1,715	2,083	6,134	19,380	34,251	36,223	40,000
Store and Forward (S&F)				1,894	7,489	16,000	35,000
Total	1,715	2,083	6,134	21,274	41,740	52,223	75,000

Source: Allen & Grigsby, 1998, p. 19.

E-Health, Telehealth, and Telemedicine

The escalation in development of telemedicine programs was in large part spawned by widespread state and federal funding. Budget allocations for telemedicine in the combined years 1994 and 1995 exceeded $100 million. In 1994, due to broad support, Congress established a bipartisan Steering Committee on Telehealth and Health Care Informatics. The committee was charged with researching how the rapid growth of information technology could be used to achieve maximum improvements in health care access, especially for rural populations (Deleon, Vanden Bos, Sammons, & Frank, 1998). With rare exceptions, the U.S. telemedicine programs begun in the early 1990s were funded, at least initially, by federal grants for equipment and infrastructure.

In 1995, the Department of Health and Human Services (DHHS) set up an interagency group called the Joint Working Group on Telemedicine (JWGT) to foster cost-effective clinical applications. The JWGT coordinates telemedicine activities and ensures that there is no overlap in federal funding. Members contribute their unique telemedicine expertise, making the JWGT a sort of forum for the discussion and sharing of information, member education, and ideas for reducing barriers to the effective use of telemedicine technologies.

Changes in Telemedicine Since 1995

Perhaps the most important contributors to our current understanding of telehealth have come from seminal "second-generation" projects initiated in the 1990s. During the mid- and late 1990s, federal and state governments allocated of hundreds of millions of dollars toward building projects that proliferated throughout the United States and internationally. Informed and creative clinicians viewed telehealth as an opportunity to develop new service delivery formats. Both rural populations and specialized urban populations were targeted in these second-generation projects to identify additional benefits of telehealth.

In the interest of coordinating federal government activities, DHHS in 1998 created the Office for the Advancement of Telehealth (OAT) to aid in the promotion of health care services using telecommunication technologies by fostering partnerships within the Health Resources and Services Administration and with other federal agencies, states, and private sector groups. Its purpose is to create telehealth projects, administer telehealth grant programs, provide technical assistance, develop distance learning and training programs, assess technology investment strategies, evaluate the use of telehealth technologies and programs, develop telehealth policy initiatives to improve access to quality health services, and promote knowledge exchange about best practices in telehealth.

Despite significant federal funding for start-up, certain second-generation programs were unable to sustain themselves when grant funding ended. However, numerous other programs (for example, East Carolina University, Marquette General Hospital in Michigan, University of Arkansas, and the Eastern Montana Telemedicine Project) have successfully demonstrated the long-term feasibility and sustainability of telehealth systems.

The newest waves of telehealth programs entering the scene at the end of the 1990s have graduated from pilot project status and have now entered a realm that should provide valuable information regarding clinical efficacy and cost-effectiveness. Among these sites are the California Telehealth Initiative, the Nova Scotia Telehealth Initiative, and the Children's Memorial Hospital (Chicago) Telecardiology Project.

The Space Bridge to Russia project has also evolved since the 1980s into a more comprehensive program that currently serves as a test bed for evaluating e-health-based infrastructures and applications (Garshnek & Burkle, 1999a, 1999b; *Internet Tools,* 1999). Electronic medical records have been made available on the Internet for practitioners to consult on clinical cases. The project also uses e-mail and interactive video supported on the Internet to provide physician education and consultation.

At present, the most significant and widespread telehealth activities involve international activities. The most active participants are the United States, Australia, Canada, France, Germany, the United Kingdom, Greece, Italy, Japan, Malaysia, Norway, the Netherlands, Sweden, Switzerland, and Finland (Garshnek & Hassell, 1997). As of 1999, there were in excess of 170 interactive video-telehealth programs in the United States alone (Grigsby & Brown, 2000). These programs will most likely continue as self-sustaining stand-alone projects, merge with similar programs to form larger private networks, or expand into Internet-based e-health companies.

Important lessons were learned from a number of telehealth programs initiated using internal or state-initiated (as opposed to federally funded) resources (for example, the University of Kansas, the University of Texas, the Ohio State University, University of Iowa **Teleradiology**, IN-PHACT Teleradiology, and Kaiser Permanente). A reliable model has been tested in many settings. Preliminary evidence suggests that these self-funded projects have enjoyed earlier success in attaining higher numbers of patient consults and financial sustainability (Grigsby & Allen, 1997). Their success may result from operating on leaner budgets with missions that extended beyond testing feasibility or providing a demonstration project. An interesting exception to this trend is the Norwegian Telemedicine Project centered in Tromsø, in northern Norway. This nationwide project has emerged as perhaps the most active program in the world, and has been developed with strong federal support since its inception in 1988.

Current Uses of Telecommunication Technology in Health Care

The combined effect of several decades of national and international experimentation with telecommunication technology in health care is an increasingly integrated system of synchronous (or same-time, **real-time**) and asynchronous (store-and-forward, such as e-mail) technologies designed to deliver the optimal care at any given moment for any given patient.

The typical telehealth model involves a **hub** hospital with satellite hospitals or clinics. The hub hospital is staffed with specialists twenty-four hours a day. Nurse-practitioners, physician assistants, or mental health counselors staff satellite hospitals or clinics.

When a specialist is needed, the professional and the patient place a videoconference call from the satellite hospital to the hub hospital and interact with the specialist. Remote practitioners and patients have access to specialized consultation, often within a few hours. No longer must physicians leave their practice, home, or office to deliver services to people in remote areas. Rather, they establish "on-call hours" and have professionals in remote clinics or hospitals call them via videoconferencing or, in the case of teleradiology, store-and-forward equipment. Some of these services are now delivered via the Internet.

Technology has had profound effects on many aspects of the health care system.

Clinical applications have a beneficial impact on all areas of patient care, such as diagnostic, treatment, and monitoring services. They are provided by real-time or store-and-forward technologies that range from the telephone to fax machines, e-mail, **chat rooms,** discussion boards, and audio- and videoconferencing. As we will discuss in subsequent chapters, the choice of technology and mode of transmission depends largely on the limitations of the setting, the needs of the patient, and the preferences of the practitioner.

Administrative applications include the recording and sharing of billing summaries, electronic connections to pharmacies for prescription ordering and cross-checking for conflict between prescription drugs, checking medical records for inconsistencies between past and current treatments, research, and public health record keeping and administration.

Remote medical instruments include various types of imaging technologies, pressure sensors, haptic feedback devices, and robotics used in special applications such as telesurgery. They include remote blood pressure cuffs, thermometers, and portable EKG units with plug-ins for computer transmission of reports to professionals. More specialized applications include wireless technologies that allow for access to medical records from a distance.

Educational applications include continuing medical education for professionals, educational resources for patients, and self-monitoring devices for patients to help cue them for agreed-on behavioral changes. Other examples of educational applications include **telementoring,** in which learning is the explicit objective of the consultation. For example, if a rural practitioner uses a series of case consultations with a consulting specialist to learn how to diagnose or manage a clinical problem, this form of training may obviate consultation in subsequent cases. Practitioners in developing countries also are able to keep informed of the latest medical information. Health care providers in these countries have traditionally suffered from limitations in their ability to share health information, participate in disease tracking through databases, and track emerging diseases. Using high-tech tools and the Internet, physicians in these countries can now connect with each other and other professionals (Dertouzos, 1997; IOM, 1996; Mitka, 1998).

BENEFITS OF TELECOMMUNICATION TECHNOLOGIES

Many sectors are in a favorable position to gain from advances in health care telecommunication technologies. These technologies promise to address three of the leading problems faced by the U.S. health care system:

1. Maldistribution of health care resources, including facilities and practitioners

2. Limited access to health care resources for specific segments of the population, including people living in rural or geographically isolated areas and those who are physically confined or who are not well enough to travel

3. Continued rise in the cost of health care, including the costs paid by the public and private sectors (Bashshur & Lovett, 1997)

This section will first briefly examine the many contributions of telehealth programs toward solving these problems, and then look at how the Internet is increasingly contributing solutions to these problems as well. The remainder of this book will look in much greater detail at benefits of and challenges to telecommunication technology in health care.

Telehealth Solutions to Health Care Problems

The early years of telemedicine funding helped identify technology-based health care solutions. The early focus on telemedicine and telehealth feasibility studies helped identify budget justifications for these pilot projects and helped researchers expand and crystallize the body of information needed to identify workable technology-based solutions to clinical, administrative, and educational problems and problems with medical equipment. The following solutions have been determined to be most relevant to telecommunication technology applications for health care.

Enhanced Health Care Access. Patients served through telehealth are likely to experience a higher level of care. A simple example of how medical problems are effectively addressed via technology can be found in the program at the Comanche County Memorial Hospital in Oklahoma. A young woman with a speech problem made remarkable progress with her disability by simultaneously watching her own image and that of her speech pathologist. In addition to the benefits she accrued during her sessions, the interactions were videotaped so she could take them home and learn by watching herself (Siwicki, 1996).

It is an axiom of preventive health that the earlier the symptoms of a disease or illness are detected, the better the chance of prevention or preemptive treatment. Another benefit to patients served by telehealth systems is faster, easier access to higher-quality, more specialized health care. This is particularly needed in settings such as prisons (Brecht, Gray, Peterson, & Youngblood, 1996) and the military (Blakeslee & Satava, 1998). Patients can be given immediate and more convenient care when a local practitioner has immediate access to a specialist. Patients in remote settings are able to remain with their friends and family and avoid the expense, social isolation, and travel required to stay in distant hospitals (Thompson, 1997).

E-Health, Telehealth, and Telemedicine

Enhanced Information and Training for Health Care Providers. Tele-health provides continuing education for medical professionals. Video-conferencing and **audioconferencing** can help keep practitioners up-to-date no matter where they are, without their taking time from home or office. Practitioners often find they can use the same technology for both continuing education and consultation in their specific area of expertise. By using remote expert systems and online databases, practi-tioners can educate themselves regarding rare or obscure symptoms or conditions (Kassirer, 1995; Montgomery, 1998).

Improved Information and Support for Patients. Patients are also using non-Internet telehealth services to help cope with social isolation. Certain groups of people, such as senior citizens with neurological and mobility disorders, those living in high crime areas, and other homebound individuals with psychiatric disorders such as agoraphobia, may find it difficult to obtain adequate health care. Such medical problems make it difficult to travel, regardless of weather conditions and geographic distance. Technology offers a range of practical tools to close the gap between the medical resources currently being offered and the health care needs of these populations.

Support for Families

Michelle Gailiun, Director of Telemedicine, Ohio State University
One of our pulmonary fellows had a patient who was dying. He was on a ventilator, confined to his bed, and his son was graduating from law school several states away. The patient asked us if we could somehow rig something up so he could see his son graduate, and we did. He was thrilled, and so was the rest of his family. During the ceremony, they announced that he was watching from his bedside, and everyone cheered (personal communication, September 28, 1999).

Warren B. Karp, Ph.D., D.M.D., Coordinator of Telemedicine and Distance Learning Activities, Department of Pediatrics, Medical College of Georgia

Patients and families value telehealth technologies tremendously. One unexpected finding is that both health care providers and technologists consistently undervalue the importance of the technologies to patients and families (personal communication, November 15, 1999).

Reduced Health Care Costs. Telehealth is also relieving some of the burden placed on family caregivers. At times of a health crisis, family members have traditionally left their jobs and homes to travel to hospitals to assist the hospital staff and provide emotional support for the patient. Because of the changes in health care, patients are given shorter hospital stays, and family members are often entrusted or burdened with a patient's care after discharge. Whether or not they feel equipped to handle the task of caregiving, they often have no choice but to learn to cope with an ailing relative. Telehealth equipment and services can often alleviate some of these burdens by offering training for caregivers, group support through e-mail discussion groups for caregivers, and direct e-mail contact with staff at the practitioner's office.

In describing some of his experiences as the coordinator of telemedicine and distance learning activities for the Department of Pediatrics at the Medical College of Georgia, Dr. Warren Karp named these experiences as examples of the benefits of telehealth (personal communication, November 15, 1999):

Allowing a terminal AIDS patient to virtually attend her GED graduation while in the hospital, which she could not have done otherwise

Watching a respiratory therapist coach a young child with cystic fibrosis—at home over the family's television set—on the proper use of the "puffer vest"

Watching a child in a distant hospital waiting for a heart transplant keep in contact with his family and friends

Watching a child undergoing a stem cell transplant and feeling less
isolated thanks to videoconferencing technology

Walking by a bassinet in the neonatal ICU and listening to a mother read
a story to her premature baby from her hometown 150 miles away

Teaching the parent of a developmentally delayed child how to position the child while parent and child are in their own home and
using the child's own crib

Watching two deaf parents with a hospitalized child communicate with
their health professionals by videoconferencing in the child's hospital room, working with an interpreter for the deaf somewhere
else in the community

Improved Distribution of Resources. Telehealth enables a more effective allocation of health care resources between regional and urban medical institutions. By providing access to medical experts, rapid diagnosis, and appropriate
treatment, telehealth makes health care accessible wherever a patient may reside, and thereby allows for a greater continuity of care (Balas et al., 1997).

Reduced Professional Isolation and Stress. Telehealth can bring needed
consultation to the rural practitioner and thereby relieve some of the
stress associated with practicing in a rural or remote environment. Many
rural communities are working together to create a "televillage" (a virtual
community of people or organizations that share telecommunication networks and related services) to help reduce their isolation, improve access,
and refine the overall health care offered to people in their area (Puskin,
Brink, Mintzer, & Wasem, 1997).

Unexpected Benefits of Telehealth

Robert Cox, M.D., Hays Medical Center, Kansas

Our state's Blue Cross/Blue Shield endorsement of telemedicine reimbursement has been a benefit. Developing relationships has been

another significant benefit (personal communication, November 16, 1999).

Michelle Gailiun, Director of Telemedicine, Ohio State University

The telemedicine program has fostered many friendships and relationships that would never have come about otherwise. The level of comfort with our doctors and technology has been another unexpected benefit. They now think about using telemedicine for their patients (personal communication, September 28, 1999).

Steven W. Strode, M.D., University of Arkansas for Medical Sciences

One of our greatest benefits in developing our telehealth program has been developing great friendship with our "champions." Some are in the remote communities and some are on our academic health science center campus. I do not think I would have developed these friendships with these great people unless telemedicine had happened to bring us together (personal communication, November 12, 1999).

Peter Yellowlees, M.D., Department of Psychiatry, Royal Brisbane Hospital, Australia

One benefit is the development of positive attitudes toward the use of technology from practitioners. A number of clinicians have been turned on to other forms of technology, having started with videoconferencing. Another benefit has been that clinicians are empowered to be quite clinically innovative because they have been allowed to make decisions about equipment and applications (personal communication, February 10, 2000).

New Business Opportunities for Health Organizations. Currently, space and time constraints hamper health care organizations in their ability to deliver health care services outside their traditional catchment area. Telehealth technologies can eliminate some of those barriers. An extreme example is the telehealth link currently being established between the University of Vermont's Fletcher Allen Health System and a health care setting in Vietnam.

Enhanced Efficiency. Telehealth also has the potential of decreasing administrative costs by facilitating patient scheduling and medical records acquisition and through rapid transfer of patient information. Telehealth also allows a specialist to do some of the workup of a complicated case beforehand, which saves time, money, and frustration for all parties. Tests and x-rays traditionally are taken at least once at the primary practitioner's office and another time at the specialist's office. Telehealth makes such duplication unnecessary.

Although telehealth offers many potential benefits, most have yet to be demonstrated by empirical research. The challenges of the next decade include evaluation to determine what the true benefits—and costs—really are.

Internet Solutions to Health Care Problems

The Internet is uniquely suited to provide low-cost, universal access to information (Rice, 1995). Although the Internet's utility is yet to be fully explored, the following uses have already been identified:

Greater Access to Health Care Information. Resources that have hitherto been available only to researchers are now available to anyone with Internet access. These include the National Library of Medicine's incomparable MEDLINE <http://igm.nlm.nih.gov/>, with over nine million medical references from 1966 to the present; professional and patient-oriented sites, sponsored by professional organizations, federal agencies, and private companies (for example, the American College of Radiology <www.acr.org> and the National Cancer Institute's "Information for People with Cancer" <http://rex.nci.nih.gov/PATIENTS/INFO_PEOPL.htm>). Increasingly, Web-based initiatives for providing health care information are also coming from private, for-profit sources, such as <http://healthatoz.com> and <http://lifescape.com>.

Increased Support for Administration of Health Care. It is quite possible that in the next few years the Internet will become the most commonly used information backbone of increasingly dispersed "integrated delivery networks." Using virtual private networks that provide **security** and **confidentiality** through **tunneling** technologies, hospital information systems will be able to extend their **local area networks (LANs)** into what amounts to a **wide area network (WAN)** that spans the planet. Anyone with a Web **browser** and the proper identification (a password, fingerprint, iris scan, or the like) will have access to administrative, pharmaceutical, billing, and clinical information. Companies already offering such services through the Internet include <www.Asterion.com> and <http://elixis.com>.

Improved Nontextual Communication. The Internet is being used for transmitting radiographs, echocardiograms, dermatology images, and so on. It is also being widely used for videostreaming, a technique for providing store-and-forward audio and video over low bandwidths. As bandwidth access improves, the Internet is beginning to be used for interactive video as well. This shift may render expensive, **dedicated** leased lines relatively obsolete.

Improved Communication Among Patients and Professionals. Patients are forming online communities to help themselves through e-mail discussion groups and bulletin boards. Increasingly, patients are interacting with their health care providers through secured specialty Web sites that cover disease management, personal health records, self-monitoring, and communication. They are using encrypted e-mail to communicate with nursing staffs and other professionals.

CHALLENGES WITH TELECOMMUNICATION TECHNOLOGIES

Although early work in telemedicine and telehealth has gone far in revealing the potential benefits of using telecommunication technologies in health care, many concerns still exist. Although the distinction we draw is imperfect because areas overlap, we will look at the challenges from two perspectives: those related to professional practice and those related to technology. Once again, we will be discussing these issues in much greater detail throughout the remainder of this book.

Professional Practice

Issues of professional practice in various aspects of telehealth and e-health are hotly debated. Pulled in opposite directions by mavericks who brandish a "Let's do it because we can" attitude and by conservatives who demand a decade of empirical validation before offering new services to consumers, most professional groups are moving ahead, but cautiously. Although the following list is not exhaustive, it covers the issues most often discussed among professionals contemplating the use of technology to better serve their patients.

State Licensure. As technological capacity surpasses the currently understood boundaries of geographical and professional practice, state licensing boards are beginning to pass laws to regulate practice in their own states. As a reaction to the resulting differences in state laws and their potential areas of conflict, several groups, including the Federation of State Medical Boards, are developing options to allow professionals to practice telehealth across state lines. Proposals have focused on the concept of national licensure, whereby practitioners would hold a license in a system similar to that in operation for driver's licenses.

Guidelines for Appropriate Use of Technology. Issues having to do with the practitioner-patient relationship, such as communication, abandonment, **informed consent,** and liability, are always present, but they are complicated by the use of telecommunication technology. Liability can exist when there is a breach in the quality of care delivered to a patient, perhaps as the result of a confusion of roles between the referring and consulting professionals. Indeed, the exact definition of *professional relationship* in the context of teleconsultations is vague. The consulting physician may or may not be responsible for the actions of the referring professional, who clearly has a relationship with the patient. The consulting professional could argue that he or she was providing services only to the referring professional and not to the patient and therefore did not have a relationship with the patient. Nonetheless, it is conceivable that the consultant in a telehealth delivery system could be held partially responsible and liable for abandonment if the referring physician has failed in this duty to the patient (Cepelewicz, 1998).

Electronic Medical Records and Related Issues of Confidentiality. Given the widespread problem of security in the health care arena as well as on the Internet, the transfer of electronic medical records poses a serious risk of breaching patient confidentiality (IOM, 1994). There is increasing concern about the security of medical records as the trend toward data warehousing and centralization of medical records grows. How medical records will be "data-mined" in the future also raises serious concerns, and it is often unclear how to responsibly communicate such concerns to patients as well as to colleagues.

Meanwhile, international health and business leaders are forming new entities and using old ones to issue statements about the international regulation of electronic communications. Several groups, including the World Health Organization, various branches of the U.S. government (DHHS, 1997a, 1997b; IOM, 1994; Ryboski, 1998), and professional associations such as the American Health Information Management Association and the American Medical Informatics Association (Kane & Sands, 1998), are providing suggestions and leadership with regard to the protection of patient records.

Malpractice Issues. If a professional crosses state lines to deliver service, jurisdictional issues related to a malpractice claim may arise. In telehealth service delivery, jurisdictional issues may become even more complicated. It is conceivable, for example, that a patient could file a malpractice claim both in his or her own state of residence and in that of the professional (Cepelewicz, 1998). Furthermore, liability could conceivably be extended to a telecommunication company or equipment manufacturer if a patient holds the quality of the transmission responsible for an adverse outcome of the **telediagnosis** or treatment. These possibilities could create a litigious environment in which patients are encouraged by the legal system to shop for the jurisdiction that will maximize their potential financial return if granted a favorable decision in a malpractice suit (Physician Insurers Association of America, 1996).

Reimbursement. The number of reimbursement plans for telehealth has increased significantly in the last few years. Many states and the federal government are considering or have enacted legislation to regulate and reimburse telehealth services.

Most states restrict both the use of communication technologies and provider services with respect to reimbursement (Health Care Financing Administration [HCFA], 1998b, 1999) by using specific codes and related definitions of services. Because reimbursement policies fluctuate from one year to the next, refer to the following Web site for legislative updates regarding Medicare reimbursement policies: <http://thomas.loc.gov/>, and search for bill S. 2505, the Telehealth Improvement and Modernization Act of 2000.

Staff Training. Training and maintaining staff in new areas of technology can be expensive, time consuming, and frustrating. In training the often unwilling clinical and clerical staff, their reluctance can be exacerbated by overly harsh or overly lenient policy decisions made by well-meaning but uninformed administrators. Equipment maintenance poses another challenge. Accurate diagnosis and treatment abilities must also be developed when training staff to use new telehealth equipment (Nitzkin, Zhu, & Marier, 1997; Phillips et al., 1997; Ruskin et al., 1998).

Practitioner and Patient Acceptance. Many "human factors" are limiting the wide adoption of service delivery through technology and of computerization of health care records. For example, clinicians may fear a loss of rapport with patients or the intrusion of inaccuracies in the transmission of information (Puskin, Morris, Hassol, Gaumer, & Mintzer, 1997). There is a general reluctance among some practitioners to use new technology at all (IOM, 1996; Weil & Rosen, 1998).

Inadequate assessment of needs and preferences by software and hardware developers can lead to other problems related to the acceptance of technology by professionals. Technology may not work well with already established professional practice routines and referral patterns (IOM, 1996; Puskin, Morris, et al., 1997). Many professionals' schedules are already overbooked; taking the time to learn new technology and programs is difficult. Other factors, such as delays in transmission of clinical information (Thompson, Ottensmeyer, & Sheridan, 1999) and problems with the ability to accurately quantify information transmitted remotely (Xiao et al., 1999), may pose further hindrances.

Publicized breaches of the security and privacy of personal health information may cause patients to lose faith in the technology. Patients often feel a strong bond with their physician and pharmacist; they may feel that telehealth services will disrupt the relationship. A Cyber Dialogue study revealed that one-third of all adults surveyed felt that they did not need these new services (Reents, 1999c). Reportedly, patients also feel uncertainty about the quality of information online and about online security and privacy. All of these factors may negatively affect the adoption of e-health, telehealth, and telemedicine.

Concerns with Technology

Technology-related concerns involve the lack of empirical research establishing the overall validity, reliability, and compatibility of technology, and the availability and affordability of such techniques are still in flux. These technical worries are amplified by concerns in the human arena as well. Licensing, ethics, and credentialing boards and committees are being pressed to regulate service delivery mechanisms before the impact of technology has been fully assessed by practitioners or decision makers. Payer organizations may need costly technological upgrades and retraining for their employees. Staffing across multidisciplinary groups is either rekindling or bringing resolution to turf wars between professions, depending on how administrators in various institutions handle these issues. Slow-moving bureaucracies are thwarting decision-making bodies in a fast-paced technological world in which the next generation of equipment arrives every eighteen to thirty-six months. In many settings, diverse professionals are banding together to fight the bigger foe, that of technology itself.

While professionals debate legal, regulatory, patient, and personnel issues, the advancement of technology is often overwhelming to administrators and practitioners. As is true in other areas of the economy, as health care becomes increasingly dependent on telecommunication technology, the stark reality of the damage caused by this dependence is also of great concern to many. Balancing the need to adopt new technology with the need to be fiscally responsible is indeed a challenge. The difficulty of this challenge is increased when one considers the many forms this technology can take and the multiple purposes each may serve. This topic is discussed further in Chapter Three; the following paragraphs serve as an introduction to issues that are typically considered central.

Affordability and Reliability of Technology. Health care organizations are facing decreasing budgets, and technology can be a relatively expensive investment. This expense can be aggravated by the expense and headaches of building network and telecommunication infrastructures. Utility costs can be an additional obstacle. Without grants or other outside funding, such "hidden" costs can be prohibitive, regardless of how much funding is available to purchase telecommunication equipment.

Industrywide Cohesion. The rapid evolution of technology has created difficulties with formats and standards. Integrating all the technologies required for telehealth services can present a number of challenges. The broader the range of functions performed by technology, the greater the possibility of incompatibility. These kinds of problems can cause the transition to electronic services to take a considerable amount of time. Although platforms are being standardized through networks such as the Internet, it will take some time before industrywide cohesion emerges. Nonetheless, technology will continue developing, and health care as a whole will ultimately benefit.

CONCLUSION

Telecommunication technologies have had a relatively short but remarkably steep growth curve. From radio messages to Antarctica in the early 1900s to instantaneous satellite transmission around the globe at the turn of the millennium, technology is here, and here to stay. Current uses of many different technologies are exciting to contemplate, with all their benefits and challenges. Certainly it is too early to make risk-free investments or plan for anything but the next decade. One thing is certain, however. Telecommunication technologies will be a dominant force in health care delivery. Chapter Two looks at how the Internet is expanding the role of technology in the world health care marketplace.

CHAPTER 2

From Telemedicine and Telehealth to E-Health

Ruth lived in a small, rural town in a midwestern state. She received a diagnosis of breast cancer from her doctor on a Monday. Ruth was determined to fight this disease with every tool she could find. The first thing she did was to search the Internet for as much as information as possible about her illness and treatment options. Armed with this information and several ideas, Ruth visited her doctor on Wednesday with a stack of printouts from her search. She and her physician went through them and jointly decided on a treatment plan. While Ruth was undergoing treatment, she continued to gather information through the Internet on a weekly basis. Another treatment option opened for her. Through her Internet research, Ruth had read that breast cancer patients live longer if they participate in support groups. But she was the only person in her town currently diagnosed with breast cancer. Ruth once again turned to the Web and found a support group that gave her encouragement and advice well beyond the formal course of her treatment.

The term *e-health* refers to Internet-mediated access to health care services, products, and capabilities (McLendon, 2000). Internet-based e-health operates anywhere, anytime, and with anyone. A direct outgrowth of telemedicine and telehealth, e-health is closely allied to its predecessors. Many clinical activities that traditionally characterized telemedicine and telehealth (for example, interactive consultation, monitoring, and home health from a distance) will be subsumed into services that are Internet based. As we discussed in Chapter One, federally funded telemedicine and telehealth pilot projects have documented many lessons learned through the use of telecommunication technology in health care. As the Internet has developed and become commercialized, the transfer of this knowledge to the Internet was inevitable. The hard work that has gone into developing appropriate telemedicine and telehealth outcome measures of efficacy, satisfaction, and cost-effectiveness are directly applicable to Internet-based health care. The transition to e-health is not as easy as many would like to assume, however, and it is most likely that e-health will complement rather than replace many specialized applications developed in telemedicine and telehealth.

With movement to the Internet, health care is not just more accessible; it is being revisited, revised, and revolutionized. Many time-tested concepts and approaches are being discarded and replaced with newer applications, much to the chagrin of many traditionalists and the satisfaction of many innovators. The tension between these two groups, like the stock market tension associated with e-health companies, is certain to experience many ups and downs over the next few years. Although our discussion here does not have room for a detailed analysis of the fiscal vagaries of e-health companies, we must acknowledge the reality of such tensions before embarking on a discussion of how e-health can benefit health care in general.

Despite the vicissitudes of concepts, approaches, and the e-health-related stock market over time, as health care delivery is increasingly shifted to the Internet, e-health will become part of our daily routine, and as a result our lives will be changed forever.

The remainder of this chapter will examine why e-health is growing so rapidly, what its emergence will mean to the existing health care system, what the principal applications for e-health might be, and what aspects of e-health might raise some concerns.

THE INTERNET AND THE CASE FOR E-HEALTH

The Internet has made access to information, products, and services inexpensive (sometimes free), instant, and universal. With immediate access to worldwide databases, libraries, conference proceedings, records, support communities, and many other resources through the Internet, people can now retrieve updated information from their own homes rather than seeking professional advice. E-health may also serve as an acceptable alternative channel for obtaining health care for people who feel they cannot access traditional face-to-face consultations due to cost, inconvenience, or social stigma. In one survey, the Center for Clinical Computing and Sapient Health Network reports that consumers of these services rate them as much more useful than their personal doctors in a number of areas, such as referrals, convenience, cost, coping strategies, and information (*Net Payoff,* 1998). E-health empowers individuals by allowing them to make their own decisions regarding their health (Spielberg, 1998). Because patients are more informed, they may practice healthier habits, which could help them reduce utilization of the health care system in general. For instance, e-health can reduce unnecessary and costly emergency room visits and instead redirect informed patients to their doctors' offices.

The **point-to-point** restrictions of telemedicine and telehealth have been reduced or eliminated as computers share previously proprietary standards and develop compatible operating systems. Using the Web browser interface and common programming languages and transmission **protocols,** anyone will be able to build—and make universally available— his or her next great concept.

The Internet will provide a common data communication channel. In essence, the world will become an immense wide area network (WAN). Through this WAN, fueled by free enterprise and directed by proper legislative support and regulation, the Internet can significantly improve upon the learning obtained through early telemedicine and telehealth programs and deliver quality health care to the global marketplace. By increasing access and affordability of products and services, the Internet can bring improved health care to local, national, and international regions that are currently underserved.

Basic Internet Demographics

In contrast to traditional telehealth populations, the Internet has a unique consumer population. Internet consumers are highly educated, relatively affluent, and predominantly middle aged (baby boomers). Of all college-educated adults, 59 percent are online. Of adults earning over $75,000 annually, 63 percent are online. Internet-based health care, then, is correlated with individuals with higher economic status who have more discretionary income and therefore can afford services and products offered electronically (Bard, 2000). The U.S. population is living longer, thanks to modern health care, and is also becoming more accustomed to using the Internet. In the coming years, the Internet consumer population will increasingly extend to seniors (Institute for the Future, 2000) and, one hopes, to many of the ethic minorities that are currently underrepresented online.

Internet Growth

Between 1991 to 1999, the number of domain names rose from almost zero in 1991 to forty-five million by 1999 (Office for the Advancement of Telehealth [OAT], 1999b). Over fifteen thousand health care sites already exist online, offering unprecedented services and benefits to their users, and the number of sites is growing rapidly. Consumer demand is very high. Cyber Dialogue, Inc., an online demographic research group, projects that the population of e-health consumers will reach 88.5 million by 2005 (Bard, 2000).

The same research group estimates that the number of consumers searching for health content online will grow from 23.6 million in the second fiscal quarter of 1999 to 79.4 million in 2005. The number of consumers connecting with payers and providers online is expected to grow from 2.7 million in the second fiscal quarter of 1999 to as high as 64.5 million in 2005 (Bard, 2000).

Cyber Dialogue estimated that over the twelve months between July 1998 and July 1999, a total of $340 million was spent online on health and beauty products, or approximately 0.2 percent of the total spent in the United States (Reents, 1999c). The number of consumers shopping

E-Health, Telehealth, and Telemedicine

for health and beauty products online is expected to grow from 6.7 million in the second fiscal quarter of 1999 to as high as 55.2 million in 2005 (Bard, 2000).

Various factors can influence these projections. On the one hand, investment in e-health applications by health insurance companies and providers could accelerate growth. Increased Internet access by yet untapped populations also could accelerate growth. On the other hand, publicized breaches of sensitive online health information and slow adoption among payers and providers who are struggling with liability issues related to security, confidentiality, and privacy could slow growth. Legislative and regulatory decisions by state and federal lawmakers will undoubtedly also have a significant impact on e-health in the next few years.

The Case for E-Health

The amount of "buzz" associated with e-health has been impressive. Many business executives have taken notice of the benefits, such as reduced back office expenses, improved patient care, and greater information accessibility that the Internet has to offer. More than 90 percent of top managers cite the Internet as a major force affecting the future global marketplace (Weber, Yang, & Capel, 1999). E-health will continue to grow once these benefits have been tested and standardized. Already we are witnessing a major interest in e-health. At an e-health conference in New York City in November 1999, there were 140 exhibitors—and 60 had to be turned away because of a lack of space. This was only the third e-health conference held in the United States. Such large amounts of energy and money have not been associated with traditional telemedicine conferences.

Moreover, private industry has taken a keen interest in bringing much of the $1.3 trillion per year health care industry to the Internet (Trafton, 1999), rather than relying on federal telehealth funding as with previous telehealth projects. Already the U.S. Internet economy totaled $301 billion in 1998 and created jobs for 1.2 million workers (Nua Internet Surveys, 1999). Large technology corporations—for example, Lucent Technologies and Intel—have teamed up with medical groups such as Johns Hopkins

Medicine and the American Medical Association to create the infrastructure for e-health.

This huge health care market includes hospital care, physician services, dental and other professional services, and home health and nursing care. Much of that market—about $400 billion of it—comprises administrative, "back office," and information-processing functions that have little to do with health care itself (Trafton, 1999). With an increasing demand for prescription drugs, consumer spending for online health products alone is estimated to increase from $1 million in 1999 to $800 million by 2004, an 800 percent increase (IntelliHealth, 2000).

E-HEALTH AND THE CHANGING HEALTH CARE ENVIRONMENT

Fueled by legislative and commercial support for the transition of health care to the Internet, e-health is a primary engine for three significant changes now occurring in the health care environment.

1. *Patients are becoming better informed.* Patients are becoming more capable of self-care, leading to significant changes in the patient-clinician dynamic. As Figure 2.1 illustrates, the classic separation of patient and clinician (physician, nurse, or other health professional) roles is blurring, and the locus of control of the medical interaction is moving strongly toward the person now commonly referred to as the consumer.

Web resources and services fueling this shift include National Library of Medicine resources <www.nlm.nih.gov/databases/freemedl.html>, disease profile and management <www.Accordant.com>, images <www/adam.com>,

Figure 2.1. The Shifting Locus of Control

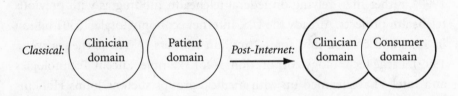

E-Health, Telehealth, and Telemedicine

finding and rating physicians <www.HealthStreet.com>, news <www. OnHealth.com>, prescription information <www.Allscripts.com>, and general health care fact finding <www.HealthAnswers>.

2. *Patients are becoming more active in their health care.* People can do things now that they could not do, or even imagine, in the past. Online disease-prevention programs such as <www.RealAge.com> automatically compute morbidity profiles tailored to the individual, recommend behavioral or lifestyle changes, and provide automatic follow-up notices for screening tests or reassessment. Elderly people can stay out of nursing homes longer because of the preventive and socialization services provided by community-building sites such as <www.Asterion.com>. Direct online health care has begun, independent of the location of the patient and physician <www.DiabetesWell.com>.

3. *Health care is becoming more efficient.* Successful health care dot-com companies are maximizing the power of the Internet by creating products that could not exist without the interconnectivity of the Internet. They are rethinking how the bricks-and-mortar health care industry can be improved. For example, patient records are being revolutionized by companies such as PersonalMD. PersonalMD offers a comprehensive personal medical record (PMR), which allows a high degree of customization for both customers (health care organizations, self-insured employers) and end users (consumers). Information tailored to each member's personal preferences and profile is delivered to the member's home page on a daily basis. Patients also receive weekly e-mail newsletters.

Once a PMR has been established, the member can automatically store paper-based documents, including EKGs and lab reports, directly into the PMR without human intervention. Unlike traditional medical files, which remain unavailable to patients, the PMR empowers members to organize, audit, and control their medical data. Members also receive an "emergency card," which provides medical personnel with crucial medical data and instructions on how to automatically access a comprehensive patient history via the Internet or fax twenty-four hours a day. Other sites offering PMRs include <www.lifechart.com> and <www.medicalrecord.com>.

Other examples of dot-coms offering increased efficiency through Internet-based approaches to health care include specialty sites offering

Medical images <www.Amicas.com>

Communication channels <www.Alteer.com>

Lab results <www.CompuLab.com>

Billing <www.Claimsnet.com>

Back office tasks <www.Cybear.com>

Scheduling <www.Healinx.com>

Differential diagnosis <www.TreeAge.com>

Evaluation and outcomes <www.Elixis.com>

Specialty information <www.Radiology.com>

Prescriptions <CVS.com>

Products and services <www.Medibuy.com>

Marketing <www.Caredata.com>

Education <www.CancerEducation.com>

CONSUMER PROTECTION: QUALITY AND ACCURACY OF INFORMATION

An area of serious concern in health care over the Internet is the quality of medical information available to consumers. Indeed, the amount of data available on the Web is so vast that the user's problem is not so much finding information as it is sifting through it (Hubbs, Rindfleisch, Godin, & Melmon, 1998). Another problem is the varying reading comprehension levels of patients. Some medical information online may be difficult to understand or easy to misinterpret (Graber, Roller, & Kaeble, 1999). Medical information on the Internet is often inaccurate or misleading (McLeod, 1998). Unlike most print resources (such as magazines and journals) that undergo a filtering and editing process, information on the

Web is often not screened according to any systematic criteria. Research conducted to analyze the content of medical information on the Internet has found that it may not be as reliable as some would like to think. For example, Impicciatore, Pandolfini, Casella, and Bonati (1997) used various search engines to systematically study forty-one parent-oriented Web sites that provided advice for the management of childhood fever. Surprisingly, only four adhered closely to published guidelines for home management of childhood fever, and some pages even proposed potentially dangerous remedies.

Other researchers are proposing solutions to guarantee Internet medical information quality. Silberg, Lundberg, and Musacchio (1997) argue that authors and publishers must be accountable for material posted on the Internet. They suggest that health information should be dated and should clearly disclose authorship and credentials, post site ownership, and cite all references and sources for the presented material.

Concerns about varying content quality have led government bodies, such as the U.S. Food and Drug Administration (FDA), to consider regulating pharmaceutical advertising and promotion on the Internet in a manner similar to the regulation of traditional print and broadcast media. The difficulty is with the FDA's attempt at global regulation, which may require an international committee to focus on Internet content (McLeod, 1998). Because these regulations may take some time to formulate and enforce, a number of health care providers have established public education sites for their patients, including Swedish Medical Center <www.Swedish.org> in Seattle, Washington, and Pinnacle Health Care System in Harrisburg, Pennsylvania (McCormack, 1999).

Groups offering criteria for evaluating health information on a Web site include Miltrek systems (Ambre, Guard, Perveiler, Renner, & Rippen, 1997) and the American Telemedicine Association (ATA) (1999). More recently, several consumer e-health sites have also begun to set up ethical guidelines to protect consumers and to govern online advertising, content, sponsorship, and privacy. These efforts were initiated in response to increasing public concern over the reliability of health information available on the Internet, the ways personal data collected from consumers may be used, and the fear that some e-commerce activities may actually be endangering consumers' health (Chin, 1999).

The American Medical Association has joined with the American Academy of Ophthalmology; the American Academy of Pediatrics; the American College of Allergy, Asthma and Immunology; the American College of Obstetricians and Gynecologists; the American Psychiatric Association; and the American Society of Plastic and Reconstructive Surgeons to produce a comprehensive health information and communication Web site called Medical Empowerment <www.medem.com>. These physician associations will own and control the new entity established to maintain the Web site. Other groups offering suggestions for ethical online health care information, products, services, and practice are discussed in Chapter Eight.

CONSUMER PROTECTION: PRIVACY OF INFORMATION

While patients are accessing e-health sites on the Internet, site operators may be gathering personal information about them without their knowledge. Web sites are indeed processing an unprecedented amount of personal information about consumers. In early 2000, DoubleClick, an Internet advertising company, raised controversy by planning to use personal information gathered from the Internet and match it with **click stream data.** This business plan caused a significant number of lawsuits and inquiries to be brought against the company. It is likely that such public events will lead to the establishment of standards from government organizations such as the Department of Commerce and the Federal Trade Commission as well as some online groups, such as the American Association of Advertising and the Internet Advertising Bureau (Whiting, 2000).

Members of these concerned organizations are asking questions like these: How have e-health Web sites constructed their policies about the privacy of patient information? How easily can consumers find and understand these policy statements, particularly if they are distressed and looking for specific information related to the cause of their distress? Are

Internet disclaimers effective? Do disclaimers or policy statements afford sufficient protection? Most important, do the actual practices of the health sites reflect their publicly stated policies? Technical issues related to privacy are covered in detail in Chapter Seven.

THE PROLIFERATION OF E-MAIL SERVICES

E-mail is the lowest common denominator on the Internet, and therefore the most widely used communication tool. It is available to people with **modems** through low-cost or no-cost Internet service providers. Patients and providers have relatively easy access to e-mail and are beginning to use e-mail for health care in various ways.

E-Mail Support Groups for Patients

As mentioned at the beginning of this chapter, the Internet is also providing a low-cost and convenient vehicle for peer support. Internet users are forming virtual communities that focus on a range of issues and common problems (Bruckman, 1996; Jones, 1995; Rheingold, 1993; Shields, 1996; Turkle, 1995; Wellman, 1997). Community members send messages via modem to a common computer that distributes the message to other members of the community. They typically want support and information about a particular illness, or to share a life circumstance, such as divorce or the birth of a child with a disorder (Lavoie, Borkman, & Gidron, 1994).

The number of participants worldwide is enormous. Developed as grassroots connections, these groups now offer unprecedented resources to people living anywhere accessible by modem. Groups range in focus from Friends of Bill W. and Alcoholics Anonymous meetings, to parents of children with diabetes. Some groups, such as <alt.support.depression>, claim to have tens of thousands of members logging on monthly (Salem, Bogat, & Reid, 1997).

E-Mail Contact with Patients

The appropriateness of communicating via e-mail with patients is hotly debated at professional conferences (Maheu, 1999a), and research supporting both the pros and cons is beginning to find its way to scientific journals (Borowitz & Wyatt, 1998; Maheu & Gordon, in press; Reents, 1999a; Spielberg, 1998).

Advantages are numerous. Trying to get a provider or patient on the telephone can be difficult, but using asynchronous e-mail can eliminate telephone tag by allowing the caregiver and patient to communicate at personally convenient times (Kane & Sands, 1998; Nettleman, Olchanski, & Perlin, 1998). Patient and practitioner may have the opportunity to devote greater thoughtfulness to communication, potentially leading to greater clarity in communication and more precision with interventions. Practitioners interacting with patients via e-mail have the advantage of being able to make sure their replies are factual and complete. This resource also gives them time to review lab results and investigate an unfamiliar condition prior to contact with patients (Nettleman et al., 1998). E-mail is ideal for certain types of store-and-forward telehealth, whereby **multimedia** files can be transferred along with textual messages (Della Mea, 1999).

E-mail can be printed or archived into an electronic database for later retrieval (Kane & Sands, 1998; Suler, 1998). Unlike the telephone, it provides direct evidence of patient-practitioner interactions. Another feature is that it can be filtered automatically by keywords and stored by specific subject (Nettleman et al., 1998; Spielberg, 1998). Research has shown that e-mail-enabled patients are being supplied with information in a timelier manner and that both practitioners and patients report high satisfaction rates (Borowitz & Wyatt, 1998; Spielberg, 1998).

In a study performed at two medical institutions in Charlottesville, Virginia (Borowitz & Wyatt, 1998), an average time of four minutes was required to answer an average e-mail consultation request. In the same study, parents reported being comfortable communicating electronically to an unfamiliar practitioner about specific clinical details concerning their children's health. E-mail can allow practitioners to follow up with a patient to clarify advice, or to direct the patient toward educational materials on the Internet (Borowitz & Wyatt, 1998; Maheu, 1997). Practitioners can easily include links in a message to direct a patient to educational resources on the Web, or they can compile educational materials and send them as attachments. They can also e-mail reminders to alert patients of preventive health measures (Nettleman et al., 1998), appointments, or compliance schedules.

Disadvantages are also numerous. E-mail slows the communication rate to the point that in some cases, using the telephone simply is more efficient and can supply a wider range of diagnostic cues (rate of speech, voice amplitude and tone). Due to e-mail's restriction on visual and auditory cues, conducting diagnosis and treatment using e-mail may be too ambiguous for accuracy when practitioners are working with unknown patients.

An important drawback to e-mail communication is that the Internet is not yet secure. Messages may be read by unauthorized persons and stored on a variety of systems prior to delivery, and the recipient can make copies and forward the message to anyone. In addition, the Supreme Court has recently ruled that e-mail is not confidential and thus not protected by normal privacy protection laws.

E-mail delivery is also unpredictable. Messages may be delivered in minutes or days, further risking violations of the patient's privacy. For example, e-mail messages to patients can be inadvertently directed to their place of employment, where they are subject to review by their employer. Therefore, many organizations using e-mail for communication with patients require patients' consent in writing. Policies governing the use of e-mail should be developed and communicated to all Internet users in the organization (Miller, 1996). Recommendations regarding responsible e-mail procedures for increased security are given in Chapters Seven and Nine.

Conscious of the potential liabilities that might arise, professionals are often at a loss as to what to do when contacted by a patient via e-mail. One study documented a lack of consensus about the handling of unsolicited patient e-mail (Eysenbach & Diepgen, 1998). Approximately one-third of the fifty-eight practitioners responding to a survey refused to answer fictitious diagnosis requests, stating a belief that a diagnosis must be made with an examination. The other two-thirds of the respondents attempted to help the patients individually, and five respondents gave detailed treatment advice.

The usual response time was one to two days, but the researchers documented response times of up to ten days, even though the requests were presented as life-threatening emergencies. Researchers concluded that fear of misdiagnosis accounted for refusals to respond, although at the time of the study, the legal consequences of misdiagnosing were unclear. Since then, several states have set precedents by legislating mandatory face-to-face contact with patients before professionals are allowed to deliver any medical service through e-mail.

The use of e-mail with established patients is increasing in popularity, however. E-mail is well suited for communication with home health practitioners, for example. These constant communications can help keep updates on blood pressure monitoring, glucose readings, and functional status. E-mail is also suitable for patients who require terminal care and may not wish to travel to an office, but still require professional attention (Nettleman et al., 1998). Other technologies can be combined with e-mail to render a complete service. For example, video images can be attached to messages to help the practitioner follow the status of a wound or the progress of other procedures.

E-Mail Contact with Colleagues and Students

Practitioners are directly contacting each other with increasing frequency through e-mail. They have formed e-mail-based peer discussion groups (Stamm & Pearce, 1995). A typical message to a professional discussion list might be a request for research material or clinical advice (Miller, 1996).

These professional forums can help expand the size of professional communities by establishing "threads" (sequences of responses to a posted message) organized by specific topics, such as oncology, psychology, or pediatrics. In addition, these lists disseminate information, such as announcements of topic-related professional conferences, job openings, requests for proposals, and calls for papers (Stamm & Pearce, 1995).

E-mail lists provide forums that can be managed by software programs that redistribute e-mail postings, known as listservs. Listserv membership is usually flexible and can be adjusted to suit members' needs. Many have no requirements for joining; others require that participants belong to a professional association or group. To protect groups from mismanagement of information, the list owners or administrators may establish and enforce charters or subscriber guidelines for members who wish to participate (Maheu, 1998). Joining a group usually requires agreeing to uphold these guidelines and sometimes requires completion of a form through e-mail. Some owners and administrators will remove participants from their mailing lists for violating agreed-on rules.

E-mail can be used to provide training for practitioners and supervision of projects (for example, student dissertations). When working in rural settings, practitioners can use this resource as a valuable tool to keep in touch with a specialty hospital. In addition, e-mail may enable practitioners operating as solo professionals in rural areas to resolve a wider range of problems when they need to go beyond their expertise. In these situations, e-mail forums and communication can be important training tools (Stamm & Pearce, 1995).

INTEGRATED INTERNET SERVICES FOR PRACTITIONERS

Although e-mail serves as a basic unit of communication, Internet technology has much more to offer professionals. Hospitals, insurance companies, and private practitioners are already beginning to use multiple channels of the Internet to maximize connectivity and protection of patient information. Integrated e-health services, which will make use of this connectivity and link various services, are likely to fall into one or more of the following basic categories.

Automation of Basic Business Processes. These services, often included under the umbrella term *connectivity,* include authorization of referrals, determination of eligibility for specific patients, coordination of benefits, and submission and adjudication of claims.

Clinical Support and Information Services. These include decision support systems, **voice recognition** software, and the maintenance and transfer of computerized patient records. Despite the difficulties with provider adoption of these services, as discussed in Chapter One, a combination of younger, computer-savvy clinicians, lower equipment prices, the movement of professionals into provider groups, and the "Webification" of managed care and other insurance companies will increase adoption of clinical support and information services over the Internet.

Data Analysis. Once patient protection criteria are in place, administrative and claims data sets can be "data-mined." This extraction of nonidentifiable patient information will be used positively to gain a better understanding of public health issues, medication reactions, and risk adjustment for health plans and capitated providers.

E-Care. Using combinations of these services to deliver direct patient care (e-care) is the ultimate goal of telehealth, whether delivered in a closed hospital network or over specialized areas of the Internet. For example, nurses in centralized call centers sitting in front of a Web-enabled system often serve as system gatekeepers. In a typical program, nurses are connected to a decision support system to help them triage or diagnose a caller's complaint. One such configuration can include fax servers (to direct faxes to hospitals, doctors' offices, insurance carriers, and drug stores), integrated telephone systems (to help nurses collaborate easily with doctors and each other), and back-end databases (to update medical and billing records). With a Web browser, nurses and other authorized users can access various modes of clinical information, including text data (for example, echocardiogram reports), graphical tracings (EKGs), images (radiographic films), and sound recordings (practitioner dictation) (McDonald et al., 1998). Advice nurses working with patients using a combination of the telephone and the Internet are likely to become commonplace (Institute for the Future, 2000).

MARKETING OF E-HEALTH

The flurry of e-health activity seems to be developing noticeable trends in various sectors. Consumers are primarily flocking to e-mail and health care Web sites to acquire information, participate in virtual communities, and purchase health care products. Hospital administrators and professionals are sorting through the legal and ethical ramifications of online health care to establish Web sites and remain competitive in the marketplace. Legislative leaders are untangling decades of state and federal turf wars to offer supportive yet responsible legislation.

Entrepreneurs are knocking on investors' doors to seek funding for innovative ways to tap into the mass purchasing power promised by e-health. Of the marketing plans investors are considering, the three following approaches seem to be predominant. Each has its own strengths, and each has its optimal timing.

Business-to-Business (B-B) E-Health

The highly competitive health care industry is witnessing a convergence of care suppliers, payer sources, providers, and consumers. With this emerging interdependence comes the heightened need for ubiquitous access to information and services that help industry members confront the pressures to reduce costs, the complexities of managing information as people and companies integrate, and the ongoing need to gain and retain a competitive advantage through growth and diversification (Ernst & Young, 1997). As the lines distinguishing the various health sectors begin to blur, e-health emerges as a strategic resource for both the purchase and sale of products and services between health providers.

Hundreds of e-health companies are springing up to address existing inefficiencies and to offer new ways of improving access to health information and services. These business-to-business (B-B) dot-coms (see Chapter Five for some examples) promise to help businesses stay competitive, but there are some concerns associated with them. Many B-B companies are finding it difficult to predict what products are needed by the industry, and some analysts are skeptical as to whether B-B dot-coms will provide the Web-based solutions promised.

Business-to-Consumer (B-C) E-Health

In a number of Internet activity studies, health care was found to be the number one area of interest for Internet users—at least in some studies. In a survey of 3,269 Internet users, e-health browsers reported that finding disease-specific information was the primary benefit of Internet services (Intel, 2000). Estimates of the number of U.S. adults who accessed the Web for information on health matters in 1999 ranged from 10 percent, or 24.8 million people (Reents, 1999a), to 25 percent, or 60 million people (Harris Poll, 1999). These numbers are predicted to increase significantly, at a rate of more than 18 percent a year, constituting a possible American e-health market of as many as 100 million people by 2002 (De Nelsky, Haspel, & Lam, 1999).

Consumers' demand for Internet solutions to their health information problems is driving the e-health industry. This "bottom-up" push ensures a dependable market. Thousands of e-health business-to-consumer (B-C) dot-coms have emerged in the past few years to exploit the efficiencies offered by the Internet. Advantages include low overhead, twenty-four-hour access, and the reduction or elimination of printing and mailing costs. Telephone bills are greatly reduced, payments are instantaneously processed, and health information and products are delivered directly to the consumer, thereby eliminating third-party costs (Solovy & Serb, 1999). At the March 2000 Healthcare Information Management Systems Society conference, the number of dot-com vendors was 35 percent higher than just one year earlier. A shakeout will occur once consumers realize which companies make legitimate and useful promises and which are only "blowing vapor" (Tieman, 2000).

Meanwhile, thousands of hospitals, tens of thousands of clinics, and many health care practitioners are scrambling to integrate Internet technologies into their strategic plans. Most U.S. hospitals and health systems now have Web sites, but very few have opened these sites to communication and interactivity with patients. At the same time, some estimates indicate that physicians are rapidly taking to the Internet, with over 80 percent estimated online at the end of 2000 (De Nelsky et al., 1999). These estimates may be high, but it is obvious that consumer demand is there. The July 1999 American Internet User Survey (Reents, 1999b) reported that 50 percent of online users would be interested in using a Web site operated by their doctor's office, and 33 percent of patients say that they would consider switching providers if Internet access is not soon to be offered (Baldwin, 1999). It

E-Health, Telehealth, and Telemedicine

is clear that physicians and other clinicians are feeling besieged and confused by the pace of change in health care. A recent survey has come to startling conclusions (Dishman & Sherry, 1999): doctors report that they are unable to access the people, information, or other resources they need in order to provide quality care in a time-constrained environment, and they also feel increasingly powerless in the midst of the changing organizational and business environment of medicine. It is clear that professionals will need to decide whether they will deliver services directly to consumers or leave service delivery to others (Reents, 1999a).

Due to the difficulty in finding products and services that consumers will purchase online, B-C companies are finding that profits are slower than anticipated. Indeed, the Internet has become a hearty challenge for some and a dismal failure for many. The stock market slump in early 2000 left overvalued companies that had poor business plans badly shaken (Schwartz, 2000). Financial predictions are difficult to trust. Investment firms, who have the most to lose by pouring their financial assets into poorly planned dot-com business ventures, are predicting that B-C companies will not see a significant profit for several more years (Lee, Conley, & Preikschat, 2000).

Consumers of Internet-based information have become accustomed to accessing information at no cost. The transformation of the Internet into a marketplace for transactions involving payment is a significant shift, one that is being met with resistance from many Internet users. Considering the reluctance of professionals to offer services beyond simple health information over an untested medium and consumer uncertainty regarding purchasing medical care over the Internet, there will undoubtedly be a lag in direct consumer purchase of health care from providers in the short term.

Considering the various tensions associated with B-C e-health companies, many investors and entrepreneurs intent on survival are seeking new distribution outlets. They see the greatest opportunity in recruiting businesses with existing large consumer bases. In essence, they are wholesaling their consumer products through businesses that already cater to groups of health care consumers.

Therefore, many companies originally intent on developing B-C services and products are marketing to employer groups, employee assistance programs, and insurance companies so as to take advantage of these existing distribution outlets. They are reverting to developing business-to-business-to-consumer (B-B-C) marketing plans, selling their products to consumers indirectly, and waiting for the much larger B-C market to develop over the next few years.

Business-to-Business-to-Consumer (B-B-C) E-Health

As just noted, some companies are servicing both businesses and consumers. Often the same sites offer information and medical services to the consumer and products and services to health care systems, businesses, insurance companies, practitioners, and educational institutions. Lifescape <www.Lifescape.com> is one such company, serving both the public and private sectors. Its Web site is focused on consumers, offering behavioral assessment tools, clinical information, and news articles. Lifescape Advantage is a business unit that serves public and private sector organizations by offering customized online and Web-enabled products and services to businesses, health plans, affinity groups, insurance companies, universities, and schools. LifescapePro offers clinical and practice management tools and education products to behavioral professionals in various settings, including private and group practices, integrated delivery networks, and community mental health centers.

CONCLUSION

The Internet has brought the world to the desktop. In the health care arena, suppliers, payer sources, providers, and consumers are converging through e-health startups to share information, education, and health care services. Unlike its telemedicine and telehealth predecessors, e-health will define its success in the worldwide marketplace. Given the unpredictability of that marketplace, only one thing is certain: the opportunities are as great as the risks. Chapter Three summarizes major telecommunication technologies and proposes considerations for purchasing telecommunication equipment.

CHAPTER 3

Telecommunication Technologies in Health Care

A hospital located in the Southeast wanted to start using telecommu-nication technology to deliver care to remote patients. A hospital rep-resentative contacted a nationally known equipment vendor, and a sales representative promptly flew to the hospital to make equipment recommendations. Knowing nothing about telemedicine equipment or telecommunication solutions, the hospital administrators pur-chased the recommended equipment from the vendor. After the equipment was installed, the hospital staff experienced equipment failure. They tried to call their vendor, but it took weeks for their phone calls to be returned. They were told that they had not pur-chased the service plan that would allow the vendor to go back to the hospital to diagnose the problem. Frustrated, the hospital hired an in-dependent consultant to analyze the situation. The administrators learned not only that part of the problem was incompatible equip-ment but also that for their needs, they could have purchased less ex-pensive, lower-end equipment using lower bandwidths. Because of poor decisions related to technology, they lost thousands of their hard-won dollars.

There is an ever-increasing range of equipment options from which to choose to deliver health care over a distance. This chapter will help you make decisions about equipment used to conduct clinical consultation.

(Due to space limitations, we will not be discussing other types of tele-health technology.)

Two broad categories of technology currently exist: synchronous and asynchronous. We define these terms and give an overview of these two modalities in the first section. Next, we outline the factors to consider when making equipment or telecommunication purchases. In the third section we provide an overview of telemedicine equipment, and telecommunication solutions. Finally, we offer some tips for selecting a vendor.

SYNCHRONOUS AND ASYNCHRONOUS COMMUNICATION

The telecommunication technology system spans the globe with satellite, telephone (copper wire), **fiber-optic**, and cable networks (switches, lines, and software). One of the primary uses of this system is the delivery of health care information and services. The system needs to be understood from two perspectives: (1) the telecommunication technology itself and (2) the communication hardware and software. These two complementary facets of technology are used in various combinations to provide the two basic types of electronic communication previously mentioned: synchronous and asynchronous.

Synchronous Services

Synchronous connections are also known as *real-time* or *live*. Data, audio, and video synchronous file transmissions are available to the recipient almost immediately. Synchronous interactions allow simultaneous review and discussion of a file, situation, condition, or patient. Examples of interactions using synchronous technologies include a standard telephone conversation, the walkie-talkie-like interaction prevalent in Internet chat rooms (commonly referred to as near-real time), and an interactive video-consultation from a specialist in an urban area to a patient in a rural area.

The most common type of synchronous equipment is the telephone, which is often neglected when discussing technology, despite the many advantages it already offers to both patients and practitioners. Internet audio services have also become popular modes of synchronous communication technology for the Internet-savvy individual who wants to bypass the cost of regular telephone long-distance service. These services are also increasingly being used by dot-com companies for nursing care delivered through the Internet, such as in the disease management e-health company <www.Accordant.com>.

Interactive televideoconferencing (ITV) is the traditional form of synchronous communication for telehealth programs. Using ITV, two or more parties are physically present in front of video equipment. They can thus see and hear each other and even share documents in real time. Of course, the quality of these interactions varies with the type of technology and the type of bandwidth connecting the technology.

The advantages of ITV for health care are obvious: the specialist can directly interview and examine a patient. The referring professional can also be present to help with the workup or participate in the course of treatment recommended by the specialist. By participating in the examination of the patient by the specialist, referring professionals can also benefit by learning to diagnose and treat problems that they previously referred to specialists. Referring providers can thereby use such referrals as training experiences that will eventually allow them to expand the scope of their own practices.

Telephone, Internet audio, and ITV applications are also used for education; they enable health providers or residents of the community to access health information through distance learning classes. As opposed to satellite **downlinks** or videotapes, all these applications are interactive; the participant is able to ask questions or contribute to the discussion during the actual event. Real-time technology is appropriate for services requiring extensive communication between a patient and clinician, as in psychiatry (IOM, 1996).

Asynchronous Services

Asynchronous communication through store-and-forward (S&F) technology provides great flexibility, as it does not depend on the simultaneous presence of parties at the sending and receiving ends. S&F services compile health information and send it to another party, who can retrieve it whenever convenient. Any disadvantages of S&F technology may be more than offset by the convenience of avoiding the need to schedule a same-time meeting of sender and receiver. Common health care applications of this technology include e-mail; the transmission of teleradiologcal, telepathological, and teledermatological images; and distance learning material used in professional continuing education, research, and administration. For example, a film clip of the tremor in a patient with Parkinson's disease can be sent to a neurologist for evaluation.

Radiology is the discipline with the most highly developed telemedicine applications (Allen & Wheeler, 1998a); it simply requires a digitized version of a film to be transported over a telecommunication medium and retrieved by a radiologist for review. The radiologist then sends a report to the referring physician. This is actually quite similar to traditional radiology, except that the radiological image is handled in a new way. Teledermatology is another growing S&F application. A primary care physician or nurse can capture digital images of a person's rash and transmit them to a dermatologist (accompanied with a history and physical examination information) for diagnosis and treatment recommendations.

If a small amount of bandwidth is used, images can be transmitted almost instantaneously. If a great deal of bandwidth is used, transmission may take hours. The goal of the service dictates bandwidth requirements. Because S&F information is rarely time sensitive, it usually requires lower bandwidths than real-time exchanges. (If used for emergency diagnoses, for which rapid turnaround is essential, more bandwidth would be required.) S&F technology typically uses existing phone lines to transmit data, which translates into lower telecommunication costs. Information can also be re-sent, if needed. Table 3.1 summarizes both synchronous and asynchronous telecommunication technology needed for different telehealth applications.

CATEGORIES OF TELECOMMUNICATION TECHNOLOGY

Falconer (1999) describes two categories of telecommunication technology to deliver health care services synchronously (at the same time) and

Table 3.1. Synchronous and Asynchronous Communication

Types of Applications	Types of Technology
Synchronous	Real-time videoconferencing with specialists
Real-time examination of patient data (for example, ultrasounds, heart and breath sounds, EKGs)	Various videoconferencing tools (for example, room-based, PC-based, POTS-based tools)
Computers and medical peripheral devices capable of transmitting real-time data	
Asynchronous	Store-and-forward still images or video clips of patient visit
Online health information	
E-mail correspondence	
Store-and-forward examination of patient data (for example, radiological image, dermatological images, pathology slides)	
Faxes	Computers with videostreaming capability
Computers with Internet access	
Computers, teleradiolgy equipment, telepathology equipment	

Source: "Telemedicine and the Healthcare Executive," by A. Allen & D. A. Perednia, 1996. Adapted with permission.

asynchronously (not at the same time): (1) communication devices and modalities used to transmit information between sites; and (2) the equipment used to capture the clinical information and then display, store, and archive the information at the relevant sites. For the purposes of this chapter, we will refer to these categories as transmission and capture/reception technologies.

Transmission Channels

There are two means by which data are transmitted: dial-up (or dial-on-demand) services and dedicated connections. Dial-up services use standard telephony, integrated services digital networks (ISDNs), cellular services (mobile phones), and some satellite connections. Dedicated connections, in contrast, are those that provide a permanent connection between specific locations. These include leased lines, digital subscriber lines (DSLs), cable, **microwave links**, and satellite.

Providers have a variety of choices when selecting a transmission channel. The first factor to consider is the type of information needing transmission: text, audio, still images, or video. Each type of information requires a specific form of transmission. For example, text-based information may require only a plain telephone connection, whereas surgical training may require the transmission of video information over more sophisticated technology.

Other considerations for choosing transmission technology include the required access and flexibility, the reliability of the telecommunication technology, and the quality of service available from the telecommunication provider. For example, rural telephone service providers are often unaware of the limitations or capabilities of their own systems, so rural service developers may need to conduct a thorough investigation of statewide or regional service rather than relying on reports by rural telephone service providers (Glueckauf et al., in press).

Another important factor to consider is the speed at which the information needs to be transmitted. Different forms of transmission technology operate at different bandwidths. Bandwidth is the measure of a communication channel's ability to carry information. Most important to the telehealth industry, which is largely focused on video transmission, bandwidth ultimately constrains video **resolution** and motion handling. The lower the bandwidth, the less capable the system is of delivering high-quality resolution or motion. This is why videoconferencing on a PC at 128,000 **bits** per second (expressed as 128 kilobits per second, abbreviated "128 Kbps") looks inferior to television signals received over cable lines into one's home; it's a matter of the bandwidth used to transmit the signals. Obviously, the higher the bandwidth selected, the higher the quality.

Some clinicians, such as psychiatrists, need less detailed visual information to conduct consultations and thus require a lower amount of bandwidth. Other clinicians, such as surgeons, may require a great deal of information and need higher-bandwidth telehealth systems to enable the use of diagnostic instruments and medical imaging technologies that show precise detail. Radiologists and pathologists require very high quality still images, but because they do not usually require video, transmission speed (which is much more important for high-bandwidth video applications) is less important, and they can use S&F systems. The following sections serve as a general overview of the various transmission technologies available.

Plain Old Telephone Service **(POTS).** This is a low-bandwidth medium with maximum transmission rates approaching 56 Kbps. Although it cannot support business-quality videoconferencing, it is quite adequate for audio transmission. Some practitioners are satisfied with limited video and data applications sent via POTS. It is the most widely available medium for home health care. Once a connection is made, the line does not have to be shared with other users. POTS also allows for limited asynchronous, as well as synchronous, data transmission.

Integrated Services Digital Network (ISDN). A widely available, relatively inexpensive technology that supports higher bandwidth is basic rate interface (BRI) ISDN. This is a set of digital transmission standards developed from telephone services over the last ten years. All information is digitally transmitted over the public **switched network**. (*Switched* or *dial-up* refers to the fact that the transmission goes through the phone company's switches, which are designed to route information from one dial-up unit—classically a telephone—to another.) Each line consists of multiple channels capable of simultaneous interactive transmission. Typically, ISDN transmission runs at 128 Kbps and can be **multiplexed** up to 1.54 megabits (million bits) per second (**Mbps**). ISDN is the most common modality for doing interactive video over a distance (that is, not within an enterprise). Once ISDN is installed, a monthly fee is paid to the ISDN service provider.

Broadband ISDN (B-ISDN) is a much faster form of the traditional ISDN that uses ATM switching networks (to be discussed shortly) to transmit data at speeds up to 2.4 Mbps. B-ISDNs were proposed by the Consultative Committee for International Telephony and Telegraphy (CCITT), a Geneva-based organization responsible for setting standards for international communications among 150 countries.

Switched 56. Switched 56 is a low-bandwidth switched data service with a two-channel call option. It can transmit at speeds of 56 or 64 Kbps per channel over the public switched telephone network. Applications for switched 56 include videoconferencing, data transfer, and digital audio broadcasting. This method uses the same physical infrastructure as ISDN. However, it is an older technology with decreasing relevance.

Asynchronous Transfer Mode (ATM). This is a data-encoding, **packet**-based technology that typically transmits over higher bandwidths, at speeds from 45 Mbps to 622 Mbps. It is a low-delay switching and multiplexing technology. Its primary use is in **backbone networks**. ATM allocates bandwidth on demand, making it a nice solution for high-speed connection of video, voice, or data services. It offers high levels of functionality and flexibility, which make it attractive for many hospitals and integrated delivery networks that require transmission speeds of 64 Kbps or less.

Digital Subscriber Line (DSL). The most common current DSL deployment is asymmetric DSL (ADSL). ADSL converts regular copper **twisted pair** phone lines into high-speed communication channels without interrupting the voice traffic on these lines. It allows transmission speeds of up to 9 Mbps. It is about ninety times faster than ISDN and requires special modems. ADSL operates through a special switching and line-conditioning service at the phone company central office, and is "always on"—in other words, it is a dedicated, rather than switched, service. Very high speed ASDL (VHSADSL) is a faster version of basic DSL. Although VHSADSL transmits at speeds at least six times faster than DSL, its range is restricted to only a few hundred kilometers.

Cable Modems. These devices are becoming widely available and compete directly with DSL services. Cable modems, which are simply modems designed for use on a TV **coaxial cable** line, provide Internet **uplink** and **downlink** services. This means that one could download and watch a health-related video clip off the Internet with minimal loading or delay time. Because coaxial cable is used with cable modems, the speed is significantly faster than traditional POTS or ISDN. The transmission speed is at least ten times faster than traditional dial-up modems. However, users must share the bandwidth on it, which means that the more people subscribe to cable modems, the slower the link for all people sharing the cable in a region. Despite this disadvantage, many cable modem users report that they would have great difficulty tolerating a return to traditional dial-up modems (Newton, 1998).

T-1. This is a dedicated (nonswitched) digital transmission link with a capacity of 1.544 Mbps. A T-1 line can normally handle the equivalent of twenty-four voice conversations, each of which is digitized at 64 Kbps. T-1 can be broken down into smaller transmission units (referred to as fractional T-1). Currently the most common transmission rate for telemedicine programs using interactive video in the United States is one-quarter to one-half T-1 (384 to 786 Kbps) (Allen & Wheeler, 1998b). Many telemedicine programs have found that fractional T-1 is adequate for their

teleconsultation needs. For larger programs, T-3 lines provide a digital transmission system for high-volume voice, data, or compressed video traffic, with a transmission rate of 44.736 Mbps.

Wireless Technologies. These different technologies enable subscribers to access services without the use of any physical wires. Cellular wireless is perhaps one of the fastest-growing forms of wireless service and employs cell-switching technologies to hand off a call from cell to cell. Cellular wireless can operate via traditional **analog** modalities or via cellular digital packet data groups. Microwaves are yet another type of wireless technology. They employ electromagnetic waves in the radio frequency spectrum above 890 MHz. Microwave is a common means of transmitting video, audio, and data conversations by common carriers as well as private networks. Microwave is commonly the frequency used to communicate to and from satellites. In essence, satellites are microwave receivers, repeaters, and regenerators that orbit above the earth. Currently, satellite transmission is provided via geostationary units. However, low earth orbit (LEO) satellites are currently in production and may eventually be an alternative to the traditional geostationary satellites. LEO satellites are discussed further in Chapter Twelve. Table 3.2 is an overview of the various transmission channels we have described.

More Transmission Terminology. When working with technology, be prepared for the alphabet soup. A local exchange carrier (LEC; pronounced "leck") provides services from a central office (CO) where the telephone service switching equipment is located. A LEC can be either a regional Bell operating company (RBOC; pronounced "ar-bock"), such as Ameritech, Bell South, or US West, or another company, such as Verizon. The LEC handles calls that begin and end within a local access and transport area (LATA); an inter-exchange carrier (IXC), such as AT&T, Sprint, or WorldCom, would handle long-distance and overseas calls. More recently, local competitors to these old monopolies—known as competitive LECs (CLECs; pronounced "see-lecks")—have arisen (Hawkins, 1997).

Table 3.2. Overview of Transmission Channels

	POTS	Switched 56	ISDN	T-1	Cable	DSL	ATM	Satellite
Definition	Plain old telephone service	Switched data service that transmits over the public switched telephone network (PSTN)	Integrated services digital network	T-1 carrier system	Cable modem	Digital subscriber line	Asynchronous transfer mode: high-bandwidth, low-delay, packet-like switching and multiplexing technique	Wireless
Bandwidth	64 Kbps	56 or 64 Kbps	Two 64 Kbps channels; one 16 Kbps channel for signaling; total 144 Kbps	1.544 Mbps	10 to 30 Mbps downstream and 128 Kbps to 10 Mbps upstream	ADSL: 1.5 to 8 Mbps downstream, up to 1.544 Mbps upstream	155 to 622 Mbps	16 Kbps to 92 Mbps downlink, depending and receiver dish size

(Continued)

Table 3.2. Overview of Transmission Channels

	POTS	Switched 56	ISDN	T-1	Cable	DSL	ATM	Satellite
Accessibility	Available to every home, including remote rural areas	Available to consumers via local exchange carriers	Available to individual homes in major cities	Available for businesses	Available to 85 percent of U.S. homes	Available in limited areas	Can be ordered in almost all geographical regions	Varies by area
Frame rate	7 fps; audio not synchronized	7 fps	15 fps with synchronized audio	30 fps; full T-1 enables close to broadcast-quality audio and video	30 fps with broadcast-quality synchronized audio	30 fps with broadcast-quality	Synchronized audio	30 fps with broadcast-quality synchronized audio

Advantages	Quick installation time; easily installed	Offers high degree of flexibility, redundancy, and scalability; often used as an alternative or backup for private, leased-line networks	Real-time audio; a "switched" service that accesses the public switched telephone network (PSTN)	Dependable	Cost-effective	Real-time audio and video; takes advantage of current twisted pair infrastructure	Real-time audio and video; allocates bandwidth on demand; high speed	Real-time audio and video; wireless solution not dependent on land-based technologies
Disadvantages	Small picture; additional line installation may be required for auxiliary equipment	Considered to have limited lifespan due to competing solutions with greater bandwidth	Complex installation and usage fee structure; installation time dependent on local phone service	Expensive; not always available; not "switched," that is, it does not access the public switched telephone network (PSTN) without special bridging equipment	Subscribers must share finite cable bandwidth; readiness dependent on local cable system	Standards not universal across different "flavors" of DSL technologies; cost structure is still undetermined	Cost structure; complex to install and maintain	Delays in deployment by certain companies; cost structure is still undetermined

Capture/Reception Equipment: Videoconferencing

The equipment selected to receive (capture, display, store, and archive) information should also be chosen based on the type of information needed: text-only, audio, still images, or video. Given space limitations, we will only discuss various types of interactive videoconferencing equipment and **peripherals,** their primary uses, and some of their technical specifications. (The room used to house video equipment is also very important. To help you make better decisions regarding equipment purchase and setup, Appendix C gives direction regarding videoconferencing room requirements.)

Specialized Telemedicine Rollabout Units. These interactive video units are specially designed to support clinical telemedicine consultations and peripheral devices, according to ITU standards. Typically they include a clinic-grade washable cabinet, a **codec,** at least one monitor and one 1-**CCD** color camera, a microphone and speakers, a control panel, and bandwidth support of at least 384 Kbps (fractional T-1 or multiplexed 128 Kbps ISDN) at a **frame rate** of 25 or more frames per second (fps).

Interactive Video Room Systems and Rollabouts. These versatile units have one or two large monitors and are used for meetings and education as well as clinical interactions. Typically they include a cabinet, a codec, one or more monitors, a 1-CCD color room camera, a microphone and speakers, a control panel, near- and far-end camera controls with presets, the capacity to send and receive captured images, operation software, and bandwidth support of at least 384 Kbps (fractional T-1 or multiplexed 128 Kbps ISDN) at 25 fps or more at full common intermediate format (full-CIF, pronounced "full sif"; 352 **pixels** by 288 lines of resolution). Products that are PC based may be more adapted to **whiteboarding,** LAN connectivity, and image storage and integration into a hospital network.

Computer-Based Desktop Videoconferencing Units. Technology has been converging on the desktop for several years, and prices have been dropping dramatically. Most computer-based units are designed to operate over standard ISDN lines. They range from a simple board set with small camera and microphone (priced under $400) to **turnkey** videoconferencing systems (priced under $5,000) to true desktop telemedicine platforms with supporting multimedia management software and support for multiple peripheral devices. These include devices that assist a clinician in conducting a physical exam and in providing care. For example, an electronic stethoscope can be added to enable the physician to listen to heart and breath sounds while conducting a physical examination. Other devices include electronic dermascopes, otoscopes, and pulse oximeters. (These devices may be used on other systems as well.)

Videophones. These stand-alone products are designed for extremely simplified, touch-tone dial-up use over POTS or digital ISDN lines. They include speaker phones integrated with color screens and are not PC based. Other versions connect standard touch-tone telephones to standard televisions. The telephone carries audio information, and the television carries video information. Typically, they are compliant with ITU standards, and the POTS units transmit images at the speed of 8 fps or greater at quarter CIF resolution (QCIF, pronounced "Q sif"; 176 pixels by 144 lines). Although providers generally consider this image resolution poor, patients reportedly prefer the convenience of using this technology to the inconvenience of traveling distances to see their practitioner for routine follow-ups. Some recent videophone technologies combine ISDN lines with standard touch-tone telephones and can be used with computer monitors (with or without an Internet connection).

Set-Top Videoconferencing Systems. These dial-up systems sit atop or beside a standard television set. Using included cables and jacks, video and audio are routed through the television system or desktop computer, saving the cost of a monitor and speakers. The high-end ISDN-based systems can rival the capabilities of more expensive rollabout units.

Internet-Based Video Transmission. Internet applications are continually improving. They currently consist of videostreaming technologies that can deliver both S&F and one-way live videoconferencing options. The quality of these services depends on a number of factors, including the quality of the video output from the sender, the quality of service purchased from the sender's ISP, the available bandwidth over the public Internet at the time of transmission and reception, and the recipient's transmission and reception technology. See Chapter Twelve for more information about Internet options soon to be available.

Special Applications: Radiology Equipment

To be effective, the transmission and viewing of radiology images require special systems that provide very high resolution. Radiology equipment therefore differs significantly from the technologies described for other clinical applications.

PACS Providers. A picture archiving and communications system (PACS) incorporates elements of mini-PACS, in-house image distribution, central reading, and at-home teleradiology to offer enterprise-wide solutions for the acquisition, distribution, viewing, and storage of images and patient information. Although PACS have classically been used for radiology applications, they increasingly are being used for other image-intensive specialties, such as cardiology.

Teleradiology Systems. These systems are designed to capture, process, store, and transmit images and patient information to support central reading networks and point-to-point transmission for at-home teleradiology.

Workstations and Viewers. There are several classes of workstations and viewers found in most PACS and teleradiology systems that are tuned in price, performance, and features to meet the needs of a broad range of medical professionals, including radiologists, clinicians, subspecialists, and referring physicians.

Connectivity Systems (Middleware). Software, hardware, or a combination of both that provides connectivity for data and image exchange between information systems, printers, modalities, and various PACS- and teleradiology-related devices, components, and subsystems.

Frame Grabbers. Devices and systems for capturing the video output from various modalities (computed tomograpy, magnetic resonance imaging, ultrasound, nuclear medicine, and so on) and converting it to a digital form for transmission, storage, and viewing.

Film scanners. To meet standards set forth by the American College of Radiology (ACR) and the National Electrical Manufacturers Association (NEMA), a diagnostic-quality plain-film scanner should capture at least 2K by 2K by 12 **bit depth.** Optical density is a measure of contrast; the greater the range the better. The spot size is the minimum pixel size; for digital mammography this should be under 100 microns (0.1 mm)—one hopes well under.

There are two types of teleradiology scanners: laser and charge-coupled device (CCD). Although experts disagree, there is an emerging consensus that, for most purposes, both technologies are adequate for doing diagnostic interpretations. Laser scanners are about three times the cost of a CCD scanner with similar specifications, and they require considerably more maintenance (Harris, 1999).

Computed radiography *(including direct radiography providers).* The technologies of storage phosphors, amorphous selenium, silicon, and CCDs form the base of systems designed to eliminate the use of film, chemicals, or processors in the production of images from general radiography. There is universal agreement that one or more of these so-called filmless technologies are fundamental to the concept of a fully filmless or enterprise-wide PACS.

General Telemedicine Equipment

Many other types of electronic equipment have also been developed for various medical purposes. Many are currently in production. The following are the types of equipment commonly available at this time.

Video display units. These specialized monitors are designed for high-resolution display and include features enabling adjustment of image parameters. Unless otherwise stated, they can display 256 shades of gray (bit depth of 8) and are **DICOM** compliant.

Mass storage systems. These systems provide multiple-gigabyte and -terabyte storage for medical images, video clips, and medical records. In a PACS environment, these large DICOM-compliant systems typically offer both reversible **compression** (for short-term storage) and nonreversible compression (for long-term archiving), pre-fetch capabilities (bringing a data file to the workstation prior to the time it needs to be read), and off-site backup along with network security and data **encryption.** They also include software interfaces to other hospital systems.

Store-and-forward systems. These systems are designed to bundle patient data, still images (including radiographs), and video clips so that they can be transmitted as a multimedia patient record for review by a remote specialist. These systems are typically software-only or include an audio-video capture card or computer, camera, microphone, and image management software.

*General **telemonitoring** systems.* These nonvideo, usually transtelephonic systems are used for remote electronic monitoring of multiple physiologic parameters (vital signs, EKGs, and so on). They may be used on a continuous or intermittent basis. They often involve a central tele-nursing station where nurses oversee monitored patients in their homes, and include case management software and protocols.

Blood pressure monitors. These are transtelephonic units (that is, units that transmit digital data over a regular phone line) used for remote blood pressure monitoring.

Pulmonary function monitors. These transtelephonic units are used for remote monitoring of asthmatics and patients with chronic obstructive pulmonary disease.

Electronic stethoscopes. These are designed for transtelephonic use or for digital transmission with a dedicated or switched transmission system. Because of the different frequency requirements, most have separate settings for cardiac and pulmonary sounds.

Tele-EKGs. These are transtelephonic units used for remote monitoring of EKGs.

Tele-echocardiography and ultrasound systems. These systems capture and transmit echocardiograms and sonograms.

Integrated light and video camera platforms. A base platform with a video camera, a light source, a video processor, and a universal adapter (C-mount) that serves as a light and video source for other peripheral devices, such as ophthalmoscopes, dermascopes, and dental scopes. These platforms eliminate the need for and expense of separate cameras and light sources for each peripheral device.

Dermascopes. These are used for close-up viewing of skin lesions. These typically include a light source and a 1-CCD camera with manual focus, automatic iris, color adjustment, and white balance.

Dental cameras. These sterilizable cameras may also be used for examining skin and wounds. Units typically include a light source and a 1-CCD camera with manual focus, automatic iris, color adjustment, and white balance.

Graphics stands and dataconferencing equipment. These "document stands" and computer-based dataconferencing platforms typically include a color camera with auto focus, white balance, RGB (red, green, blue) output, and table illumination that is backlit, lit from above, or both.

VENDOR CONSIDERATIONS

As you make decisions regarding equipment and telecommunication choices, it is likely that you will be contacting vendors. There is no magic formula for selecting a vendor. However, selecting a poor vendor can cause innumerable headaches and roadblocks. Not all vendors offer the same services and deals (upgrading, technical support, equipment breakdown, and backup systems), so you must carefully consider the particulars of your program when selecting the most suitable vendor. (See Appendix B for further information related to vendors.)

Choosing a Vendor to Meet Your Needs

First, review the services your company or program wishes to provide, and draw up a list of its requirements to deliver those services. Your service director should speak with all department heads to get an adequate idea of these needs. Every company and program has unique needs for technologies and services—such as bandwidth requirements or precision information transmission devices. The technology used at each site must be coordinated and **compatible** with that used throughout the system (Puskin, Mintzer, & Wasem, 1997).

Once this needs assessment is completed, research a variety of vendors, and match the requirements of the company to the capabilities of each vendor as closely as possible, keeping budget restrictions in mind. Contact the prospective vendors to inquire about installation timelines and products that are compatible with your existing system.

Negotiating and signing an agreement with the vendor is the next step. Because dealing with a vendor is so critical, information related to vendors is included elsewhere in this book. Chapter Nine outlines risk management considerations for dealing with vendors, and, as already mentioned, Appendix B includes both an overview of some specific vendor types and the services they can provide, and details about negotiating a vendor agreement.

Tips on Working with Vendors

Robert Cox, M.D., Hays Medical Center, Kansas

- Check the relationship between sales and service within the vendor company.
- Carefully review perceptions held by all parties.
- Put agreements and expectations in writing.
- Review the status of the relationship on a regular basis (personal communication, November 16, 1999).

Warren B. Karp, Ph.D., D.M.D., Coordinator of Telemedicine and Distance Learning Activities, Department of Pediatrics, Medical College of Georgia

- You should be interested in functionality, not a product. What are your needs and applications for the technology in your specific settings?
- Always talk about your needs rather than "features" of specific equipment.
- Do not be sold into buying more technology than dictated by your needs.
- Remember that the most significant limitation on using telecommunication technology is people, not the technology itself. The simpler the technology, the better. It is much better to have an easier, less sophisticated piece of equipment than to have options that result in better-quality pictures and sound but that are perceived as too complicated to be easily used by the health care providers, patients, and families.
- Although it is fine to have a company representative give demonstrations of equipment, always arrange a way of "field testing" the equipment with your own people and in your own environments. Make sure sales representatives are not present when you are doing this. This is the only way you will get to know whether the equipment will function under your exact conditions. Anyone can set up a "wow!" demo; that is not what you want (personal communication, November 15, 1999).

Rosa Ana Tang, M.D., MPH, Professor of Ophthalmology, University of Texas Medical Branch, Galveston

- Ensure that technical support is available and ask other clients about their experiences with the vendor or telecommunication company.
- Make sure that technical support policies are clearly explained in the contract—before finding out that support is unavailable at an important time (personal communication, November 11, 1999).

Peter Yellowlees, M.D., Department of Psychiatry,
Royal Brisbane Hospital, Australia

- The first step is to establish the types of standards you want to work with and the specific applications you plan to use.
- Be clear about your expectations of the vendor.
- Work only with contacts who have been with the company for a long time.
- Insist on trials—that is, being able to test the equipment before buying it.
- Check out vendors who will lend equipment either for demonstrations or for agreed periods.
- Do not tie yourself to one specific vendor. When we want to buy more equipment, we organize a "shoot-out" between the various vendors and let the clinicians who will use the equipment actually make the final choice, rather than making it ourselves (personal communication, February 10, 2000).

Technical Considerations

Your system will require technical support, repair service, and preventive maintenance. Vendors offer several levels of support, including

Toll-free telephone technical support

Emergency assistance for failed systems

Spare parts kept in an accessible warehouse

Twenty-four-hour dispatch for on-site services

Standard factory repair service

Vendors will usually provide some of these services at no cost, but after a designated period, they will charge for them. Charges can be substantial if there is a serious problem. Ongoing technology maintenance and repair is often best managed through an in-house technical support center (Reid, 1996). In addition, a tool kit should be kept on-site for routine maintenance, adjustments, and repairs (Hodges, 1997).

Supporting the system is particularly important. One approach is to double-check all the equipment at the source location before sending it to a remote site, where access to technical support might be limited. This ensures that the software and the medical peripherals all work properly together. It also might be wise to locate and contract with a local service company to do on-site installation, repair, and maintenance.

It is important that you project the support potentially needed in terms of maintenance, upgrading, and training for each program. This support may vary considerably, depending on the rate of technological change related to the particular equipment purchased. On the basis of this projection of needed support, negotiate with the vendor to establish a contractual agreement detailing the service, fees, and price breaks over time. If you anticipate requiring substantial ongoing support services, weigh this factor heavily when choosing a vendor.

Upgrading Versus Purchasing. Software-based technology needs to be continually updated. Updates are important because they eliminate glitches and provide new functions previously not available. The advantage to using software technologies is that they can be updated relatively inexpensively with simple software revisions. The disadvantage is that such upgrades can be costly. Some vendors update their software without additional fees within twelve months of purchase. Thereafter, they may require revisions to be purchased. Vendors should specify details of their upgrade policies at the time of purchase.

An alternative might be to lease rather than purchase equipment. On the positive side, lease contracts often include maintenance service. The negatives are that newly leased equipment may not be compatible with the older equipment in the system and that leasing can cost more in the long run (Reid, 1996).

Surviving Equipment Breakdowns. Planning for potential equipment failures is essential. Telehealth services can range from routine care to dealing with life-or-death emergencies, and if the video connection fails, the results can be disastrous. Backup plans include the use of other equipment to replace the software or hardware used. For example, speakerphones may be used until the video comes back online. Ideally, other video equipment should be available to provide backup if needed (Hodges, 1997). For some programs, these backup systems will be critical (and possibly expensive). A vendor should be able to provide all backup systems, as well as primary systems, to ensure compatibility and adequate service.

CONCLUSION

Knowing the basics of interactive technologies will save much time, frustration, and expense. Facility design and equipment options vary in many ways, and options will only continue to expand. When planning a health care service to be delivered through telecommunication technology, be sure to identify needs, design the facility on paper, and compare equipment carefully before purchasing. You now have an overview of telecommunication technologies; Chapter Four focuses on some of the clinical advantages brought by telecommunication technology.

CHAPTER 4

Clinical Applications

Nancy, a cancer patient in a rural town, was tired. She had been fighting cancer for years, all the while putting on a brave face. One autumn day, she simply had enough; she began to cry during her teleconsult with her longtime oncologist hundreds of miles away. Her husband warmly embraced her, comforting her as she sobbed. Her sons shared the experience as they sat by her in front of the video monitor. The trusted physician offered words of comfort and advice for the family. Nancy thanked God for the support that her family provided in these trying times. She was also grateful for the technology that made it possible for her to stay with her family, knowing that the four children would never have made the six-hour trip to the oncologist's office. Telemedicine not only enabled Nancy to have access to vital cancer care in her small town but also enabled her whole family to play a more active role in her well-being.

Telecommunication technology comes in all shapes and sizes and can deliver health care for a wide range of specialties, including dermatology, cardiology, pulmonology, ENT, primary care, oncology, neurology, rheumatology, infectious diseases, and endocrinology. Because it is often helpful to look into detail at specific applications to draw ideas for new services, we devote this chapter to an examination of three clinical applications of technology-mediated health care: radiology, behavioral health, and home care. We chose these clinical areas because they offer a sense of the diversity of technical applications; they also show how deeply and specifically patients' needs can be served when the best of health care and technology combine to help those who otherwise might not receive adequate treatment.

RADIOLOGY

Teleradiology is defined by the American College of Radiology (ACR, 1999) as "the electronic transmission of radiological images over a distance for the purposes of interpretation and/or consultation." It is distinct from a radiology PACS (picture archiving and communications system), which is deployed within a hospital or integrated delivery network and enables images to be viewed at workstations scattered throughout the enterprise. A PACS involves very sophisticated **digital image** storage and retrieval technologies that are not usually part of a simple teleradiology system. Nonetheless, as the cost of computing and telecommunication technologies drops, and as their functionality increases, the distinctions between teleradiology and PACS are beginning to blur (Alvarez, 1998).

Clinical Applications

Teleradiology is needed in many rural communities, especially in emergencies. Trauma care often requires critical on-the-spot decisions that involve interpreting x-ray images. Teleradiology allows a practitioner in a rural location to transmit high-quality images to a remote specialist for an instantaneous interpretation.

Typically, a radiologist will receive radiographs at home, after hours, for a preliminary interpretation. This avoids the old-fashioned and wearisome alternative of driving to the hospital for an on-site reading. Except in rare cases, this preliminary reading is sufficient to cover the clinical situation until the morning; the radiologist makes the official interpretation upon arrival at the hospital reading room the next day. Today, the number of interim-read studies dwarfs the number of traditional diagnostic studies. Teleradiology is the most studied of all telemedicine applications. The first teleradiology project began in Montreal, under the direction of Albert

Jutras, in the mid-1950s (Jutras & Duckett, 1957). Since then, hundreds of studies have been conducted to evaluate the diagnostic quality of transmitted images and clinical benefits.

Real-time emergency teleradiology has been shown to have significant benefits for patients and practitioners. For example, the emergency department of rural Chatham County Regional Hospital and the University of North Carolina Hospital established a real-time emergency teleradiology fiber optic network. Lee and colleagues (1998) assessed both the turnaround time for each teleradiology consultation and the effect of the consultation on diagnosis and treatment. The emergency department practitioners recorded their satisfaction and comfort levels with the system by using a Likert scale of one to seven, with seven representing the highest satisfaction and comfort. Over the one-year study period, a total of 123 separate cases comprising 460 radiographs were interpreted. The average turnaround time for a teleradiology consultation was calculated to be 1.3 hours. The study found that the teleradiology consultations led to changes in the emergency department practitioner's initial diagnosis in 30 percent of the cases and resulted in treatment changes in 26 percent of the cases. Furthermore, the emergency department practitioners reported an average satisfaction score of 5.4 and a comfort level of 5.6 with the teleradiology system. The results indicate that real-time teleradiology consultation is feasible and beneficial.

Issues of line and gray-scale resolution and minimum requirements for ensuring diagnostically complete information have been extensively examined (Brown, 1996). Leading many other professional groups in the adoption of professional practice standards for telemedicine, the ACR (1999) has developed standards for the proper choice of equipment to ensure high quality. There is now widespread consensus that given the proper equipment, teleradiology can provide diagnostic-quality information that is equivalent to hard copy, with one possible exception: telemammography. Due to the very high resolution requirements for mammograms, which must be able to detect microcalcifications smaller than 100 microns, there is concern that teleradiology technology may be inadequate in its ability to transmit or display this critical information (Abdel-Malek, 1996). However, more recent research suggests that telemammography may achieve diagnostic reliability (Murphy et al., 1999).

The Importance of Image Resolution

Health care organizations are looking to match the level of image quality with the particular application, while maintaining cost-effectiveness. Because image resolution is a key determinant of the quality of an image used in both real-time and store-and-forward applications, teleradiology must adhere to strict standards of image resolution. High-resolution (and high-cost) monitors are crucial to teleradiology, which depends on the ability to display images as close as possible to those yielded by conventional or laser-printed film (Ruggiero, 1998). Images are ideally transmitted immediately by using lossless compression (that is, none of the original data are lost when the image is reproduced).

An effect of digital imaging systems, unlike conventional hard-copy systems, is that the displayed image is not necessarily identical to the original image or the digitally stored image. The stored image may be very vivid in contrast or detail and may exceed the capacity of the display device to convey such contrast or detail. If that is the case, the image data are processed selectively before being displayed (Ruggiero, 1998).

Another important factor is that the displayed image be presented such that it can be perceived accurately by the examining physician. From the practitioner's viewpoint, the displayed image has three important attributes: *fidelity* (affected by spatial resolution, gray-scale resolution, gray-scale linearity, and noise), *informativeness* (the capacity of the image to convey clinically important information), and *attractiveness* (the aesthetic properties of the displayed picture) (Kundel, 1986; Dwyer, Stewart, Sayre, & Honeyman, 1992).

The pixel characteristics of the displayed image must also be considered. The visibility of pixel boundaries interferes with perception of the overall picture and contrast (Ruggiero, 1998). The sensitivity to contrast and detail of the display image also depends on the display luminance (Swartz, 1998). The shades of gray that occupy the luminance region between black and white are critical to radiologists, because they help determine accurate diagnosis (Levens, 1996). Therefore, depending on the medical application, some display systems should be designed to allow for maximum contrast in all portions of the image (Sund, 1997).

Resolution tests also include what are known as multiburst tests. The lines on the test screen get closer together as they proceed to the right. Therefore, the farther to the right on the test screen the viewer is able to distinguish individual lines of black and white, the better the resolution. This is extremely important for teleradiology, because the radiologist must be able to resolve very small bone and vascular structures (Levens, 1996).

Together, the American College of Radiology (ACR) and the National Electrical Manufacturers Association (NEMA) have developed specific standards for teleradiology that fall under the larger set of Digital Imaging and Communications in Medicine (DICOM) standards. DICOM is a standard for transmitting medical images and related information. It has evolved steadily since its implementation in the 1980s and has come to define how electronic medical imaging devices should transmit information (Levens, 1996). DICOM standards have already been developed for radiology and are now being developed for cardiology and pathology imaging. Details about the current ACR-NEMA standards can be found at the ACR Web site <www.acr.org/f-standards.html>.

Utilization and Cost-Effectiveness

Radiology is by far the most active application of telemedicine, and accounts for about 80 percent of all telemedicine interactions. In 1998, about three hundred thousand diagnostic teleradiology interpretations were done in the United States, most of them through private, for-profit teleradiology providers (Allen & Wheeler, 1998a). This figure does not represent the actual number of teleradiology interactions, for it ignores all nondiagnostic teleradiology interactions that are completed each year. So-called at-home teleradiology, which includes interim-read and preliminary studies, is becoming commonplace, and there is no accurate way of tracking utilization.

There is a modest consensus that teleradiology can significantly reduce radiology services. Due to the predominant use of radiology in telemedicine, this application has been studied for cost-effectiveness more than any other telemedicine specialty (Allen, 1998). Although fewer than twenty such studies have been published to date, most show a reduction in cost, which will only become more significant as the price of equipment and telecommunications continues to drop.

BEHAVIORAL HEALTH CARE

Behavioral telehealth and e-health involve the use of telecommunication and information technology by professionals from many disciplines to provide behavioral health services. A wide variety of behavioral telehealth services are currently offered in a number of contexts, including hospitals, community mental health centers, nursing homes, schools, and jails (Gibson, 2000; Oberkirch, 2000; Smith, 1998; Stamm, 1998; Whitten, Cook, Shaw, Ermer, & Goodwin, 1998; Whitten, Zaylor, & Kingsley, 2000; Zaylor, 2000). The services offered by these organizations involve almost every aspect of traditional behavioral and mental health care delivered face to face. They include assessment and evaluation; mental status examinations; neuropsychological evaluations; crisis intervention; psychotherapy with individuals, groups, and families; accessing patient histories; fine-tuning diagnoses; monitoring patient progress; medication support; remote biofeedback; patient education; patient and family support; case management; preadmission and discharge planning; court commitment hearings; and case conferences (Deleon, Folen, Jennings, & Willis, 1991; Deleon & Wiggins, 1996; Lamberg, 1997; Smith & Allison, 2000). Additional emerging applications include activities related to telehome care with nurses, administrative functions, research, teaching, supervision, staff training, and continuing professional education (McCarthy, Kulakowski, & Kenfield, 1994; Stamm & Pearce, 1995).

The first use of telecommunication technology for psychiatric consultation and treatment was in 1959, when a two-way television link was established in Omaha at the Nebraska Psychiatric Institute (Maxmen, 1977). Limited mental health interventions have therefore operated via videoconferencing technologies for several decades. They were initially housed as experimental projects in specialized telemedicine programs developed for other disciplines such as cardiology, dermatology, and pediatrics. The number of behavioral and mental health interactions has steadily increased throughout the years. In 1998, behavioral health care accounted for about 18 percent of all telemedicine consultations in the United States (Allen & Grigsby, 1998). In 1999, the Association of Telemedicine Service Providers surveyed 132 telehealth programs and found that 42 percent involved mental health services (Grigsby & Brown, 2000). This high utilization rate makes behavioral telehealth the fastest-growing aspect of telehealth.

Behavioral telehealth nevertheless continues to represent an untapped opportunity for many psychologists, social workers, and counselors because psychiatrists and psychiatric nurses have delivered the bulk of these services. This trend is likely to change as e-health education for psychologists, social workers, and counselors increases and new opportunities emerge as e-health companies offer services to clinicians through the Internet.

Types of Technology

As detailed in Chapter Three, many types of technology are available to clinicians.

Telephone. The first technology developed for the audio channel was the telephone. Although neglected as a primary telecommunication device for psychotherapy, the telephone has had a significant place in the development of behavioral health care for several decades. Telephones are instrumental in giving referrals, scheduling appointments, and conducting intake assessments, emergency sessions, follow-up sessions, alternate sessions, and crisis intervention (Liebson, 1997). Nonetheless, the telephone has been discounted as an important vehicle for conducting psychotherapy.

Moreover, the use of telephones has generated very little interest in the scientific community. As with most new areas of practice, much of the research in this area consisted of subjective, inconclusive case reports. The next group of studies improved the research design by increasing the number of subjects, employing control groups, and examining different patient populations (Aneshensel, Frerichs, Clark, & Yokopenic, 1982; Baer, Brown-Beasley, Sorce, & Henriques, 1992; Evans, Smith, Werkhoven, Fox, & Pritzl, 1986; Fenig, Levav, Kohn, & Yelin, 1993; Swinson, Fergus, Cox, & Wickwire, 1995). Nonetheless, most of these studies were still inconclusive and did not provide definitive evidence for or against the use of telephones as primary service delivery vehicles for psychotherapy to previously unknown and undiagnosed patients.

In 1992, the American Psychological Association formed the Telephone Therapy Task Force to address the appropriateness of using telephones for psychotherapy. An article by Haas, Benedict, and Kobos (1996) outlined pros and cons but, owing to the lack of studies in this area, were unable to cite conclusive empirical findings to support or refute their statements regarding clinical utility. Nonetheless, their analysis of ethical issues may be of assistance to practitioners considering the use of a variety of behavioral telehealth and behavioral e-health programs in the future. Haas and colleagues identified a number of areas of key importance related to the requirements of ethical practice using telephones. These included the responsibilities to deliver competent service, avoid patient harm, protect patient confidentiality, obtain informed consent from the patient, and make explicit financial arrangements in both primary and adjunctive treatment by telephone. The authors took the stand that telephones were most appropriate for the delivery of adjunctive services, and their use as a primary treatment vehicle was most appropriate when face-to-face services were not otherwise available.

Studies in recent years have begun to identify with greater accuracy specific patient groups and clinical services with potential for delivery via the telephone (Cukor et al., 1998; Kobak et al., 1997; Rhode, Lewinsohn, & Seeley, 1997). These studies suggest that the telephone may indeed be useful to consumers and practitioners for convenience, desirability, cost-effectiveness, and enhanced outcomes. Research has not yet clearly delineated why the public does not regard the telephone as a primary choice for psychotherapy, however. Findings related to increased social presence as established through videoconferencing may hold some answers to this question.

Meanwhile, telephones are evolving into applications that include teleconferencing with hundreds of participants, Internet applications that offer connections for conversations between two or a thousand people, and audio broadcasting, which parallels radio broadcasting. As the use of audio channels evolves, the audio role in behavioral e-health will undoubtedly gain in importance.

Computer-Assisted Self-Help Programs. Other types of behavioral health services that may involve both assessment and treatment of patients directly includes computer-assisted self-help programs available via the computer, telephone, and Internet. These services are sometimes developed as stand-alone interventions that can be used with or without therapist involvement. Inexpensive, automated telephone technologies have been developed and successfully implemented for a variety of behavioral health care needs (Bruderman & Abboud, 1997; Friedman et al., 1996; Mahone, Tarlow, & Sandaire, 1998; Penk et al., 1999). The fields of computerized assessment (Newman, Consoli, & Taylor, 1997; Pasveer & Ellard, 1998; Sampson, 1995) computerized self-monitoring (Newman, Kenardy, Herman, & Taylor, 1997), and computerized treatment (Newman, Kenardy, et al., 1997) are growing rapidly. Other groups have developed interactive programs based on empirical research offline to work with consumers online. Topics already developed online include weight management (<LearnEducation.com>), tobacco cessation (<NicotineFreedom.com>), stress management (<Stress-Management.com>), and depression management (<CopewithLife.com>).

Other forms of self treatment are available through Web sites for download onto personal computers, such as the Behavioral Self-Control Program for Windows (BSCPW), a program to help individuals who want to moderate their drinking, therapists working with clients with alcohol problems, and trainers who work with other counselors and therapists. BSCPW is available through <BehaviorTherapy.com>.

Video. Behavioral health requires a minimal level of technological sophistication and has been easy to incorporate into telehealth projects that required videoconferencing for more specialized applications. Videoconferencing has thus led the movement toward remote behavioral health care delivery, both in the field and in the scientific literature. Text-based environments have recently come to the forefront and are raising many questions about the nature of behavioral health care and appropriate technologies to be using with patients. Computerized assessment and intervention programs are also gaining status, proving to be effective with and without the involvement of a clinician.

E-Mail and Chat Rooms. Despite the public demand for e-mail and chat room contact with practitioners, empirical analysis of appropriate ethical and diagnostic procedures for use over the Internet is clearly needed before behavioral e-health services based exclusively in textual environments should be offered to unknown consumers worldwide. A number of researchers have attempted to document the experience of working with patients via e-mail, but empirical findings are still difficult to locate (Gustafson et al., 1993, 1994; Jerome, 1997).

More specifically, the therapeutic requirements of obtaining consent, determining diagnosis, and planning appropriate treatment in psychotherapy are complicated. Offering such service online to unknown patients worldwide is fraught with hazards for both patient and clinician. Therefore, the wise practitioner may wait until more empirical studies demonstrate the viability of e-mail, chat room, audioconferencing, and videoconferencing technologies delivered to consumers via the Internet. Specific protocols for delivering direct diagnostic and therapeutic services to unknown patients worldwide must be drawn up and thoroughly tested.

For those who choose to deliver services to the public without waiting for empirical validation of methods, the trend seems to be to offer behavioral e-health services by defining such services as "giving advice," "moderating a chat room," or "coaching" rather than as practicing psychotherapy. As with telephone service delivery, ethical and legal requirements may

E-Health, Telehealth, and Telemedicine

complicate matters to the point of making such benign definitions irrelevant if a situation results in a suicide or homicide. For example, given the broad definition of psychotherapy codified by many state licensing laws, advice given in e-mail and chat rooms may simply be a trap for the unsuspecting practitioner who is eager to participate in the latest technological trend but has not considered the rigors and precise requirements of state law mandated by professional licensure.

Moreover, consumer protection issues are also in question. Patients may be unaware that Internet behavioral health care practitioners may be unlicensed and unregulated, leaving the consumer without recourse if harmed by treatment (Maheu & Gordon, in press).

Even if the majority of consumers visiting Web sites may be well served by alternatives to psychotherapy such as online advice giving, coaching, and moderated chats, one tenet of behavioral health care remains to identify and help patients who are mentally ill. Licensed practitioners have a responsibility to assess and diagnose patients properly before agreeing to deliver service within the context of a professional relationship. Although some developers of dot-com companies believe they can provide valid consent agreements and disclaimers through Web sites, the efficacy of such an approach with mentally ill patients is questionable until proven effective through empirical research. Likewise, until technology can provide tools demonstrated to be comparable to face-to-face assessment and diagnosis, licensed professionals are likely to be held to the face-to-face standard of care set by community norms when agreeing to work with new patients. These issues remain unresolved; they are discussed in more detail in Chapter Eight and Nine.

Implications of E-Mail and Chat Rooms for Behavioral E-Health. The use of e-mail and chat rooms may be an extension of psychotherapy by correspondence, as conducted by Freud at the turn of the twentieth century. Nonetheless, text-based communication technologies may be transforming human communication as well. An examination of the similarities between the research in the use of telephones may be helpful to clinicians looking to the possibilities of using e-mail and chat rooms for contact with behavioral health care patients. (See Chapters Seven, Eight, and Nine for more information related to privacy, security, confidentiality, ethical and legal issues, and risk management.)

Telephones, e-mail, and chat rooms all offer the possibility of anonymity, eliminate visual cues, provide immediate access to a professional, and can be terminated within seconds by a disgruntled patient without the effort needed to walk out of a clinician's office. Therefore, ethical standards identified by Haas and colleagues (1996) for the use of telephones need to be addressed in e-mail and chat rooms. As noted, these include, but are not limited to, the responsibilities to deliver competent service in an area unproven by empirical research, avoid patient harm, protect patient confidentiality, obtain informed consent from the patient, and make explicit financial arrangements (for more on this topic, see American Psychological Association, 1997, 1998).

It is also easier for a patient or practitioner to be distracted while on the telephone, reading or writing e-mail, or typing in a chat room. And all three means of communication are subject to eavesdropping. Clinicians need to be aware of these attentiveness, distraction, and privacy issues. These same concerns are also relevant to use of the video channel.

The Video Channel as the Preferred Technology

It is interesting to note that videoconferencing has become the preferred vehicle for behavioral telehealth rather than the use of telephones. In fact, the terms *telemedicine* and *telehealth* have become synonymous with videoconferencing. The traditional definitions of telepsychiatry and other forms of behavioral telehealth have also equated such service delivery solely to videoconferencing equipment. Furthermore, the early behavioral telehealth literature does not mention the significant use of the telephone as a service delivery vehicle. Such a heavy focus on videoconferencing is considered unfortunate by some researchers (Cukor et al., 1998) yet inevitable by others (Glueckauf, Whitton, & Nickelson, in press). In a review article examining the effectiveness of telephone versus videoconferencing assessment of cognitive state, Ball and McLaren (1997) concluded that telephones could be effective more often than their current use would suggest but that videoconferencing "allows for a much wider range of assessment than the telephone" (p. 126).

The video channel seems to create a social presence, or **telepresence** (Anderson, Newlands, & Mullin, 1996; Cukor et al., 1998; Prussog, Muhlbach, & Bocker, 1994; Sellen, 1995). Telepresence apparently allows the parties to feel comfortable discussing emotional issues, as often crop up in psychotherapy. For example, the visual channel can allow the sender of a message to know if the listener is smiling in agreement or looking skyward in exasperation. These reactions would be lost on the telephone, in e-mail, or in a chat room.

Other potential benefit of using a joint video and audio channel as available through videoconferencing, rather than an audio channel alone as available through telephones and some audio technologies mediated by the Internet, is increased accuracy for delivering information commonly used in assessment and diagnosis. This information includes shifting gaze, facial expressions, and other bodily movements. Nonverbal cues are commonly used in diagnostics, medication consultation, and some psychotherapies. For example, diagnosis of patients with obsessive-compulsive disorder (OCD) was shown effective using videoconferencing technology by Baer et al. (1995). These researchers found that remote video diagnostic assessments resulted in near-perfect interrater agreement when compared to in-person assessment.

New uses of videoconferencing technology are opening the door to new ways of conducting diagnosis and assessment. For instance, videoconferencing's ability to focus in on a scene with added precision using a zoom lens has been found superior to face-to-face consultations when closely examining a patient's reaction to psychotropic medications (Smith & Allison, 2000). Other researchers have found that facial expressions can give information about mutual level of understanding (Whittaker & O'Conaill, 1997). Thus the additional information provided by the video channel may be the most basic of potential technologies to fulfill ethical requirements related to the need for behavioral telehealth and e-health practitioners to ensure comprehension of communication by all parties involved in a psychotherapeutic exchange.

Video Considerations in Behavioral E-Health

As would be expected, some assessment and treatment protocols will require more sophisticated technology than currently available through POTS-based videophones (Squibb, 1999). As broadband capabilities become increasingly available over the Internet, near-television-quality transmission speed and resolution can be expected. Vendors for various types of videophones include Connectix, CU-SeeMe, Intel, InnoMedia, Leadtek, Microsoft, Philips, Smith Micro, Tandberg, and Video Con. Improved Internet, POTS videophones, ATM, or ISDN technologies might be deemed appropriate, based on patient and practitioner satisfaction, cost-effectiveness, access to higher-speed transmission, and patient needs. (See Chapter Three for more details regarding these particular technologies.)

It is interesting to note that initial research using a variety of technologies for videoconferencing, comparing face-to-face, audio-mediated, and video-mediated psychotherapy, shows little difference in outcome between groups studied (Day & Schneider, 2000; Glueckauf et al., 1998; Glueckauf et al., 1999; Glueckauf, Whitton, & Nickelson, in press; Hufford, Glueckauf, & Webb, 1999). Other recent programs are combining the use of videoconferencing and the Internet. For example, a program in rural Australia is combining videoconferencing, videotaping, printed materials, and the Internet by allowing patients who could not attend video-conferenced sessions to obtain videotapes or portions of sessions by means of videostreaming over the Internet (Mitchell & Robinson, 2000). As such research expands to larger groups, different patient populations, and more consistent use of the same technologies to facilitate effective comparison, practitioners will be in a better position to make decisions regarding how to offer behavioral health care most responsibly via these technologies to various populations accessible over the Internet.

Looking to the very near future, broadband capabilities are paving the way for complex video interactions and multimedia services to be delivered simultaneously. The video transmission speeds required to create telepresence are minimal by today's standards. These speeds are achieved with a variety of technologies, including low-cost videophones that use standard telephone lines or the Internet (Croweroft, 1997). The development of specific applications for various behavioral and mental health populations, as well as for specific legal and ethical requirements for service delivery via the broadband Internet, is the next step. The combination of clear video messages and multimedia capabilities over the Internet will allow the practitioners and patients to show and discuss material located on the World Wide Web, simultaneously analyze and view videostreamed information for suggestions regarding behavior change, take advantage of **whiteboarding**, and much more.

Some public Internet Web sites are already beginning to deliver such clinically oriented services for behavioral e-health practitioners and patients. We can expect to see significant offerings to clinicians over the next five years. These broadband capabilities may ultimately free the practitioner and patient from the traditional office setting.

Ethical Concerns for Behavioral E-Health

With mounting empirical evidence for behavioral telehealth, professionals are beginning to accept the concept of local evaluation of a patient by a clinician and referral or consultation with a remote specialist using videoconferencing technologies. It is a leap, however, to consider both evaluation and treatment of unknown patients through technology without face-to-face contact. Such is the potential of the Internet, and many ethical questions are yet unanswered for behavioral e-health care providers.

Consumers may want anonymous psychotherapy in e-mail or chat rooms, and even over the telephone and via videoconferencing technologies, but it is the professional who must decide if such technologies are appropriate for the treatment being requested from undiagnosed consumers worldwide. The American Medical Association (1999) has stated that physicians must see patients face to face before prescribing medication over the Internet; it can be posited that it is the duty of behavioral health care professionals to set limits on demands that may be potentially harmful to consumers.

The ease with which we can communicate with potential patients clashes with the strict requirements to which most licensed professionals in the United States are subject. Even if technology allows us to make contact with unknown patients in new and unprecedented ways, we must nevertheless ask, is it appropriate for professionals to start delivering services using the advanced technologies offered by the Internet? Research has not yet conclusively proven the effectiveness or ineffectiveness of the telephone, videoconferencing, or text-based communication technologies for specific clinical groups. Does that mean professionals are at liberty to experiment on their own and hold themselves out to the public as licensed experts in these new media? Case law has not yet been determined in these areas either. Is it therefore reasonable to proceed with treatment delivery and see what happens?

Answers to these questions are unfortunately clouded by the size of the need for care outside of traditional behavioral health care models. The surgeon general of the United States has reported that almost half of the numbers of people with diagnosable mental health problems do not seek treatment (Satcher, 1999). In a survey of 326 people, researchers reported that over one-fourth of their sample would prefer to seek advice and counseling for depression via the Internet than visit their family physician (Graham, Franses, Kenwright, & Marks, 2000).

Given these types of reports, it is clear that the Internet is the next large-scale vehicle for people to find relief from behavioral health issues. It is hoped that technology will bring professional services to many people who otherwise would not seek this aid. The central questions facing behavioral e-health, which may potentially limit the services offered, are the legal and ethical ramifications, as well as the clinical utility, of each Internet technology for specific patient populations.

Many behavioral health care professionals are uncomfortable not only regarding how to integrate these technologies into daily practice but also regarding how to use them responsibly with an amorphous population that may have members who can prove dangerous to themselves or others. The need for accurate diagnosis before treatment is paramount, whether that involves one or more face-to-face sessions for accurate diagnosis or a battery of psychological assessments given in person or through technology.

While the behavioral health care literature is beginning to offer evidence of how technology can be used with specific groups of patients (Troester, Paolo, Glatt, Hubble, & Koller, 1995; Zarate et al., 1997), these studies are most often conducted in very controlled settings with small patient subgroups. Telecommunication requirements for positive outcomes in behavioral and mental health care are still largely unknown (Glueckauf, Whitton, & Nickelson, in press). Moving from these small studies to offering services to a worldwide population is a very large step and certainly worthy of more research before professionals hang their virtual signs on Web sites and open their browsers to anyone who happens to find them. Caution is in order with the delivery of behavioral health care via technology to undiagnosed consumers (Maheu, 2000a).

A more likely scenario is one that is in practice currently with many military and rural telehealth projects, that of a referring practitioner being present in the room with the patient and using videoconferencing technology to link to a specialist at a remote site. Both the referring clinician and the specialist conduct the assessment, and the patient is thereafter treated by either the referring clinician or the specialist, depending on a number of issues, including the diagnosis of the patient and the licensure of the specialist. This model provides local professional care for the patient, with emergency backup services available through the referring clinician, as well as access to whatever specialized care the patient needs. B. Hundall Stamm also described a scenario encountered in frontier areas, when "there are times when the specialist is on call for a remote area, even when there is no provider in that area. These are nonetheless formal relationships, arranged by a village with a clinician, so there is a level of oversight" (personal communication, September 11, 2000).

It is also important to keep in mind that specific patient populations may respond differently to different technologies. As indicated by the telephone studies previously cited, telephones may be more effective with some patient populations than with others. It is also likely that each type of patient population will benefit from a blend of various technologies at different points in time. For example, patients who have a fear of judgment or interpersonal contact, such as those with agoraphobia, social phobia, anorexia, or schizophrenia, may be treated optimally through a combination of telecommunication technologies and face-to-face sessions. Research will be needed to determine the validity of this hypothesis.

Similarly, some clinicians may work best or be more comfortable interacting with particular patients using a combination of technologies and face-to-face contact. It is also important to note that self-help technologies may be optimal for some patients and that a combination of professional and self-help approaches would be optimal for yet others. Obviously, much research still needs to be conducted to determine the optimal technologies for specific patient-practitioner combinations.

As discussed in Chapter Eight, issues of the professional's linguistic and cultural competence are also relevant to such discussions. Emergency backup for suicidal, homicidal, or duty-to-warn cases is also a necessity. The impact of local events, such as natural disasters, wartime conflicts, local festivities, and traditional holidays, can also influence a patient's mood and therefore must be known to the practitioner offering services to a worldwide population. It is also the responsibility of the professional to explain patient consent agreements verbally and in writing to all potential patients before delivering behavioral service of any type (Maheu, Callan, & Nagy, 1998; Maheu & Gordon, in press).

Furthermore, issues of technology must also be considered by the professional offering services to an Internet population. Reliability of the therapeutic connection is important when establishing rapport and delivering services, yet reliability is all too often problematic when delivering services through telecommunication technologies. Similarly, the confidentiality of patient information, and therefore the security of technology, is a concern of patients and professionals alike. This topic is more thoroughly discussed in Chapter Seven.

However, based on the limited models of behavioral telehealth and telemedicine to date, it is premature to determine appropriate practice guidelines for the use of technology with consumers (Joint Working Group on Telemedicine, 1998; National Telecommunications and Information Administration, 1997). Until such practice guidelines have been developed and are in effect, it may be necessary for face-to-face contact to occur for proper assessment and consent can be obtained before the onset of formal psychotherapy with the majority of behavioral health patient populations.

Organizational and Practical Considerations

While behavioral telehealth and e-health offer promising services to patients, much work still is needed in the practical aspects of delivering such care. In fact, traditional programs still lack basic organizational structures. Research by Whitten, Zaylor, and Kingsley (2000) reports that even formal telepsychiatry programs developed along traditional telemedicine formats are not well organized. This analysis of sixteen active telepsychiatry programs around the world found that programs almost universally did not possess a business or strategic approach to delivering their services. The researchers found an overall lack of formal goals, future strategic plans, and budgetary details in the programs investigated.

On a positive note, data from this same study also point to an interesting direction for telepsychiatry. Both hospital and freestanding programs have traditionally delivered telepsychiatry with the aid of an assistant. These programs have demonstrated that a remote provider can eventually deliver telepsychiatry without the need for an assistant at the local site. In other words, as the learning curve stabilizes for both professionals and patients, the need for telecommunication technology support staff diminishes. In fact, Tracy, McClosky, Sprang, and Burgiss (1999) found that less than 5 percent of all of telehealth consultations involve physicians at both ends of a transmission. As behavioral telehealth care becomes more widely used, it will most likely follow this trend. These findings suggest that delivering mental health services via telecommunication technologies will eventually be a ubiquitous option for providing behavioral and mental health care and that direct video connections from clinician to patient over the Internet will be an increasingly viable approach to delivering behavioral health care.

Cost-Effectiveness

Compared to cardiology and radiology, for which fidelity of digital images is critical, behavioral telehealth requires less complicated technology and therefore can be more cost-effective.

In Australia, a telepsychiatry rural outreach service was compared to traditional face-to-face consultations in terms of cost effectiveness. In that study, health services were delivered to a mining town six hundred miles from the regional hospital in Townsville. The results of the study showed considerable savings from reduced travel by patients and health care practitioners (Trott & Blignault, 1998).

Other studies are showing that behavioral health care services can be offered to existing face-to-face patients inexpensively and conveniently through low-end technology, such as videophones over regular phone lines without the use of computers. As discussed in Chapter Three, these inexpensive videophones connect telephones and televisions. They have been shown to serve as adequate vehicles for patients to feel emotionally connected to their therapists in mental health applications using technology (Cukor et al., 1998). Videophone technology is migrating to the Internet and offering added benefits of multimedia and real-time video to the home-based consumer market. Research is needed to provide a cost-benefit analysis of these broadband services for enhancing the therapeutic alliance, proving clinical utility by improving treatment outcomes for behavioral e-health.

HOME CARE

Telehome care can be defined as providing monitoring (telemetry) and home health care services at a distance, using advanced telecommunication and information technology. It includes a variety of services, such as physiologic monitoring, patient education, compliance reminders, and social support to isolated individuals. Cost is now a limiting factor for home care, but as practitioners and health plans become more knowledgeable about the potential of telehome care, they will be able to provide cost-effective services to patients (California Telehealth/Telemedicine Coordination Project, 1997).

Clinical Applications

Telehome care provides service for the elderly, the chronically ill, patients who have been recently discharged from the hospital, and many others restricted to their homes. The advantages of telehome care include easier accessibility to health care and more frequent social and clinical interaction with providers. It can decrease costs by enabling close monitoring of patients who have a chronic or deteriorating condition. The practitioner also has an opportunity for more timely interventions. It can allow convalescent patients to continue living at home instead of relocating to expensive nursing facilities. Patients remain in their communities to access care, which has far-reaching benefits to both patients and the businesses serving them. Telehome care also enables improved responsiveness and higher frequency of visits by nurses, thereby reducing unnecessary hospital visits (Burdick, Mahmud, & Jenkins, 1996).

Telehome care has enormous potential. The need for such care is increasing because of several factors. Demographic trends show an increasing population of people living in rural areas, where it is not convenient or feasible to get to a hospital. And as the baby boom generation ages, there will be a growing population of elderly people who will need health care. As the first generation extensively exposed to Internet technology, these people are more informed about e-health services. In addition to demographic changes, there has been a decade-long movement from hospital-centric health care to clinic- and home-based health care.

Research into the benefits of telehome care is yielding positive results. The Office for the Advancement of Telehealth grantees have found that telehome care has been largely successful and can allow greater access to care, particularly in rural settings where a nurse may have to travel two hundred miles one way for a twenty-minute face-to-face visit with a homebound patient. With telehome care, a home health nurse can "visit" multiple patients in one day using interactive video (Office for the Advancement of Telehealth, 1999b).

Properly structured telehome care systems that directly interface with computer-based medical reporting and case management software will increase staff efficiency for treating the cases with the highest clinical priority. Telecommunication technology provides better documentation of patient care services and thus can decrease omissions and exposure to risks associated with negligence and other forms of human error.

The American Telemedicine Association has recognized the need for standards and clinical guidelines for home health care. The association has outlined important criteria for patients and practitioners to consider, along with recommendations for developing technical criteria when using telehealth technology to provide telehome care services. The guidelines are available at the ATA Web site <www.atmeda.org>.

Cost-Effectiveness

The potential savings from telehome care are enormous. The average on-site home visit by a registered nurse costs about $90 in the United States. Much of this cost is to cover the nurse's travel time, which limits the average visiting nurse with respect to either the number of patients visited or miles traveled. Because the average telenurse can complete up to fifteen to twenty visits per day (Goldberg, 1997), telehome nursing visits cost only $15 to $25 per visit, including the cost of the nurse's time. This significant leveraging of a nurse's time is a compelling impetus for developing the telenursing option.

A published study (Allen et al., 1999) quantified the activities home health care nurses undertook during their home visits, and from this information estimated the percentage of home health care visits that could have been delivered using the electronic technologies available in 1996. Home nursing charts of 906 patients in four states were reviewed for relevant data. The study estimated that 47 percent of the home health care visits could have been delivered through telehealth technologies.

Another study from the United Kingdom (Wootton et al., 1998) using the same methodology contrasted significantly with the former study. It concluded that only about 15 percent of home health care visits could have been made using telehealth technologies. Although the reason for the discrepancy is not completely clear, it appears to be related to differences in the acuity of care for the respective countries (higher acuity in the United Kingdom) and to social factors.

Cuts in U.S. home care reimbursement are making the use of technology to leverage the process of health care delivery a necessity—especially in rural communities where travel can be very costly (Russo, 1999). Garnering the support of nurses for such drastic changes to their pay scale is a separate challenge, however. Home health care nurses often become disgruntled after realizing a telehome visit can be conducted up to fifty-five minutes faster than the traditional method. If the intent of the organization is to reduce overall costs associated with skilled nursing visits (SNVs), creative problem solving may be helpful. For example, reimbursement structures could be modified to make the field more attractive to nurses using telehealth technology, or the organization could contract with a health management organization to create a more comprehensive disease management program and thereby share costs and cost savings with the payer (K. Rau, personal communication, October 6, 1999).

Sample Telehome Care Programs

The following sections present accounts of some successful home care programs that incorporated telecommunication technology.

Senior Care. Initial studies of a telehome care program in Kansas that provides nursing services to elderly people in four rural areas indicated that telehealth was an adequate means of delivering nursing services into the home. Researchers have examined patients' and nurses' perceptions of a variety of related issues (Whitten, Collins, & Mair, 1998).

The program used a cable television–based interactive video system that transmits video pictures at 30 fps. According to the patients, the technology was not an important issue. They did not describe any difficulties in adapting to its use or function. Use of telehealth technology also did not appear to have any negative effects on communication. Results also show that overall, patients perceived the system as a valuable resource that offered great potential, and they were very enthusiastic about the project. An issue that did arise were the types of illnesses that could be treated (Whitten, Collins, & Mair, 1998). Later, this project added ISDN and POTS-based technologies to the repertoire of technologies used to bring nursing services directly into patients' homes.

Kaiser Permanente Medical Center in Sacramento, California, launched a telehome care project to evaluate satisfaction and cost-effectiveness. Kaiser's project involved newly referred elderly patients diagnosed with congestive heart failure, chronic obstructive pulmonary disease, or cerebral vascular disease. With 212 subjects, this study (Harris, 2000) is unique in having enough statistical power to actually prove the benefits of telehealth. The research concluded that more than 90 percent of patients were satisfied with telehome health care services. In addition, the researchers concluded that the average direct costs for home health care services were $1,830 for the nontelehome health patients and $1,167 for those receiving telehome health services.

Senior Health Online, created by Crozer Keystone Health System in partnership with Community Transit of Delaware County, Senior Community Services Inc., and the Delaware County Office of Services to the Aging, provides seniors living in Delaware County, Pennsylvania, with in-home connections through their televisions, giving them access to community services, contact with their health care providers, and Internet service. This interactive network helps older adults remain independent. Using this simple technology, participants can, for example, arrange transportation services, order home-delivered meals, speak with a case manager, retrieve information on community events and activities, and receive medication reminders (Russo, 1999).

E-Health, Telehealth, and Telemedicine

Public Health. Various public health programs have begun identifying and tracking community needs. Through a project at the University of South Florida called Comprehensive Assessment for Tracking Community Health (CATCH), program developers have created a data warehouse of health status information that is available to local communities for health assessment and planning. This information clearinghouse creates a single source of data necessary to evaluate a community's health status. It makes the information available to multiple end users. For the first time, sixty-seven counties in Florida can access an objective and systematic profile of the health needs and problems of their communities. The project developers hope that this will result in focused programs aimed at decreasing or eliminating the identified community health problems (Russo, 1999).

In yet another approach to serving communitywide needs, the Every Block a Village Program, a partnership with the PCC Community Wellness Center, West Suburban Hospital, and Loyola University's Center for Urban Research and Learning in Illinois, has successfully trained citizen leaders to use in-home technology (WebTV) to help their neighbors obtain timely health information and services. The program provides access to an electronic doctors' office center, health and safety information, and a twenty-four-hour triage and information service (Russo, 1999).

Comprehensive Programs. Many programs offer a comprehensive range of services. For example, the Dakota Telemedicine System at MedCenter One Health Systems represents an electronic lifeline between rural patients and the support they need. MedCenter One's telemedicine consults include orthopedics, radiology, mental health, dermatology, emergency and trauma, pediatrics, neurology, critical care, plastic surgery, cardiology, internal medicine, and physical therapy (the most prevalent consults being in the areas of orthopedics, mental health, and trauma) (Russo, 1999).

In fall 1995, Sauk Centre Home Care and St. Michael's Hospice in Minnesota integrated telehome care technology into both home care and hospice using American TeleCare's MCI flip phone system. This program was initiated in what was at the time a highly competitive home care and hospice environment that was moving toward a prospective payment system for patients receiving medical assistance. The ultimate goal was to realize an overall reduction in associated skilled nursing visit costs (mileage, travel time, and direct time) as a means of surviving fluctuating Medicare reimbursement policies. Primary nurses were asked to select patients based on the patient's and caregiver's cognitive ability to use the equipment, the diagnosis, the number of miles from the agency, and the patient's need. Specific diagnoses included terminal illness, rheumatoid arthritis, diabetes, and congestive heart failure. Preliminary data suggested that patients found the equipment easy to operate; that nurses displayed an adequate ability to capture appropriate and necessary data; and that mileage, time, direct time, overtime, and bonus pay were all reduced. Problems associated with the program were that the available technology required installation of a costly second phone line for the use of the stethoscope. In addition, video and audio transmission was slow, with the equipment operating at only 4 to 7 fps. The Minnesota Department of Health became actively involved by reviewing policies and procedures related to staff and patient orientation, trouble-shooting techniques, patient consent forms, infection control, standards of practice, and more (K. Rau, personal communication, October 6, 1999).

The telehome care project of the University of Minnesota is using a combination of the Internet, videophones, and physiological monitoring devices (handheld devices with peripherals) that connect to a client's television and telephone lines to supplement traditional home health care visits. The project focuses on three health states: heart failure, chronic obstructive pulmonary disease, and wound care (Russo, 1999).

Disease Management

Although much of the telehealth focus has been on radiology and home health care, a promising area of development is disease management (Schlachta, 1998). Disease management extends beyond home health care by focusing on education and preventive measures. In pilot programs, various professionals and nurses (who follow approved protocols) use tele-

conferencing equipment to instruct patients in disease management techniques, such as following dietary and behavioral programs. More specifically, they teach, monitor, and assist patients to change existing behaviors
related to illness and recovery. Such remote disease management systems
can reduce total health care costs of chronically ill patients by reducing the
number of emergency room visits, pharmacy costs, and ICU and hospital
admissions (Rauber, 1999).

The model for telehealth-based disease management systems was previously tested and proven effective with chronically ill patients in the 1996
Georgia-based Electronic Housecall Project (Jerant, Schlachta, Epperly, &
Barnes-Camp, 1998). It was focused on prevention as opposed to typical
acute care delivery. The system developers concluded that the disease management model requires a shift in the thinking and actions of providers.
Physician resistance to disease management in general is often a barrier to
the design and implementation of telehealth-based disease management
programs. The situation is also further complicated by software that con-
fuses rather than encourages physician involvement. The active presence of
physician champions in both the development and implementation of user-
friendly and timesaving software are vital to the success of such an initiative.

A successful program was developed by Pennsylvania State University,
the Visiting Nurse Association of Greater Philadelphia, and American
TeleCare, Inc. The three combined efforts to use information technology
to provide home disease management services to insulin-dependent dia-
betics in Philadelphia County. The project continues to provide valuable
information on the use of technology in disease management and to improve its program design and applications to other chronic diseases beyond diabetes (Russo, 1999).

Another successful disease management program is CHESS, in Madison, Wisconsin. Patients diagnosed with AIDS, breast cancer, and a number of other conditions are given a PC-based home health workstation by
their insurance companies. The workstation comes loaded with up-to-
date information specific to the patient's condition and serves as a sort of
electronic support group that allows patients to talk directly to their

health professionals, to connect with local community groups, or to confer with people with similar diagnoses.

Gustafson and colleagues (1999) report that these patients take more responsibility for their own recovery, demonstrate an improvement in their overall quality of life, require less clinical care, are hospitalized for a shorter time, and cost much less per day. In a number of studies, researchers concluded that computerized health support systems can offer the benefits of specialized professional expertise to various patient populations while providing depth and specificity of individual information, social support, and decision-making tools (Rolnick et al., 1999).

CONCLUSION

Clinical applications of telehealth technologies are limited only by the imaginations of the organizational leaders, practitioners, and patients using them. We most certainly have only glimpsed the world of possibilities to be experienced in our own lifetimes. Chapter Five looks at the movement of these early clinical telehealth programs to special settings and broad populations using the Internet.

CHAPTER 5

Special Settings

A boy bounced around his seventh grade classroom, just as he had done for the past several years. Even though he had a long history of behavioral problems, his mother had never been able to leave work or find transportation to take him to a psychiatrist. This year was different. This year the child was able to go to his school nurse's office to have his medical visit. The psychiatrist never left his office. Instead, with the mother's written permission the school nurse made an appointment with the psychiatrist, who conducted a visit via telecommunication technology with the boy in the school nurse's office. The diagnosis was attention deficit hyperactivity disorder. The child received follow-up telecare on a regular basis, coordinated with his regular pediatrician, and there was noticeable improvement within three months. The mother later stated, "I wish this service had been available for my son when he was younger. If it had, he might not have had to repeat a grade in elementary school."

Telehealth applications have expanded to broader points of service, such as correctional facilities, the military, rural health settings, personal residences for home health and long-term care, schools, overseas countries for international projects, and the Internet. Telecommunication technologies are used at all these points of service, for particular purposes. The goal of this chapter is to provide an overview of telehealth applications in these various special settings.

CORRECTIONAL FACILITIES

Prisoners make up the only population in the United States that has a constitutional right to health care. However, this population is considered medically underserved, because prisoners have generally not received appropriate and timely medical attention. This is true in part because the provision of health services is subordinate to the missions of maintaining the security of the institution and custody of inmates. Addressing prisoners' health care needs is a demanding task that sometimes requires the transport of inmates over hundreds of miles to receive specialty care.

Pursuant to the federal lawsuit *Ruiz* v. *Texas* (1981), primary care physicians must be available to inmates on-site and provide primary care and specialty services consistent with those in the surrounding community. This is a daunting task. The United States is the world leader in the rate of incarceration, which is six to ten times that of other industrialized nations (Sentencing Project, 1995) and an inmate population approaching two million (Huling, 2000). Providing community-comparable health services to such a large number of inmates puts a great strain on the correctional facilities. Telemedicine has been researched to discover its potential to relieve some of this strain.

Advantages Provided by Telehealth

The first correctional telemedicine system in the country began in 1973 in a project funded by the National Science Foundation. Led by Dr. Jay Sanders at the University of Miami School of Medicine, the telemedicine system linked the Dade County Jail with Jackson Memorial Hospital (J. Sanders, personal communication, May 29, 2000). Despite the program's local success, enthusiasm for the concept in correctional facilities did not reappear for two decades. In 1996, the federal government formed a Joint Program Steering Group to study the feasibility of using telecommunication technologies within the military and the federal prison system. The first task of the group was to identify and develop technologies of interest to law enforcement and the military. In September 1996, a hub site at the United States Medical Center for Federal Prisoners in Lexington, Kentucky, was connected with remote sites at the U.S. penitentiaries (USPs) in Lewisburg and Allenwood, Pennsylvania.

The majority of the physicians and patients involved in the demonstration project reported that teleconsults were effective substitutes for face-to-face consultations for psychiatry and dermatology. However, other medical needs of the prisoners, such as cardiology and orthopedics, seemed to be best served within the institution. Because of the high success and satisfaction with telepsychiatry, a nearly complete substitution of teleconsults for in-person psychiatric care took place very quickly (U.S. Department of Justice, 1999).

In another study (Mekhjian, Warisse, Turner, Gailiun, & McCain, 1999), prisoners consistently gave favorable satisfaction ratings when using teleconsults. In this study, prisoners preferred the use of technology, for example, because it allowed them faster access to general health care as well as to specialty care. The improved referral system also led prison administrators to hypothesize that the improved psychiatric care available through technology helped calm the prisoners and led to fewer incidents of violence. More specifically, after the telehealth demonstration began there were fewer assaults at USP-Lewisburg and USP-Allenwood than in the previous year (U.S. Department of Justice, 1999).

Some correctional facilities have inmates representing more than forty different nationalities. Many of these inmates speak obscure dialects of their native language as well. Language is often a barrier to health care in prison systems with highly diverse populations. Telemedicine can provide specialists or translators to communicate with these inmates (R. Ax, personal communication, March 16, 1999).

Another advantage to using telecommunication technology is related to provider satisfaction. Many correctional facilities are built in rural areas where clinicians often do not want to practice. As we have noted elsewhere, having access to other professionals via technology reportedly reduces practitioner isolation by increasing consultation and social support. Technology also provides opportunities for distance learning, which can enhance the role of the on-site health care personnel.

Another potential benefit of using telecommunication technology in larger systems is the optimization of specialized staff and resources. For instance, even if only one in ten prisons has a neuropsychologist, practitioners may not need to consult a specialist outside the correctional system for a neuropsychological consult. Technology allows practitioners to obtain consultation from experts in other geographical areas (Magaletta, Fagan, & Ax, 1998).

Cost-Effectiveness

As correctional facilities are being built and populated at unprecedented rates, there is increased pressure from both the general public and system administrators to minimize costs and devise more efficient ways to deliver health care to prisoners. Options for reducing costs for these facilities are available through technology by developing partnerships with major medical centers and managed care companies (Rabinowitz, 1997).

The potential cost-effectiveness of using technology for prison teleconsults has wide appeal for administrators (Magaletta, Bartizal, & Pratsinak, 1999). Transporting inmates and bringing specialists to rural prison sites is a costly and sometimes dangerous process. Technology cannot only reduce the cost involved in transporting inmates and allow for more specialized and timely care but also reduce the danger of ambush or simple escape related to repeatedly transporting prisoners (Zincone, Doty, & Balch, 1997). Keeping costs down and helping maintain security may also lead to an increase in the quality of inmates' health (Hipkins, 1997; Magaletta et al., 1998).

Although prison teleconsultation start-up costs can take a while to recoup, the more the system is used, the lower the per-unit cost. Equipment expenses will increase initial operating expenses, but leasing and outside funding can help offset these costs. The break-even point can range from as early as seven months after implementation (McCue, Hampton, Marks, Fisher, & Parpart, 1997) to four years (Zincone, Doty, & Balch, 1997). Savings result from the reduced use of escort personnel and from lowered medical costs due to fewer emergency room visits and less duplication of

E-Health, Telehealth, and Telemedicine

lab tests. To further reduce costs, teleconsultation equipment can also be used for legal proceedings, inmate visitations, and parole hearings (Brunicardi, 1998).

Texas, which has one of the highest inmate populations in the United States, was one of the first states to implement a large-scale approach to teleconsults for cost reduction. The Texas Department of Information Resources implemented a two-way statewide video network, called Vidnet. Delivering educational programming and medical assistance throughout the state, Vidnet aims to save the Department of Corrections 50 percent in medical transport costs annually (Wallace, 1996).

Another correctional teleconsultation pioneer is the Ohio Department of Rehabilitation and Corrections. Implemented in 1995, the project evaluated the use of interactive video for linking practitioners at the Ohio State University Medical Center with inmates from the Southern Ohio Correctional Facility in Lucasville and the Corrections Medical Center in Columbus.

The costs of providing inmate medical care were lowered by reducing or removing the need for additional security guards, vehicles, and travel time for physicians (Mekhjian, Warisse, Gailiun, & McCain, 1996). As predicted, continued use of the service after termination of the pilot project also increased savings (Brunicardi, 1998). This study also demonstrated (as have similar programs) that teleconsults enabled inmates to receive health care in a more timely fashion (Mekhjian et al., 1996).

Additional projects have addressed specific health care issues, such as those related to HIV-positive inmates. The Virginia Department of Corrections and Virginia Commonwealth University's Academic Health Center conducted a feasibility study that involved HIV specialty teleconsults (Mazmanian et al., 1996; McCue, Hampton, Marks, Fisher, Parpart, 1997). Among other things, the study evaluated the costs and benefits of such consultations. Benefits included dollar savings in transportation and medical reimbursement, more consistent and timely treatment of inmates, and reduced security risks associated with transporting inmates. Inmate and practitioner satisfaction was another key element to the success of these health care–specific programs. Over 90 percent of the treated Virginia inmates indicated satisfaction with the consultation. They preferred the convenience of not traveling and reported good communication with consulting health care practitioners.

Exemplar Prison Telehealth Project

The University of Texas Medical Branch (UTMB) and the Texas Tech Health Science Center (TTHSC) provide health care services for roughly 130,000 inmates of the Texas Department of Criminal Justice through a health maintenance organization (HMO). The HMO regularly contracts with various universities or local hospitals on a fixed-sum-per-prisoner basis. Telecommunication technology was implemented to solve some of the medical problems associated with prison health care (Brecht, Gray, Peterson, & Youngblood, 1996).

After establishing the usefulness and acceptability of the telecommunications network, UTMB linked four rural sites to its hospital via a T-1 connection in 1994, and teleconsults began at a rate of thirty to fifty a week (Dakins & Jones, 1996). The system used a range of available technologies, from two-way interactive video to store-and-forward systems for ophthalmology and archiving. The network now takes advantage of a less expensive dial-up ISDN network provided by the state Department of Information Resources. The consultant centrally controls the network. The presenter simply needs to focus the camera. Allowing a great deal of flexibility in the system, this arrangement permits a nurse, physician assistant, or prison physician to present patients. The system encompasses nearly every medical specialty. The areas of heaviest volume include orthopedics, infectious disease, and general surgery (Allen, 1995a).

Because reimbursement for practitioner services is provided through the managed care contract, the network is able to operate without grants or federal funds. For example, the managed care contract for 1996 allocated UTMB $180 million for all inmate health care, including telehealth. Operating costs for the network totaled about $300,000 in 1996, which was about the same as the previous year's expenditures on inmate transportation

(Dakins & Jones, 1996). Savings to the prison facility were one of the major benefits of the system. The managed care plan saved over $125 million over a five-year period (1994–1999). Users surveyed throughout the project indicated a high degree of satisfaction on the part of patients, presenters, and specialty consultants (Brecht, Gray, Peterson, & Youngblood, 1996).

Having reviewed the results of a demonstration project in 1992 that worked with 437 prisoners, UTMB officials concluded that teleconsults were technically viable and acceptable to patients and physicians (Dakins & Jones, 1996).

Because telehealth addresses crucial cost-benefit considerations within the capitated care environment that characterizes prison health care, and brings about a measurable decrease in the risks associated with prisoner transportation, prison care has been at the forefront of telehealth activity in the U.S. In 1997, four of the ten most active telehealth programs involved correctional facilities (Wheeler, 1998).

MILITARY SETTINGS

The U.S. military is viewed as a leader in telehealth applications worldwide, largely because telehealth has received substantial funding and is supported by numerous research and development projects. Telecommunication technology increases the accessibility of specialty care and can offer immediate care for personnel wounded in combat zones, where timely, efficient, and accurate information is necessary for quality trauma care. Technology can deliver patient information, treatment records, and medical knowledge to medics who can then properly treat wounded personnel. In peacetime, technology permits remote military treatment facilities to link with specialty clinics.

Advantages Provided by Military Telehealth

Because of the nature of medical practice in a battle zone, the primary requirements for battlefield technology are speed of transmission and ready availability of information. Issues of licensure and liability, for instance, have little bearing. Military telehealth is thus a unique setting that can push the edge of technical capabilities, unencumbered with legalities that might impose constraints on the creative development of technology. As a result, military telehealth programs have led the way in

Creating and updating electronic patient records

Efficiently transmitting electronic patient records so that medical personnel will have information about the patient and the casualty before arrival

Improving readiness by providing access to computer-aided medical instruction, collaborative mission rehearsal, and medical and surgical simulations

Enhancing health status monitoring through the development of a variety of physiological sensors

Many of the telehealth technologies developed by the military for use on the battlefield also have applications for civilian use. These include individual monitoring devices and biosensors, diagnostic ultrasound imagery, and advanced life support for trauma patients and transportation from remote locations. These applications promise to improve the continuity of care for both the military and civilian sector by providing access to specialized consultants, bringing instant responsiveness to patient needs, and reducing health care costs (Burdick, Mahmud, & Jenkins, 1996).

The ability to provide integrated health care in diverse and distant situations has long been a focus of the U.S. military. In the late 1980s and early 1990s, the U.S. armed forces implemented telemedicine technology in several natural disasters and conflicts (Garshnek & Burkle, 1999a, 1999b). For example, the U.S. military set up a telemedicine system connecting mobile army surgical hospital (MASH) units, army hospitals, and tertiary centers. The system proved useful, transmitting 749 radiological images and fifty-five other services (Jones, 1996).

During the Persian Gulf War in 1991, advanced telecommunication technology was combined with mobile health units for a variety of emergency and trauma services. The success of using computed tomography (CT) scanners to transmit CT images via satellites and of using the international telephone networks for expert consultations demonstrated that such systems can function under extreme geographical and climatic conditions, proving the value of teleradiology in combat situations.

In 1992 and 1993, telemedicine proved valuable in the United Nations humanitarian relief effort in Somalia (Garshnek & Burkle, 1999a, 1999b). The Remote Clinical Communications System was used to transmit digitized neurosurgical and neuroradiological images to Walter Reed Army Medical Center in Washington, D.C., using low-bandwidth (9.6 Kbps) telecommunication links to facilitate a variety of telemedicine services (Crowther & Poropatich, 1995).

Cost-Effectiveness

Telecommunication technology allows the military to diagnose, treat, and consult service personnel stationed in remote regions around the globe. To avoid medical evacuations (MEDEVACs) and return patients to work more quickly, the Navy has investigated various possible methods of implementing technology, including the use of telephone and fax, e-mail and the Internet, videoconferencing, teleradiology, and diagnostic instruments (Stoloff, Garcia, Thomason, & Shia, 1998).

Over a one-year period, a panel of Navy medical experts with telehealth experience reviewed a representative sample of patient visits and estimated the savings that might have occurred if telehealth services had been used to avoid MEDEVACs (Stoloff et al., 1998). The ships' medical staffs estimated the savings initially and then projected these figures to the entire fleet. The projections demonstrated that 17 percent of the MEDEVACs would have been preventable (representing 155,000 travel miles) at a savings of $4,400 per MEDEVAC. They concluded that e-mail, Internet, telephone, and fax communications services would be cost-effective on all ships (including small ships and submarines), whereas videoconferencing and teleradiology would be cost-effective only on large ships, such as aircraft carriers and amphibious ships (Stoloff et al., 1998).

The U.S. military is also investigating the cost-effectiveness of avoiding MEDEVACs in the European theater. The U.S. Military Health System commissioned a study to identify ways technology could reduce costs at each European military facility. Two thousand consecutive air referrals were examined to determine whether the use of technology could have avoided evacuation. The study reported that the potential savings amounted to $3.7 million in travel costs and twenty-five thousand working days (Navein, Arose, & Pietermich, 1999).

Exemplar Military Telehealth Projects

The U.S. military is developing the Theater Medical Information Program, designed to link the medical information systems within a battlefield or operational theater. Information gathered through this program includes environmental health data. This analysis will aid commanders in making tactical decisions that could reduce disease and noncombat injuries.

The Defense Advanced Research Project Agency is evaluating a system that alerts the nearest medic when a soldier is wounded in combat. Each soldier would have personal status monitors that include a global positioning system, communications, and vital-signs monitors that the medic can access via a handheld unit. In the case of numerous injured personnel, with such a system the medic could perform "en route triage" and go directly to the most critically injured. The medic could then relay ultrasound information from the image on the handheld device back to the MASH unit for interpretation by a physician (Blakeslee & Satava, 1998). Although these technologies are promising, they have not been fully deployed in the field.

Another program is the Pacific e-Health Innovation Center (PeIC), a Department of Defense program investigating clinically relevant applications of emerging technologies. Located at Tripler Army Medical Center in Hawaii, the PeIC focuses on prototyping, demonstrating, validating, and maturing leading-edge and emerging e-health and telecommunication technologies in the military's Pacific region health care system. The PeIC was launched to investigate the uses of advanced telecommunication technologies to augment traditional health care methods for consultation, diagnosis, and treatment at a distance in both peace and wartime situations. The PeIC has applied technology to provide consultation for such subspecialties as behavioral health, dermatology, orthopedics, and otolaryngology (L. Ierdme, personal communication, August 30, 2000). The PeIC has also demonstrated emerging technologies, such as hyperspectral diagnostic imaging that supports diagnosis of cervical cancer. Continuing technology efforts by the PeIC include creation of proctored surgery protocols and investigation of digital imaging devices. Active PeIC operations link Micronesia, Alaska, Hawaii, the Republic of South Korea, Washington State, Guam, Okinawa, Japan, Diego Garcia, and U.S. Coast Guard and Navy ships at sea to health care resources (Kerrigan, 1999). Early anecdotal indications are that e-health applications can meet consultation needs for linking patients in remote areas to subspecialists. The PeIC is conducting a formal research project to establish empirical data to support the hypothesis that consultation via telecommunication technology is as good as, or better than, a conventional face-to-face patient and provider encounter requiring travel by either the patient or provider (Garshnek & Hassell, 1999).

TRIBAL COMMUNITY HEALTH CARE

Programs for tribal communities have been evolving throughout the history of telemedicine but are slow to develop when compared with correctional and military telehealth applications. Nonetheless, tribal programs have much potential for growth. Often located in remote areas that require extensive travel from visiting health care professionals, tribal communities have benefited greatly from telecommunication technologies developed specifically for their needs. The opportunities for these communities are primarily in home care. It is of special note that funding is available from numerous sources.

Cost-Effectiveness

Properly designed studies are still lacking in this area, and generalizability of findings that do exist is often limited. Many of the projects are still in their second phase, so formal data analyses have not yet been reported (H. Russo, personal communication, October 7, 1999).

Exemplar Tribal Community Telehealth Programs

Several exceptional tribal community telehealth programs have been funded by various federal agencies. The Partners in Health Telemedicine Network (PHTN) is a partnership of health providers in Montana. PHTN has worked to increase health care access and to enhance preventive and maintenance medical education for rural frontier people. The NASA/ KRUG Life Sciences Telemedicine Instrumentation Pack (TIP) unit, initially developed for space flight applications, is being used by PHTN to adapt the unit for rural health care use. The TIP unit, a small portable medical diagnostic system, makes it possible to transmit clear images and other information obtained during a patient assessment. The TIP unit has recently been used by certified diabetes educators at Lame Deer Clinic to capture data during home assessments of Cheyenne tribe members. Due to the low penetration of telephone lines in the Lame Deer reservation, nurses visit patients in their homes and collect information that is then stored and later forwarded to a clinical physician. An additional important component of the project consists of educational programs for patients and medical staff via videoconferencing at remote sites (Russo, 1999).

Known as the Circle of Health, the Northwest Portland Area Indian Health Board Information Infrastructure for the Northwest Tribes project provides electronic communication, collaboration, and online research capabilities for forty-one tribes in Washington, Oregon, and Idaho. One of the goals of the project is to aid the tribes in the collection and analysis of epidemiology information. By tracking and analyzing data, tribes will be able to plan and react more quickly to the needs of their community (Russo, 1999).

SCHOOL SETTINGS

Telecommunication technology is bringing quality health care to children in rural and underserved areas as well as urban areas. An example of a school-based telemedicine project is located in the rural farming community of Hart, Texas (D. McBeath, personal communication, October 5, 1999). This town of twelve hundred residents is located in the Texas panhandle. The only health care provider for the entire community is the school nurse. In April 1998, Texas Tech University Health Sciences Center (TTUHSC) in Lubbock, some seventy miles away, added telecommunication technology to an existing school clinic. For several years prior, TTUHSC had conducted an on-site clinic, one afternoon a week, to give pediatric faculty and residents experience with rural health care. The use of technology allowed a second visit a week via an NEC Videoworks 5000 system, which includes a live-interactive videoconference unit and a satellite link back to the main TTUHSC campus in Lubbock.

The clinics operate only during the school year. On average, four to five children are seen via technology each week. During the first operational year (April 1998 until April 1999), seventy-two patient teleconsults were recorded. Research conducted with patients, families, and physicians indicates that all found teleconsults as acceptable as in-person examinations.

Benefits to the Hart school system have been numerous. The convenience of having access to physicians without the need to travel is a tremendous benefit to students, given that the nearest available health care professional is thirty miles away and that the nearest medical center is seventy miles away in Lubbock. Without the local teleclinic, many of the children would more than likely not seek immediate treatment. Moreover, school officials attribute a 6 percent increase in average daily school attendance to the teleclinic. (This increase in attendance has resulted in additional funds, as the state of Texas funds local schools based on daily attendance.) TTUHSC has also reported benefits, including an excellent rural training model.

There are other uses for telecommunication technology in school-based settings aside from medical consultations. Mental health professionals can meet with troubled children at school via interactive videoconferencing technology, which reduces travel time and relieves the burden of transportation for the parent. In addition, when students are absent from school for extended periods, telecommunication technology can connect the student with the classroom. This can benefit not only the student but also the child's peers, by increasing their awareness of illness and the disease process (T. Kormylo & W. Karp, personal communication, May 22, 2000).

Cost-Effectiveness

The initial investment by TTUHSC of approximately $110,000 for the remote-site Videoworks 5000 and satellite uplink antenna has not been cost-effective in terms of direct cost recovery. The connectivity cost is essentially zero, as the fixed cost of the satellite time is borne through other programs. However, cost recovery comes indirectly from its use as a research and education tool. From an operational perspective, the program is cost-effective when one considers the enhancement of community health care, the extra dollars flowing into the school budget, and the improved school attendance. Future projects, similar to the Hart school clinic, are anticipated to be more cost-effective with regard to capital expense because they will use less expensive equipment.

Other Exemplar School-Based Telehealth Programs

The Tele-KidCare project uses PC-based technology, equipped with electronic peripheral devices, to link physicians and patients for clinical visits from the school nurse's offices in eight schools in Wyandotte County, Kansas. This project increases access to medical services and enhances medical and educational outcomes for children living in this community by focusing on early intervention in the diagnosis and treatment of disease, preventing unnecessary loss of school and activity time, and engaging children in healthy behaviors and self-monitoring of their care (H. Russo, personal communication, October 7, 1999).

Research into the efficacy of a similar program in Kansas City, Kansas, has shown several positive results. Telehealth units are placed in school nurses' offices and linked to practitioners at the University of Kansas Medical Center, who are on call. A child is able to interact with a practitioner in real time without having to leave the nurse's office. The goal is to overcome socioeconomic barriers related to health care for disadvantaged children at their schools (Whitten, Cook, Shaw, Ermer, & Goodwin, 1998).

The preliminary results of the pilot test in four schools with 187 consultations indicate that the most common reason for consultation was ear, nose, and throat problems. The average elapsed time between a request for a consult and confirmation of appointment was twenty-three minutes. When immediate service was requested, 85 percent of consults were completed the same day. The results from the pilot program indicate that technology is able to deliver immediate, adequate service to children in need of health care (Whitten, Cook, et al., 1998).

The Children's Medical Center at the Medical College of Georgia is connecting students with their teachers, classrooms, and homes, thus enabling children who are absent from school due to medical conditions to keep up with their education. The child attends the class and interacts with the teacher virtually using a standard thirteen-inch monitor, videoconferencing equipment, and a telephone and speaker. The student can participate in discussions with the class and complete assignments on the computer. The technology also allows the hospital educator to consult with the teacher instantaneously instead of traveling to the school, saving time and money. The program has proven to be cost-effective (T. Kormylo & W. Karp, personal communication, May 22, 2000).

PROJECTS WITH INTERNATIONAL SETTINGS

In nations in which standards of health care are lower than in the United States, technology can deliver sorely needed and previously inaccessible specialized services. As you might expect, the use of telecommunication technology for international applications is growing, particularly in preventive medicine.

The primary device for improving the world's health is through preventive public health measures such as immunization, maternal and child health care, improved sanitation, and modification of risk factors for disease. The main goal of prevention is to reduce the incidence of disease, be it infectious or chronic (La Porte et al., 1994). Because timely access to quality health care is a need that extends beyond all political borders, technology can be a solution both domestically and internationally. As health departments improve their technical capacity, interactive health communications (IHCs) may become a central strategy for community health education, community outreach for services, and social marketing for positive health behaviors. In fact, some health departments are already developing applications that serve these functions.

In addition, IHCs may have a positive impact on disease surveillance and monitoring of community health indicators. In the future, the idea of disease surveillance may be blended into a larger system of health surveillance, and a substantial proportion of health information and data may be generated by routine collection of data from many community settings rather than be driven by reports from clinical encounters (Eng & Gustafson, 1999). This may lead both to more accurate community health monitoring and to improved detection of disease outbreaks (O'Carroll, 1997).

The development of a global health network offers a unique opportunity to yield improved health and a reduction of costs through preventive actions. The global health network also improves national and international community consciousness through the transfer of accurate and timely information on preventing health care (La Porte et al., 1994). In addition to its monitoring features, the global health network provides almost instantaneous access to information needed for diagnosis and treatment. Furthermore, practitioners can obtain a consult from peers across the globe.

Working in concert toward economic, political, health care, and education goals, the G8 nations (England, France, Canada, Germany, Italy, Russia, Japan, and the United States) are also involved in the deployment of telemedicine. As one of the United States representatives for telemedicine, Dr. Jay Sanders works to help developing nations adopt telemedicine. He explains, "Telemedicine using an IP [Internet protocol] platform is now being viewed by the developing nations as their mechanism for bringing health care to their citizens" (personal communication, May 29, 2000).

However, there are several barriers to implementing a worldwide telehealth and telemedicine network. The most serious barrier to the widespread use of technology in some developing countries is the lack of an adequate telecommunication infrastructure. Even telephone systems in many countries are plagued by an inability to sustain a call once initiated.

The average citizen's lack of computer knowledge also contributes to problems with developing telehealth internationally. Although this problem can be overcome by training, developing countries have not yet demonstrated an overall interest in technology investments. The cost of a telehealth system also presents problems for international developments. Most telecommunication products, including videoconferencing equipment, are more costly in countries other than the United States.

However, the Internet is quickly bringing many solutions to these problems. Successful international preventive telehealth programs have involved the transfer of low-bandwidth medical information via the Internet—more specifically, via e-mail and the World Wide Web. The Internet is rapidly opening avenues of communication to the most remote of regions. Public health workers from Ghana, Brazil, India, and many other developing countries already have access to the latest information related to prevention of disease.

THE INTERNET (E-HEALTH)

E-health can be considered the combined outgrowth of international telehealth projects and private industry expansion into the worldwide marketplace. Because e-health companies have expanded to cover many geographical and marketplace arenas so quickly, we present a typology to acquaint you with this rapidly emerging field.

Looked at in the most general way, e-health companies aim at one or more of three major target groups: the consumer (nonprofessional), the provider, or the supplier and payer. In terms of functions, e-health Web sites offer the "five C's": commerce (online sales, auctions, and so on), connectivity (serving as a link between groups), content (providing information), community, and clinical care (as discussed in Chapter One).

Some Web sites offer all or a combination of these functions. One site that offers a combination of services is Healtheon/WebMD <www.webmd.com>.

It provides a comprehensive Internet health care service for all parties involved in the industry. WebMD offers a communications channel for transactions between participating consumers, employers, physicians, and health care institutions. Consumers are provided breaking news on health care, a library of articles and resources, message boards relating to many areas of interest, chat rooms, and a list of local providers (among other services). Professionals are offered services for increasing the efficiency of office-related tasks, creating their own Web site, taking continuing education courses, obtaining research materials, and pursuing insurance eligibility and verification services. One of the big services that WebMD offers is an employer **portal** where the administration can analyze the demographics of their insured employees, and employees can review their benefits.

The following sections further define the major types of e-health services and include examples of each type. Please note that these examples are intended to serve as illustrations rather than endorsements. Table 5.1 is a snapshot view of the posited categories.

Product Marketing Sites

Insurance companies, medical suppliers, hospitals, clinics, laboratories, and even individual practitioners have created informational Web sites as an indirect marketing tool. Often these sites have articles on health problems, offer self-tests on overall health, or post the latest health news, then offer the products or services designed to cure the ailments described. Essentially, the sites serve the same role as a brochure, direct mailing piece, or newspaper advertisement. AllHealth <www.allhealth.com> offers all of the aforementioned services (articles, shopping carts, self-tests) along with discussion boards and chat rooms for members. Members with an illness can go to this site, research the topic, get recommendations for treatment, then order a related product, all without getting out of their seat.

Metasites

There are many Web sites serving as gateways to specific information, providers, and suppliers. These sites typically provide generic information about an industry or service sector and often include a special link

Table 5.1. Types of Internet Sites

Internet Category	Purpose
Product marketing	Informational sites created as indirect marketing tools, providing information about a product or service
Metasites	Gateways to specific information, support, providers, or suppliers
Patient information and education	Specific information about disease management; support and education for consumers without marketing specific products
Provider information and education	Specific health information or formal continuing education for health professionals without marketing specific products
Medication	Access to over-the-counter and prescription medications
Medical equipment and supplies	E-commerce sites for ordering equipment and supplies directly
Clinical services	Conduit for providing clinical diagnostics or assessment, consultations, office functions, and related services; includes application service providers (ASPs)
Health insurance	E-commerce solution for purchasing and managing health insurance plans
Alternative medicine	Sites for obtaining information or services related to alternative medical solution

to a directory of providers. As is true of business directories in other industries, this combination of health or product information with an online "yellow pages" capitalizes on the benefits of lowered search costs to the health care sector. For example, the American Medical Association home page <www.ama-assn.org/> includes information about the nonprofit group's mission and goals, various medical conditions, and treatments. In addition, the AMA provides an e-commerce service to its visitors through an online physician locator that directs them to the nearest specialist.

Patient Information and Education Sites

Perhaps one of the most exciting developments is an explosion of information access for patients and their families. *SelfhelpMagazine* <www.SelfhelpMagazine.com> represents the combined effort of hundreds of professionals and programmers to form an Internet community to share free information. It offers daily behavioral health care news, articles, reviews, discussion forums, cartoons, postcards, a meditation center, and thousands of links to other health care Web sites. It serves a dedicated readership from over 106 countries. Its consumer audience enjoys material from over 3,800 *SelfhelpMagazine* Web pages and participates in more than one hundred discussion areas.

Provider Information and Education Sites

Health providers are able to access a wide range of health information through OnHealth, Medline, WebMD, and other health databases. Because some patients are walking into their provider's office armed with recent medical information they have gleaned from the Internet, many health providers are feeling increasing pressure to frequently check these information sites themselves.

In addition to accessing health information, health providers are able to obtain continuing educational credits via the Web. Many health organizations offer, as a marketing tool, continuing education credits (mandated by U.S. states for ongoing licensure) for physicians, nurses, and allied health providers. For example, hospitals hope that physicians will refer patients to them for tests and procedures, pharmaceutical companies hope that physicians will prescribe their medications, and nonprofit agencies hope that nurses or physicians will maintain their membership.

A different type of information—or "edutainment," a combination of entertainment and education—is that of live surgeries being performed over Internet channels. This type of broadcast has found some success in television, and a few organizations are now considering broadcasting it with their new telecommunication technology (Thrall, 1999). Also known as Webcasting, video service via the Internet can be directed to only those people who order it (like pay-per-view), and the videos can be shown in real time. New surgeries can be routed to doctors for continuing education, or interested consumers can order them. Revenue generated from this type of service can help balance the cost of installing the technology.

Internet-based services are being recognized by some of the leading professional associations as well. For example, in the mental health field, the Psy Broadcasting Corporation <www.psybc.com/> has been approved for continuing education credit by the American Psychological Association; the National Board of Certified Counselors; the California Board of Behavioral Sciences for Marriage, Family and Child Counselors and Licensed Clinical Social Workers; the National Register of Certified Group Psychotherapists; and the American Psychoanalytic Association. In 1998, Psy Broadcasting won the Gradiva Award for Best New Medium.

Many academic institutions are viewing online continuing education as a potential revenue stream in itself. The Internet offers a way to make continuing education credits available on a continuous basis without necessitating the expense of physically bringing experts to the students. For example, for a fee Stanford University <radiologycme@stanford.edu:80/> provides continuing medical education for radiologists through its Web site. Radiologists select the topic of interest, register, and pay the stipulated fee to participate and obtain credit. Periodic questions appear on the screen to ensure that the doctor is present.

Pharmaceutical companies are also offering e-learning for professionals. A good example is Helix, sponsored by GlaxoWellcome

. Helix offers a wide range of courses on practice management and treatment, as well as career planning. Professionals can benefit from online continuing education courses and from links to audio lectures by world-renowned experts, medical databases, and associations.

Medication Sites

Medications sold on the Internet range from anything traditionally found in the health section of a supermarket or drug store to products prescribed by a physician. E-commerce sites offering medications are emerging in three distinct forms: (1) online sales of over-the-counter (OTC) medications that are delivered directly to the consumer, (2) online ordering of prescription medications that can be picked up by the consumer or delivered directly to the home or office, and (3) direct marketing with an online consultation service for a specific prescription product. These sites often display a disclaimer stating that they are not liable for negative consequences of using their services. The following are examples of sites that offer medications online.

- MoreOnline <www.moreonline.com/pharmacy/> is an online supermarket for consumers who wish to have OTC products mailed directly to their homes. Consumers can purchase a wide range of OTC medications, including but not limited to analgesics, antacids, antidiarrhea products, cold and allergy relievers, menstrual remedies, and vitamins. Clients simply load their shopping carts with these products and charge them to a credit card.

- Wal-Mart <www.wal-mart.com/stores/pharm_mail.shtml>, a national U.S. discount store chain, offers an online service for shipment of any prescription drug within twenty-four hours of receipt. Customers simply e-mail their prescription (obtained from a physician) to Wal-Mart. Clients must provide the name of the medication, their doctor's name, and their doctor's phone number so that Wal-Mart can verify the prescription.

- Medical Center <www.medicalcenter.net/> is an Internet marketing and administrative agency owned by the Pill Pharmacy. It sells Viagra, Propecia, and Claritin to clients around the world via the Web. For example, clients wishing to obtain Viagra are able to obtain an online consultation for a prescription that is then shipped directly to them. A credit card is all that is needed to purchase ten to thirty Viagra pills.

Medical Equipment and Supply Sites

Traditionally, health providers have worked through a company sales representative or distribution middleman to purchase medical equipment and supplies. The Web offers an opportunity for staff to avoid the middleman and shop for everything from hospital beds to bedpans and tongue depressors. The transition from using print catalogues to disseminate information about health commodities to using online publications is remarkably straightforward and relatively simple. Some companies are attempting to establish sites that operate in the style of a "reverse auction," in which consumers set the price they wish to pay for a product, and the different vendors try to meet that price. Priceline now operates in this format for such products as airline tickets and hotel reservations (McCormack, 1999).

There are two potential sets of clients for medical equipment and supply vendors. The first comprises industry members: hospitals, doctors' offices, outpatient health centers, home health agencies, nursing homes, and medical laboratories. The second set of clients is the direct patient population: actual patients and their family members or nonprofessional caretakers. This group directly purchases a host of medical equipment and supplies, including specialty beds and mattresses, wheelchairs, canes, glucose monitors and supplies, blood pressure monitors, or bulk items such as wound dressings and bandages. The main focus is on the baby boomers who are beginning to have health problems and are taking a keen interest in the Internet. Many of these consumers are also handling the medical decisions for their aging parents, who find health care to be too strenuous (Gillespie, 1999). It is interesting to note that the preponderance of e-commerce sites currently being developed are directed at businesses rather than at these individuals. This is logical given current trends in computer dissemination and use, but as the health care market becomes more solidly established and publicized, there may be a shift in focus. The following two sites provide such services.

• CustomerLinks <www.pssd.com> bills itself as the first Internet-based health care solution designed for medical practices. CustomerLinks claims to be a source for information and a multitude of services—including direct online ordering of medical supplies, equipment, and pharmaceuticals—accessible twenty-four hours a day.

• Able Medical Aids <www.ablemedical.com/> sells medical equipment and supplies to clients for use in their homes or in assisted living environments, and to professionals in the medical field. Thus prospective clients range from individual consumers to health organizations. Able Medical Aids' products include bathroom safety equipment, mastectomy supplies, ostomy and incontinence supplies, and medical equipment and wheelchairs. The company delivers nationally.

Clinical Service Sites

The Internet has the potential to be an important conduit for the accessing of medical care and services. The purchasing of medical diagnoses, treatment recommendations, ongoing health care management, or a simple second opinion from a licensed health provider falls in this category. These services could theoretically be purchased from a physician, nurse, nurse-practitioner, physician assistant, psychologist, social worker, or speech, physical, or occupational therapist.

Currently, the handful of forays into e-health appears to be coming from a few enterprising practitioners who have virtual offices on the World Wide Web. These practices allow patients to log onto the Internet, type in their credit card number and a description of their symptoms, and be connected to a real practitioner (Greene, 1997). This service may help solve the issues of access to adequate health care for people who are physically unable to see a professional due to various constraints. The following are examples of Web sites offering these services.

• WorldClinic <www.worldclinic.com> is a company that provides overseas telemedical support to U.S. corporate employees traveling abroad.

• Health Hero Network <www.healthhero.com> helps health care professionals connect with patients to manage chronic disease.

However, health care delivery by professionals is a highly regulated business. As we have already discussed, this modality of service raises a number of perplexing legal questions about licensure, efficacy of care, and ethics. In addition, there are worries that Internet-based care opens the door to the misrepresentation of credentials by health providers as well as the falsification of illnesses by patients attempting to obtain prescription drugs. For a more complete discussion of these issues, refer to Chapters Eight and Nine.

Office Functions

Many time-consuming office functions can be performed quickly over the Internet. Merck-Medco found that many nurses spend nearly 80 percent of the day—over six hours—handling prescriptions; pharmacies make millions of calls to providers' offices because of incorrect or unreadable prescription forms. Authorizations and referrals take up much of the remaining time. These types of inefficiencies cost the health care industry up to $280 billion dollars per year, according to some estimates. Expenditures of time and money can be reduced through the use of electronic transactions. Services that allow eligibility verification on the desktop save six hundred to eight hundred hours per year for many offices using the system (Menduno, 1999, 2000).

Hospitals are also looking into using Internet technology to improve office functions. For example, Milwaukee's nine hospitals are connected through the Internet. In emergency and disaster situations, patients can be directed to different hospitals according to doctor availability. When one hospital's emergency room has reached its capacity, it will refer other critical patients to the nearest available hospital (Pasternack, 1998).

Some companies have found that using the Internet for supply orders saves money and space. MacNeal Health Network now uses its seven-thousand-square-foot warehouse for other purposes than storing backup supplies. MacNeal relies on a materials management system that automatically tracks supplies and then places orders over the Internet for overnight delivery (Solovy & Serb, 1999).

A significant new form of service available to clinicians over the Web is integrated clinical and management software, which clinicians access from outsourced, centralized application service providers (ASPs). Emerging ASPs charge only a subscription fee and nominal transaction fees for a wide variety of services. These services free clinicians and clinical organizations from the expense of purchasing, maintaining, and upgrading software for their individual desktops. With ASPs, there is no substantial up-front investment in software, nor are there costly upgrade fees, because each upgrade is handled through the ASP's main server rather than on the clinician's computer; hardware costs are lower; and the clinician requires only a very basic computer (T. Trabin, personal communication, May 29, 2000).

Despite the obvious advantages, many issues are still to be resolved. One is data privacy in transmission and storage of confidential patient information; definitions of who owns the data; another is the guarantee of quick access and transmission power over the Internet so that transactions are reliable and expedient.

The following are some examples of ASPs:

• Healinx <www.healinx.com> provides a Web-based messaging system, among several other tools designed to facilitate physician-patient communications. Using Healinx, patients can request online consultations, fill prescriptions, schedule appointments and obtain referrals to specialists, access their medical profile, and engage in online consultations with their own physician. Physicians establish an online presence through their own Healinx Web site and can interact with patients in a secure environment that exceeds the guidelines of the HCFA and the American Medical Informatics Association. Physicians can broadcast customized prevention and wellness messages and general newsletters. Healinx also provides disease management tools for payers and other managed care organizations. Their routing capability allows messages to be intelligently directed to the physician's staff, relieving the physician of the burden of responding personally to the vast majority of messages.

- MedicaLogic <www.medicalogic.com> aims to aid patient-practitioner communication through the use of electronic and Internet-based medical records. The company, which focuses on ambulatory care, offers the practitioner an efficient schedule management program and brings patient records to the point of care. Other MedicaLogic services streamline communication between the practitioner's staff and colleagues.

- Confer <www.confer.com>, a software developer for the health care industry, provides Internet-based applications for securely managing the flow of information from patients to providers to payers to suppliers. The company has developed database security technologies that are fully compliant with the federal Healthcare Information Portability and Accountability Act (HIPAA). This information flow, combined with the company's disease management capabilities, allows it to identify at-risk patients and contact them to assess their willingness to change.

- Asterion <www.Asterion.com> develops a wide range of technologies that enable a health care community to access such services as eligibility and benefits verification, interactive clinical guidelines, referrals, concurrent review, claims adjudication and processing, and capitation disbursement. Asterion also supplies technology for use in case, disease, medication, and practice management, as well as application software, hardware, networking, integration, installation, training, consultation, and ongoing service and maintenance.

Health Insurance

Payers of health services obviously play a pivotal role in the entire health care system. Currently, most health insurance companies are using the Web for informational purposes. However, some companies are using e-commerce in one of two ways. First, following the traditional "independent agent" structure of the insurance system, insurance companies use the Web to enable agents to order policies for their clients electronically. Second, insurance companies are using the Internet to bypass independent agents and sell health insurance policies directly to the end consumer. Some sites provide consumers with electronic forms to speed up the process of obtaining health insurance. Other sites, such as the ones listed here, go a step farther and actually support the online purchase of health insurance.

• The Provident Health Insurance Agency <www.theprovident.com>, headquartered in Norristown, Pennsylvania, has a Web site that offers general information about the company's major products. The Web site also gives licensed agents the tools necessary to complete a sales transaction, including marketing updates and rate software.

• Champion Insurance Advantage Ltd. <www.champion-ins.com>, located in Bel Air, Maryland, offers several types of health insurance policies online, including travel medical insurance, insurance for students who study in other countries, health insurance for U.S. university and graduate students, and temporary health insurance for people between jobs and for new U.S. university graduates. This Web site summarizes each type of coverage, then offers links to insurance companies that offer the requested coverage, a rate quote, and a virtual location to which consumers can submit an application for insurance coverage.

• eHealthInsurance <www.eHealthInsurance.com> provides its members with a variety of services, such as instant quotes on a desired health care plan; the ability to research different companies and the plans they offer; online applications; and customer service representatives available through e-mail, chat rooms, or phone lines to answer questions on billing, claims, and enrollment. The company services individuals, families, senior citizens, and small businesses. eHealthInsurance is a licensee of the TRUSTe Privacy Program, which allows members to review the information practices of the company and will voluntarily inform members of everyone who has access to the information, how it is used, and how to correct any mistakes.

Alternative Medicine

Alternative approaches to traditional Western medical practices are increasing in popularity and acceptance. Alternative medical therapies include folk medicine, herbal medicine, homeopathy, faith healing, New Age healing, chiropractic, acupuncture, naturopathy, massage, music therapy, reflexology, aura therapy, homeopathy, and aromatherapy. The Internet is a ready source for information about alternative sources of care for a wide range of chronic and acute health conditions, such as AIDS, arthritis, cancer, and back pain. Although traditionally the patient has been the main seeker of information regarding these alternative treatments, health providers are displaying increasing interest. The November 1998 issue of the *Journal of the American Medical Association* contained several articles highlighting trends in alternative medicine in the United States. They noted the founding of a number of academic research centers for alternative medicine (for example, at the University of Texas and the University of Medicine and Dentistry of New Jersey). The following are Web sites concerned with alternative medicine.

• Enzymatic Therapy <www.enzy.com/homeo/> claims to be the exclusive distributor to health food retailers of Lehning Laboratories' homeopathic formulas, which have been available for almost sixty years through traditional channels.

• Acupuncture <www.acupuncture.com/> offers consumers information about acupuncture and sells Chinese medical supplies. This site also has links to preferred provider organizations seeking licensed acupuncturists, malpractice insurance providers for acupuncturists, and an acupuncture provider network.

• AlternativeMedicine <www.alternativemedicine.com> provides information on alternative medicine and sells related products.

• QuackWatch <www.quackwatch.com>, developed to report on Internet "quackery" (questionable and unreliable information) and to expose misinformation, offers valuable information for the consumer. Many QuackWatch reports discuss the scientific validity of alternative medicine techniques, and cover other topics, such as illegal marketing and consumer protection lawsuits.

Although the United States is leading the way for much development related to alternative medicine on the Internet, the worldwide community is also contributing significantly to this effort.

CONCLUSION

Telecommunication technologies are "busting out all over," without many constraints. An analysis of health care trends suggest that the Internet may become the common pathway for a variety of health care interactions. As higher bandwidth becomes universally available and affordable, there will be wholesale movement of all types of electronic information—medical information included—onto the Web. Chapter Six discusses how computerized patient records will be central to health care activity, what their advantages are, what changes they will force, and related crucial issues.

CHAPTER 6

Computerization of Medical Records and E-Health Services

A rural hospital in a town of less than twenty-five thousand people spent a great deal of money to develop and deploy a computerized patient record. Because it was the only large hospital within a one-hundred-mile radius, hospital administrators saw this change as a way to facilitate care for everyone in the region, including patients referred from local doctors' offices. Despite administrators' high hopes, actual diffusion and adoption of this record was extremely slow. Why?

Other health organizations in the hospital's service area had differing ideas of what an electronic medical record can do and goals for what it should be. They also had varying attitudes about how this record should have been designed and who should have access to it.

Computerized information systems have existed for over three decades. The first systems were mainly designed to support patient data systems related to such administrative tasks as billing and insurance. These programs were later followed by more advanced systems capable of supporting clinical processes. They now are used for everything from building and maintaining medical record databases to e-mail communication between practitioner and patient. The use of computers for handling on-line medical information, telehealth communication networks, and electronic patient files has enabled improved health care decisions, prevented dangerous oversights, increased access to care, and reduced costs for patients, practitioners, and insurance companies (Lindberg & Humphreys, 1995, 1998).

This chapter gives an overview of the main elements of the computerized patient record and demonstrates some of its uses. The terms *computerized patient record* and *electronic medical record* are often used interchangeably. In this book, we use the term computerized patient record (CPR) as a comprehensive term that includes all database systems capable of electronically storing information about an individual's lifelong health status and health care.

BENEFITS OF A COMPUTERIZED PATIENT RECORD

Accurate patient records are the most important patient resource in a health care facility. The advantages of maintaining accurate CPRs are numerous.

Improved Access

Well-designed CPRs provide documentation that is more easily accessible, manageable, and transmittable. CPRs become the agent that tracks a patient's or member's activity over time within an organization and across various types of health care settings (Fernandes et al., 1997). Improved access to patient data is a significant advancement in health care. Making the record available electronically enables delivery of these data to all authorized health care practitioners, independent of where the data were originally acquired. Improved access to medical records is important for the delivery of timely and efficient health care, especially when patients are not in their practitioner's office.

Even when patients are in their practitioner's office, precious time is often wasted searching for necessary patient records. For example, several

E-Health, Telehealth, and Telemedicine

studies have reported that during patient visits, practitioners were unable to find the necessary or desired information up to 30 percent of the time (U.S. General Accounting Office, 1991; Tufo & Speidel, 1971). CPRs speed access to patient information, benefiting both health care practitioners and patients (Fernandes et al., 1997); they therefore allow health care professionals to more easily track treatment, diagnosis, and intervention when needed.

By using a shared patient information directory, practitioners have access to an integrated delivery system containing information from other practitioners in the system. This **master patient index** allows confidential patient data to be shared across different types of care settings (Waller & Alcantara, 1998). In addition, CPRs also allow patient data to be electronically exchanged over regions. For example, CPR systems are used for communication with health insurance bodies, governmental organizations, medical libraries, and research institutions. They also allow orders, payments, and laboratory data or referral letters to be exchanged or e-mailed (Dick, Steen, & Detmer, 1998).

Reduced Cost and Reduced Frequency of Errors

CPR systems also serve to unify diverse clinical data, which can help reduce the cost of filing paper records, and can eliminate such problems as illegible notes, lost charts, and illegible prescription orders (McDonald et al., 1998). For example, research has shown that by entering orders by computer, more than half of serious medication errors or adverse drug interactions can be prevented—especially when dosages can be selected on an electronic entry form (Bates et al., 1998).

Outcomes Management and Decision Support

CPRs provide a more reliable and sophisticated basis for outcomes management and can used for epidemiological studies (McDonald et al., 1998). They also provide handy reminders and alerts, linkages with knowledge sources for decision support, and data for outcomes research and improved management of health care delivery.

Protection for Confidential Information

CPRs promise greater protection for confidential information than paper-based records. Although still imperfect with regard to security, CPRs allow system administrators to more easily monitor and protect information than is possible with paper-based records (Office of Technology Assessment, 1995). In fact, because the security of medical records, the pertinent legislation, and the suggested solutions to existing problems are such central elements to the development of successful telehealth programs, we have devoted all of Chapter Nine to this topic.

CONCERNS ABOUT THE CONFIDENTIALITY OF COMPUTERIZED PATIENT RECORDS

A majority of patients surveyed by Princeton Survey Research Associates in 1998 feared for the confidentiality of their medical records due to security breaches in the computer system. In California, the number one perceived threat to CPR confidentiality is computer hackers (California Healthcare Foundation, 1999). Most of those surveyed responded that they do not want outside sources—such as drug companies—to have access to their medical records, except in cases of medical research or if they were being offered a new job.

Classic, pre-CPR methods of ensuring patient confidentiality are imperfect at best. For instance, unauthorized access to files in hospital systems is commonplace. Despite efforts to protect patient confidentiality with advanced technology, many health care organizations report breaches of confidentiality with the old systems of paper-based records. It is important to avoid the pitfall of holding CPRs to an impossibly high standard, one to which paper-based systems have not adhered. Issues of patient confidentiality are examined in more detail in Chapter Seven.

As you can see from even this brief overview, the complexity of issues involved with the design of CPRs; with the understanding, tracking, and complying with relevant laws; and with the management of data to ensure their quality and integrity makes it almost imperative that the administrator of any sizable telehealth program hire a health information management (HIM) professional.

E-HEALTH AND THE COMPUTERIZED PATIENT RECORD

The field of Internet-mediated CPRs is in rapid development. When the key issues of confidentiality and security have been resolved—and they will be soon—CPRs will take their proper place at the center of the information stream that supplies the entire health care enterprise. To track developments in this area, you can refer to the Web site of the Medical Records Institute, a nonprofit group, at <www.medrecinst.com>, or check the American Medical Association's topic area at <www.ama-assn.org/med-sci/cpt/emr.htm>.

Although there are significant issues of compatibility, security, and resource allocation, the lower costs of using advanced technology will likely drive decisions in the increasingly competitive health care field. The bottom line is that, with proper security precautions, the Internet may cause the CPR to expand beyond its application as a system for recording a patient's status. CPRs may evolve into more dynamic, interactive systems for storing and obtaining health-related information by and for patients. No longer would the patient record be a static document used only by health practitioners. It could become a repository that records all on-site visits (including videotapes of telemedicine visits), e-mail correspondence between practitioner and patient, and links to additional health information. Patients could review advice provided by a physician at their own convenience or with family members.

OWNERSHIP OF COMPUTERIZED PATIENT RECORDS

With the widespread deployment of CPRs over the Internet, it is critical to determine who will own the copyright to health information databases. Clarification with respect to copyright avoids the risk that individual practitioners will be considered authors. Waller and Alcantara (1998) have suggested that database developers and organizations start using written agreements to distinguish between those who create and those who actually implement the database.

We will now derive some basic principles regarding the ownership of CPRs by drawing from the principles governing the ownership of paper-based records.

Practitioner as Owner

With paper-based medical records, a distinction has generally been made between the medical record itself and the information contained within it. Many groups, such as the American College of Physicians, have traditionally considered health care practitioners to be the owners of the paper-based medical record. However, the information contained in the record has traditionally been considered the property of the patient (Waller & Alcantara, 1998; Lazoff, 1997). The practitioner's ownership has given him or her the right to possess, access, and use the record for patient care or other legitimate purposes, but the patient's ownership of the information has prevented practitioners from having complete sovereignty over the information.

Ownership laws actually differ from state to state, a circumstance that further complicates matters. In California, the regulation concerning medical records maintained by hospitals and emergency services states, "The medical record, including x-ray films, is the property of the hospital and is maintained for the benefit of the patient, the medical staff, and the hospital. The hospital shall safeguard the information in the record against loss, defacement, tampering or use by unauthorized persons" (Cal. Code Regs. Ttl. 22, sec. 70751, 1997). This regulation specifies that the hospital does not have complete sovereignty over the record and its contents. Similarly, the practitioner's ownership is considered similar to a trusteeship. The record itself is the property of the hospital; the record is for the benefit of the patient as well as the hospital. Therefore, a practitioner's ownership of a medical record in a hospital is limited by the rights given to the patient and to the medical staff (Waller & Alcantara, 1998).

Patient as Owner

One of the essential issues in computerized record keeping is protection of patient data. Patient ownership rights specifically include (1) the right to access or obtain copies of the information contained in the record, (2) the right to request correction of inaccurate or incorrect information, and (3) the right to have the information remain completely confidential (Waller & Alcantara, 1998).

The most common agreement is that patients should have access to their own record. The following are certain exceptions to consider, however: (1) where access poses a risk of harm to the patient, (2) where access could reveal personal information about others, and (3) where access could undermine the validity or integrity of a clinical trial (Ryboski, 1998).

Multiprovider Ownership Arrangements

An increasing number of entities are claiming ownership rights to medical records. Aside from practitioners and patients, these groups and individuals include hospitals, medical groups and health care networks, managed care companies, health plans, drug manufacturers, and disease management firms (Borzo, 1999).

Entities often enter into contractual agreements whereby they arrange to share ownership of information; however, some of these arrangements may lead to conflicts with patients' rights to the data, and to problems if a malpractice suit arises. When there is more than one provider, for example, the ownership of medical records is more complex, requires more planning, and may more easily conflict with the patient's rights.

OWNERSHIP OF NONIDENTIFIABLE PATIENT INFORMATION

Health information is defined as any information, whether oral or recorded in any form or medium, that

- is created or received by a health care provider, health plan, public health authority, employer, health care clearinghouse, life insurer, school or university
- relates to the past, present, or future physical condition or mental health condition of an individual; the provision of health care to an

individual; or the past, present, or future payment for the provision of health care to an individual (DHHS, 1998).

It becomes patient-identifiable when the information contains any identifiers of the individual or there is a reasonable basis to believe that the information could lead to the identification of the individual (Cepelewicz, 1998). Health plans, health care clearinghouses, and health care practitioners must protect identifiable health care information to ensure privacy and confidentiality when health information is electronically stored, maintained, or transmitted (DHHS, 1998).

Reuse and Resale of Patient Information

One of the biggest concerns related to privacy is the reuse and resale of private health care information without a patient's knowledge. Resale in this context refers to the practice of some organizations to gather information about an individual or group and sell it for commercial profit. Blatant sale of patient-identifiable information is understood as a violation and is regulated to various degrees by enacted and pending legislation. An example of such a violation would be the sale of patient-identifiable information to pharmaceutical companies to target consumers who might be interested in their new products—for example, the use of hospital admissions data by infant formula manufacturers to solicit purchases by new mothers (Ryboski, 1998).

Data Mining

A patient's rights are usually removed when records are stripped of identifiers (Waller & Alcantara, 1998). Patient identifier codes could be computerized, which would make the removal of such codes a relatively straightforward process. Patient identifiers, then, could easily be stripped. This possibility has opened a new world of opportunity for those interested in gathering such information. As one would expect, the prospect of data-mining CPRs for profit has led to significant controversy.

Central to the debate is whether patients will be allowed to knowingly contribute to such nonidentifiable patient databases. The fact is that pa-

E-Health, Telehealth, and Telemedicine

tients are often deluged with paperwork when signing agreements for health benefits, and rarely take the time to read or understand the fine print.

Despite the obvious difficulties related to data mining, sale of some types of nonidentifiable patient information to various groups has attracted the keen interest of many parties. Public health advocates claim that it is of benefit to the patient to have researchers study the longitudinal relationship between diagnosis, compliance with medication regimens, and treatment outcomes. Similarly, when patients are offered a variety of treatment options, their choices could be tracked and correlated with such factors as age, gender, educational level, geographical location, race, culture, and primary language. By data-mining CPRs, health care groups, companies, and organizations could easily gather such information and use it for the following purposes:

To track the global spread of disease

To track the number of people with specific diagnoses, their response rates to specific medications and dosages, and their adherence patterns

To measure the efficacy of public health outreach

To develop more specifically targeted prevention programs

To identify patient choice patterns in relation to medication adherence

To help understand the clinician's choice of one treatment protocol over another

To develop more appealing pharmaceutical and alternative medicine products

Another area of interest is the data-mining of CPRs for provider behavior (using nonidentifiable patient information, in accordance with HIPAA). Data-mining CPRs to better understand provider behavior could benefit vendors of various decision support, disease management, and treatment protocols. More specifically, if a provider's choice of treatment protocol for particular disorders is inappropriate, contraindicated because of other factors, or simply a poor choice among better choices, decision support programs could be enhanced to offer better alternatives. If pharmaceutical companies could better understand why a professional chooses one medication over another, better products or product information could be developed and disseminated. These possibilities raise many concerns, however.

As is true in the case of patient information, the distinction between nonidentifiable and identifiable provider information is crucial. On the one hand, deriving previously inaccessible information about a professional's nonidentifiable decision-making practices could be beneficial to public health. On the other hand, knowledge of *identifiable* decision making could prove detrimental to an individual provider if his or her decisions were proven inadequate.

The benefits and dangers of professional accountability are complex. Whereas increased oversight of identifiable professional behavior may satisfy disgruntled patients, it may also have a negative impact on clinical decision making by forcing safe rather than creative applications of expertise to solve critical medical problems.

As providers become more acquainted with the potentials of processing such vast amounts of data about their patients and themselves, the issues related to data-mining CPRs will most certainly come under even greater debate.

SOLUTIONS TO CPR PROBLEMS RELATED TO MULTIPLE PROVIDERS

Several technological and practical solutions can provide greater security, easier access, and better data management for medical records in multi-provider arrangements. The solutions we present are simply possible alternatives, not an exhaustive list. New solutions are evolving regularly.

Clear Labeling

To minimize security problems, each party could be considered the owner of the data he or she originates. Labeling shared data is a precaution that is

E-Health, Telehealth, and Telemedicine

well worth the added effort when creating data. Such a multiprovider arrangement should also include procedures for handling a court order, steps for provider withdrawal from a patient's care, and the right to "mine" others' data. It is also important to stipulate when working with information system vendors whether a third party will be permitted to use patient-identifiable data (Waller & Alcantara, 1998).

Identifiers

Another solution to security and access problems is to develop and use a system of standard identifiers. Combining, for example, a file number with the provider's middle initial and address could create unique identification for medical records to be used within the provider group. Such standards could eliminate confusion in the sharing of clinical and administrative information between institutions (Office of Technology Assessment, 1995). Each provider or provider group (as well as payers and other users of health information) can maintain its own identification number scheme and assign its own numbers.

Some examples of standardized identifiers are those outlined by the Health Insurance Portability and Accountability Act of 1996 (HIPAA), which when enacted in the next few years promises to mandate new ways to protect an individual's health information. This and other legislation designed to protect patients will be discussed in greater detail in Chapter Eight.

Identifiers include the National Provider Identifier and the National Standard Employer Identifier (also known as the Employer Identification Number), as well as other code sets in current use. As defined by HIPAA, a code set is any set of codes used for encoding data, such as terms, concepts, diagnosis codes, or procedure codes. The following paragraphs describe whom these identifiers affect and how they will be used.

• The National Provider Identifier (NPI), an eight-digit alphanumeric code, is a unique identification number intended to be used by all health care providers and health care clearinghouses. The NPI could be used to identify health care practitioners in health care transactions or related correspondence, to coordinate benefits with other health care plans, and to keep track of prescriptions issued by other health care practitioners.

The NPI would be assigned by a National Provider System, based on information entered into the system by an organization known as an enumerator. Enumerators would enter identifying information about a health care practitioner into the system and confirm the validity of that information. The enumerator would update information about health care practitioners on an as-needed basis. Either a federally directed registry or a combination of federal programs, state Medicaid agencies, and other registries would serve the enumerator function (DHHS, 1999a).

• The Employer Identification Number (EIN) facilitates the transactions that take place between employers and health insurance practitioners. Employers already need to identify themselves in electronic transactions when they enroll their employees in a health plan or make premium payments to that health plan. The EIN consists of a nine-digit number; the first two digits are separated from the others by a hyphen. In 1998, the Internal Revenue Service agreed to adopt the EIN as the identifying number for employers in all electronic health care transactions. An employer may obtain an EIN by submitting IRS form SS-4, Application for Employer Identification Number. Any business that pays wages to one or more employees must have an EIN (DHHS, 1999b).

THE ROLE OF THE HEALTH INFORMATION MANAGEMENT PROFESSIONAL

Clinical information of all types and of any origin can be included in the CPR. These data are managed by HIM professionals, who are gaining an increasingly important role in medical staff offices (Braden, 1999). They are deploying advanced CPR systems in academic medical centers, teaching centers affiliated with universities, the Department of Veterans Affairs, and the Department of Defense. These centers have been leaders in developing protocols for handling the information associated with CPRs. For example, Clayton Curtis from Veterans Affairs Medical Center (Boston) and Susan Fenton from the Department of Veterans Affairs (Washington, D.C.) have identified a number of tasks to be accomplished by the HIM professional (Curtis & Fenton, 1999). We will discuss a few of these tasks to give you a sense of the importance of the HIM professional's role.

HIM professionals are often involved in the design and creation of the CPR, and they oversee its use. Developing a useful, comprehensive patient record needs the dedicated attention of both HIM and **information technology (IT)** professionals to supply information services to the rest of the health care enterprise. Such a partnership requires an understanding of HIM and IT domains, joint planning, and a high level of collaboration. To become better CPR "partners," HIM professionals need to understand the principles underlying today's information technology.

For example, they must decide if their organization must build or buy information systems that will capture and manage billing and support patient care. HIM professionals also will help make decisions by understanding the data elements to be used by the organization. Data elements might include identifying as well as diagnostic characteristics of patients, such as their name, identification number, and address; details of a visit or inpatient stay; the diagnosis; the location of encounter; date(s) of service; the names of the referring and consulting practitioners; the practitioner facility; status of informed consent; the type of evaluation performed; procedure codes; evaluation results; diagnosis or impression; and recommendations for further treatment (Fernandes et al., 1997; Fletcher, 1999).

Another task of the HIM professional is to decide on the amount of data to be collected. This factor is particularly important because, on the one hand, collecting too little data may render the CPR less effective. Moreover, the cost of later expanding the number of data elements can be very costly. On the other hand, unnecessary information wastes resources, incurring higher data entry and validation costs and occupying more storage space. HIM and IT staff must work together for good planning at the database design stage. This initial phase helps determine how data elements relate and can make it easier or harder to satisfy specific functionality, such as displaying patient summary information by diagnosis.

Other important issues addressed by the HIM professional are data quality and integrity. The goal of the HIM professional is to maximize several aspects of the data being stored:

- *Comprehensiveness* relates to the types of data stored. If the data elements collected by the system are incomplete, practitioners may draw incorrect conclusions.

- *Timeliness* relates to the interval of time between the collection of information and its entry into the database. If the interval is prolonged, practitioners do not have accurate or current data from which to draw conclusions.

- *Data quality* relates to both accuracy and precision.

A qualified HIM professional can also assess the requirements for privacy and confidentiality. One of the most valuable and controversial roles of the HIM professional is to develop a data system that protects confidentiality and individual privacy while simultaneously providing maximal functionality. Although this complex challenge involves human factors in addition to technological ones, the HIM professional plays an important role in the development of secure, functional systems.

Such a professional can also help by establishing appropriate organizational policy and procedures with regard to privacy and confidentiality. In doing so, the HIM professional must ensure that the organization complies with several federal rulings, such as the Privacy Act of 1974, the Health Insurance Portability and Accountability Act of 1996, and the Internet security policy of the Health Care Financing Agency (HCFA, 1998a). These laws mandate that specific regulations must be followed to ensure the privacy and confidentiality of medical data. In addition, some states recognize common law tort actions that enforce privacy protections between practitioners and patients and between hospitals and patients (Goldstein, 2000).

Although the optimal method of entering data is for the practitioner to enter data as they are being collected, in many cases surrogates enter data later (a problem by no means exclusive to CPRs). HIM professionals can play a critical role in suggesting methods for optimal data entry, in monitoring data collection processes, and in supervising data sampling and analysis for quality assurance. An important data quality function of the HIM professional is to resolve errors by isolating the source of the error, implementing the appropriate corrections, and educating the staff member or members whose actions caused the error.

CLINICAL CONTEXT MANAGER

A number of health care and technology companies have joined efforts, forming the Clinical Context Object Workgroup (CCOW), to develop Clinical Context Manager, visually integrated software that combines many of the programs used by providers. The "patient link" feature synchronizes all of these programs to a specified patient name. Thus a provider can access the personal history of a patient, prescribe medication, or obtain radiological images without logging onto multiple programs and navigating through different Internet sites (Karson, 2000). This capability significantly reduces the time required for electronic health care and increases ease of operation.

Clinical Context Manager is an outgrowth of the Hewlett-Packard Medical Products Group and Duke University Health System collaboration to develop multivendor information systems. This initial effort was crystallized by its association with CCOW, a consortium of more than one hundred leading health care providers, IT vendors, and consultants.

CONCLUSION

Technology now gives us the capability to surpass traditional and cumbersome paper-based medical records. Use of the CPR enables simplified storage, access, and transmission of information; in addition, new technologies offer the potential to reinvent information management by transforming the CPR into a centralized resource for both health practitioners and patients.

The CPR must be properly designed and maintained, however. Issues related to ownership must be clarified, and the record must use proper identifiers. Finally, the health information network itself must be designed to maximize the benefits of the CPR, while keeping it secure, confidential, and user-friendly for the provider. Chapter Seven takes a closer look at security, privacy, data integrity, and confidentiality as they relate to CPRs and to telehealth issues in general.

CHAPTER 7

Privacy, Confidentiality, Security, and Data Integrity

A young programmer worked in a large university-based medical center. Her physician was on staff at the same medical center. One day the programmer sent her doctor an e-mail asking for help with her weight problem. In her message, she explained that her weight had climbed to over three hundred pounds and that she was quite depressed. She wanted to know if she could visit him to talk about treatment options. He quickly responded to her message by simply leaving her original message within his message and adding that she should come see him the following week. However, unbeknown to the physician, the e-mail program he was using had a "universal" default for replying to messages. Almost two thousand people in the university medical center were sent the doctor's reply to his patient.

Although large computerized databases are a more efficient and integrated system of record keeping and have allowed for easy access, they have also increased the potential for error and for misuse of medical information. To optimize the quality of health services developed by new telecommunication technologies, providers and system designers must take every possible step to safeguard against misinformation and breaches of confidentiality. This chapter examines the basic concepts related to the safeguarding of information in technology-based health care programs, as well as the legislation that has arisen from deep-seated concerns with the protection of health care information.

The terms *privacy, confidentiality, security,* and *data integrity* are used in many different ways in relation to the protection of personal health information from intentional misuse (National Research Council [NRC], 1997). Although these terms are often used interchangeably, each possesses distinct attributes.

Concerns with these issues can exist in relation both to the public Internet and to proprietary **intranets**, which are owned and operated by private groups with security and privacy as their goal. According to the U.S. General Accounting Office (GAO, 1999, p. 4), *privacy* is "the specific right of an individual to control the collection, use, and disclosure of personal information." Privacy advocates insist that the individual is to be informed of how information is to be released and of its intended purpose. *Confidentiality* "is a tool for protecting privacy. Sensitive information is accorded a confidential status that mandates specific controls, including strict limitations on access and disclosure. These controls must be adhered to by those handling the information" (National Telecommunications and Information Administration, 1997). *Security* refers to the methods by which access to information is controlled and protected from accidental or intentional disclosure to unauthorized persons and from alteration, destruction, or loss. *Data integrity* refers to the accuracy and completeness of data.

Federal regulations regarding privacy, confidentiality, security, and data integrity have steadily been developed through the last several decades. This movement has been accelerated by reactions of the American public to potential breaches of confidentiality in areas related to the Internet (see, for example, Graphics, Visualization and Usability Center, 1998; Nua Internet Surveys, 1999). Because these four issues are important and distinct, we discuss each of them in depth and offer recommendations regarding each.

PRIVACY

In traditional telehealth activities, patient data are commonly maintained manually in charts and are thus not challenged by issues of privacy or confidentiality in the ways faced by electronic management of similar data. According to the American Medical Association (AMA) guidelines for medical and health information sites on the Internet, privacy "refers to the right of the individual site visitor to choose whether to allow personal information to be collected by the host site or by third parties and to know what type of information is collected and how that information is used" (Winker et al., 2000).

With respect to privacy, controversial issues abound in consumer advocacy and professional groups. Many people argue that patients have a right to know who and why others would have access to their private information. According to this view, violations of this right can destroy the trust that is fundamental between practitioner and patient. Research has shown that without trust, individuals are inclined to withhold sensitive information (Ryboski, 1998).

Electronic health information complicates the issue of privacy, because electronically stored information is available for purposes other than those for which it was originally collected. Before the establishment of computer networks, health information had a physical embodiment (for example, medical charts) and was accessible only from central locations. Computerized and networked records allow health care information to be accessed, copied, and transferred to unauthorized parties (NRC, 1997). As discussed in Chapter Six, one of the most hotly debated issues related to patient privacy is that of use and reuse of information obtained through the computerized patient record (CPR).

CONFIDENTIALITY

The relationship between a patient and practitioner includes an expectation that privileged information obtained as part of the relationship is protected. The patient's right to give informed consent for the release of that information is known as confidentiality and relates to information that is either shared or released in a controlled manner (NRC, 1997). The AMA states, "Confidentiality is the right of an individual to not have personally identifiable medical or other information disclosed to others without that individual's express informed consent" (Winker et al., 2000).

The development of electronic media has led to the need to coin a new term, *data confidentiality*. Data confidentiality refers to data that have been officially declared to be sensitive and must therefore be handled and protected as such (Institute of Medicine [IOM], 1994). This new stipulation refers to the protection of the actual electronic data themselves as primary, rather than the information obtained solely in the context of the relationship between the patient and practitioner (IOM, 1996). The focus is therefore solely on the protection of the physical data and not necessarily on the information they contain that could be found in nonidentifiable forms. In this context, confidentiality might be considered the security service that protects a patient's right to privacy (J. Wyant, personal communication, October 9, 1999).

Complicating Factors

Several factors have complicated the maintenance of confidentiality despite the best efforts of those involved. For example, practitioners have traditionally been fully responsible for maintaining confidentiality. Nonetheless, others, such as a secretary or colleague, may easily have access to confidential information if they are sharing an office space, overhearing telephone conversations, or listening through treatment room walls. With the introduction of electronic data, concern for compromised medical information has increased significantly. Although many health care organizations are developing more stringent confidentiality policies, confidentiality leaks in computerized settings have been occurring with regularity and are being noticed by consumer groups and the media.

As health management groups have computerized their services and warehoused their data, responsibility for confidentiality has become complicated. Practitioners, as employees of these companies, are required to keep the health management group fully informed of the details of a patient's condition and treatment.

When participating in managed care insurance plans, patients sign waivers of their rights to confidentiality. Similarly, practitioners sign agreements to provide patient information to managed care organizations. When enacted, laws such as the Health Insurance Portability and Accountability

Act of 1996 will help increase patient confidentiality by imposing stringent penalties on both health care organizations and practitioners who breach patient confidence electronically (Gilbert, 1999).

E-Health Privacy and Confidentiality

The privacy and confidentiality of medical information are most vulnerable when such information is transported through the public Internet system. It has already become common knowledge that the privacy and confidentiality of medical information can easily be violated without knowledge of the Internet consumer. Privacy and confidentiality are therefore expected but not guaranteed on the Internet. The following sections describe some of the ways that people's expectations of Internet privacy and confidentiality can be violated and exploited.

Forwarded Mail. Many people falsely assume that when they contact a health care provider, their personal e-mail will go only to the intended recipient. E-mail is routed through multiple servers from the point of origination to the point of receipt. All these servers are potential points where e-mail can be "tapped." For example, a practitioner might forward unencrypted e-mail from a patient to a nurse. One of the transmission servers may give e-mail access to its employees, thus potentially violating the patient's privacy and confidentiality. People so commonly experience such compromises of privacy and confidentiality that one regularly hears the admonition, "Don't send anything through the Internet that you wouldn't want to hear again in a court of law." Unexpected recipients of what was originally intended to be private e-mail include third-party vendors, hackers, public forums, the police, the IRS, rivals, and future employers.

E-Mail Address Logs. Another problem with privacy relates to Web site address logs. Web sites can automatically capture and permanently store e-mail addresses into log files. Any Web site manager can easily gather e-mail addresses from viewers, build a mailing list, and send e-mail solicitations for commercial products to every name on the list. If a patient were to surf multiple Internet sites looking for medical information, products, or counseling services, his or her e-mail address could be accumulated into many different mailing lists. That person could then be targeted by embarrassing or otherwise undesirable advertising campaigns without any easy means of removal from such lists.

Snippets of Information Compiled from Multiple Sources. A more serious problem related to capturing e-mail addresses occurs when Web site managers begin sharing information with each other and with specialized companies that compile information about specific individuals. These companies can gather detailed information about income, age, gender, profession, education, hobbies, investments, insurance benefits and usage, medical records, electronic equipment purchased, and much more from other Web sites; non–Web site mailing lists; news reports; city, state, and federal government documents; and credit card purchases. Although much of this information has been available to interested parties for years, it formerly required a significant amount of energy to accumulate and compile. Companies specializing in such database development are remarkably accurate in their tracking of an individual's preferences, spending habits, frequented locales, employment history, medical conditions, legal records, and so on. This information can be used for such purposes as market research by advertisers to identify target audiences or for gathering mailing lists of names identified with specific buying patterns or needs (Gilbert, 1999). Advertisements can then be individually directed. As discussed by Esther Dyson (1997), "The user wants a seamless experience as he explores the Web, but he wants to appear as a discrete entity to each place he visits with a legitimate identity revealed as appropriate—a credit rating, an employment record, a bank account, or a medical history. Indeed, a person's identity gets splashed all over the Net in little fragments—no problem. But then someone in particular—anyone from a benign marketer only after the customer's business, to an employer, a stalker, or a blackmailer—can start collecting these fragments" (p. 196).

Cookies. Another vehicle for gathering information about consumers from Web sites is the "cookies" file that resides in the Web browser subdirectory of the computer. This file holds personally identifiable information that is deposited by some Web sites and can be read by Web site staff members—all without the patient's knowledge. The lack of consumer choice about where and when this information is deposited is of great concern to privacy and confidentiality advocates.

The following example describes how information is typically gathered. An individual visits a Web site with banner advertisements. She clicks a banner ad, which carries her to another site, which could plant a thirty-two-digit code (cookie) into her computer. Whenever the person uses the same computer to visit other Web sites containing an advertisement from the same company, the company may record additional information from that second visit. After the computer user has made a number of visits to different Web sites, the company can have a surprisingly large amount of information. If the user gives out her e-mail address during any of these visits, the company has its missing link. It can then cross-reference the individual's name with other companies, which can sell their information on that person. This is an example of how personally identifiable information is sold on the Internet. When such information is used by health Web sites to sell health care information to third parties, privacy legislation and consumer protection groups can become involved.

Online Discussion Lists and Archives. There are other ways to learn about patients. For example, search engines often link to postings that were originally intended for a specific e-mail discussion group or **newsgroup** but that were complied and made available to the public Internet community through large Web sites. The danger with these sites that function as "lists of lists" is that many patients may not expect or may not be informed that their communication to a specific e-mail health or mental health support group will be archived and made accessible through such Web sites. The personal information they may have shared late one night about a private and embarrassing medical condition may not be information they would want a potential future employer, for example, to find when typing the employment candidate's name into a search engine three years later.

Other Types of Intrusion. Privacy and confidentiality come in many forms, as do invasions of privacy and confidentiality. Parties interested in a particular person's activities online can easily obtain several kinds of information:

A patient's real name, address, and telephone number, and other information, is often publicly available from the company from which the patient buys his or her Internet account (the Internet service provider, or ISP). Some ISPs ensure the privacy and confidentiality of this information, but most do not.

Passwords might be private, but hackers and the staff of the ISP from which an Internet account is purchased can still access e-mail and Web pages without passwords.

Transmitted files can be accessed by ISPs. In transmitting mail, ISPs can easily divert and store portions of posts (e-mail letters). Employees, who may or may not download such posts for use at some later time, can also access files.

Many Web sites adhere to the privacy guidelines promulgated by various organizations, and promise not to misuse patient information. Nonetheless, given the unprecedented access to personal information about consumers, there is growing concern that merely stating policies is not enough. The California Healthcare Foundation sponsored a study that reviewed twenty-one of the most trafficked consumer health-related Web sites as of January 2000; the study found that a surprising number of Web sites leave consumers vulnerable to privacy violations, despite those Web sites' statements regarding their privacy standards. In particular, a team led by researchers from the Health Privacy Project of Georgetown University (Goldman, Hudson, & Smith, 2000) found that because of tracking programs such as those collecting data through banner ads, click streams, cookies, and profiling, consumers are not anonymous when visiting some health-related Web sites, even if they think they are.

Many health Web sites have written privacy policies, but these policies are inadequate because they do not follow fair information practices, such as providing adequate statements and giving consumers some control over recipients of their information, and many companies do not hold their business partners to the same privacy standards. Contradictions exist between stated policy standards and actual practice. In some cases, violations consisted of banner advertising and cookies collection, but in others, the violations involved the outright transfer of personally identifiable information to third parties without disclosure to the consumer (Goldman et al., 2000).

Adequate measures often have not been taken to protect the consumer from casual hackers or others actively seeking to access company databases. And some health-related Web sites negate their own policies without notification to the consumer by actively disclaiming the actions of third parties acting within the host Web site (Goldman et al., 2000).

Moreover, violations of privacy can easily occur in the form of copyright infringement on the public Internet. For example, some Web site owners blatantly reproduce articles written by professionals and consumers, alter the language to meet their own agendas, and post such articles claiming them to be written by the original author—all without the knowledge or permission of the original author. When such misuse of proprietary information has occurred to date, the author has had very little recourse, aside from going to considerable legal expense to protect copyright, contacting the Web site owner and asking for removal of the article, or contacting the ISP of the Web site owner and filing a complaint. Unfortunately, such action does not always lead to remediation of the problem.

Patient Protection Solutions

The growing concern over patient protection on the Internet has led to numerous potential solutions. From the formation of advocacy groups to federal legislation, these attempts are likely to continue as technology offers increasingly more complex solutions to old problems and creates new problems. We describe legislated solutions in Chapter Eight; we discuss voluntary solutions in this section.

Patient education is primary. It is crucial for health care sites to inform patients about their privacy rights. Furthermore, e-health companies need to examine their stated policies regularly and ensure that all involved parties, including employees, vendors, and other third parties, are continually adhering to those policies. Individual health care providers would also be wise to read the fine print regarding privacy when signing agreements with ISPs. If privacy is not specifically ensured, practitioners should be leery and search for an ISP that has made it a point to protect privacy.

A good alternative to encouraging people to use e-mail discussion lists for health care information or psychosocial support is to develop discussion forums within private Web sites. A good example of such a site is <www.SelfhelpMagazine.com>, in which there are more than one hundred discussion areas. Patients can post messages anonymously but also receive e-mail responses directly to their e-mail boxes when someone answers their post. The site's privacy policy also ensures that e-mail addresses of consumers will not be sold or released to third parties.

SECURITY

The security of electronic information should be a top priority for all e-health organizations, including health care providers, health care clearinghouses, and health plans. Security refers to the protection of data through encryption, **authentication**, **firewalls**, **electronic signatures**, and other methods that allow only authorized personnel access to those data. Security also includes nonelectronic systems, such as alarms, standard key locks, and guards, which protect the information at the storage site.

Security is contextual, and therefore it is difficult to define the level of protection needed for different types of data. Existing regulations for security of electronic records also do not require specific security technologies. Defined security requirements could limit the development of security systems. Security is constantly advancing and should be seen as the process, rather than the state, of protecting data. These measures should be chosen based on the sensitivity of the information being protected, the cost of each security system, the liability cost of failure, and the results of a loss of public confidence (Federal Trade Commission, 2000). For example, highly sensitive personal material, such as mental health records or HIV test values, need compounded security measures (Goldstein, 2000). An organization that does not secure this type of information might be found guilty of negligence or defamation, or found to be in violation of a number of legislative acts. These judgments can lead to large expenses (even larger than the cost of security installation) for legal counsel or settlements. Some carry the possibility of incarceration.

The main goal of security systems is to prevent individuals from accessing, altering, or generating unauthorized information (Brandt, 1996). Before an organization decides to use the Internet, e-mail, or other nonsecure methods of transferring patient information, it should develop a security policy. The organization should begin by conducting a comprehensive assessment of its information security needs. This assessment should indicate the relative value of the information in question, the potential risks to which this information might be exposed, and the possible controls that might be put in place to protect this information (DHHS, 1998; Rhodes, 1997).

Security also often includes physical safeguards, such as those required for protecting computer systems and related buildings and equipment from fire, intrusion, and other natural and environmental hazards. Technical security services to guard data may also be necessary and include processes that prevent unauthorized access to data transmitted over a communication network (DHHS, 1998).

Aside from the DHHS, the **Joint Commission on Accreditation of Healthcare Organizations** (JCAHO) and the Commission on Accreditation of Rehabilitation Facilities (CARF) both require security measures as part of their accreditation processes (Fiddleman, Hawthorn, & Jones, 1997). In addition, such laws as the Privacy Act of 1974, the Copyright Act of 1976, and HIPAA (see Chapter Eight) have enacted or will enact specific requirements for security of electronic medical records.

Assessing Security Needs

Although adopting (or improving) security methods will help manage risk, doing so does not *eliminate* risk, because every security system is vulnerable in some way. Health information professionals must assess security needs by considering threats to the confidential information contained in their systems and focusing on developing an acceptable, cost-effective level of security. Security measures that go above the necessary level of risk may hinder the legitimate user, be very costly, and negatively affect system functionality (Brandt, 1996).

The greatest danger to security of medical records is from within the company or organization (Brandt, 1996). Currently or previously affiliated employees are responsible for 80 percent of hacking (Reaser, 1999). Disgruntled, malicious, or vengeful employees are a constant threat. With data warehousing and database removal programs so easily available on the open market or in hacker groups online, it is easy for almost any employee, including members of the janitorial staff, to sabotage a company's data warehouse from company computers. After retrieving the information, this person can post it to internal e-mail systems or to newsgroups and other public discussion areas on the Internet. To minimize this risk, passwords should be deleted as soon as an employee resigns or is discharged. It is also recommended that before hiring or promoting any employee with clearance to sensitive information, an organization assess the level of security threat the employee presents.

Many companies hire hackers because of their technical knowledge but ignore the possible risks associated with employing such individuals. The hacker ethic often includes beliefs that access to computers and to information should be unrestricted. Hackers feel that by working "on the inside" they can promote their beliefs about decentralization, all the while mistrusting authority figures. It is important that all managers understand this hacker ethic to minimize the threat of increased risk to security by hiring a self-identified hacker (Civello, 1999).

The Internet has supplied a new medium for economic espionage. While remaining relatively anonymous, deceitful employees can quickly copy information and forward it to unauthorized parties. A possible solution to such problematic behavior by employees is the availability of services for employees to air their dissatisfaction. For example, a well-publicized employee assistance program (EAP) may minimize this risk by defusing employee disgruntlement and offering alternative coping strategies. The Web site DejaNews <www.dejanews.com> provides helpful information on these and other insider concerns (Civello, 1999).

Whether dangers issue from inside or outside the organization, there are risks inherent to the use of CPRs that every practitioner should be aware of:

- *Unauthorized access.* A recent survey conducted by *Information Week* and PricewaterhouseCoopers of twenty-seven hundred executives, security professionals, and technology managers worldwide revealed that suspected sources of security breaches were both unauthorized and authorized users, including employees, customers, computer hackers, and terrorists (Larsen, 1999). Systems accessed by passwords and then left unattended are at primary risk.

- *Administrative failure.* Inadequate data input by employees can cause problems with storage of the material.

- *Technology failure.* System crashes, viruses or other computer contaminants, and hardware or software failure can all lead to massive corruption of data or data loss.

- *Theft.* Computers are vulnerable to theft from inside or outside the organization.

- *Physical problems.* These kinds of problems include natural disasters (fires, floods, and earthquakes), power outages, and loss of communications (Brandt, 1996; Granade, 1998).

- *Unauthorized disclosure of confidential information.*

Recommended Security Practices

Having assessed your organization's security risks, consider the following suggestions for policy approaches to improving security.

The organization should develop a centralized security mission statement. It might include a policy clearly defining acceptable e-health activities, the procedures used to investigate unacceptable behavior, and the penalties (including notification of law enforcement) determined for each violation. (Use of the phrase "no tolerance" is discouraged due to the limited response available for reprimand—namely, termination; Civello, 1999.) The organization should attempt to clearly differentiate confidential and nonconfidential information. Job descriptions and procedures should be updated to include information security requirements, and all employees should sign security agreements. Providing training, policies, and procedures that focus on ethics and information security before any new computer application is introduced can reduce security risks. After training, every user, including both staff and end users (Civello, 1999), must know what information should never be included in an e-mail message. Policies and procedures can also be coordinated with appropriate security software and hardware (DHHS, 1998; Rhodes, 1997).

Other suggested considerations include the development of hiring protocols that include risk assessments, employee threat reporting forms for internal security threats, prevention and intervention methods for discovered breaches, and termination protocols for possibly disgruntled employees (Civello, 1999).

Technical security practices and procedures may also be required. They often need to be built into information systems as the systems are developed and implemented. Partnering with local law enforcement agencies, such as the FBI, can alert a company to potential hazards; you can find local FBI contacts at <www.fbi.gov> (Civello, 1999).

In a survey of fifteen important industries (Larsen, 1999), health care ranked third after banking and aerospace for setting priorities for security. The survey identified the top five security devices among the many available for use: (1) multiple logons and passwords, (2) **access control** software, (3) basic user passwords, (4) terminal key locks, and (5) one-time passwords. Newer technology, such as biometric authentication, ranked last in the list. An increasingly popular approach is the use of virtual private networks (VPNs), which create secure, encrypted transmission channels to carry data over private and public networks, such as the Internet. The survey reported that 27 percent of organizations use VPNs to secure data. The following sections look at some of these technical practices and procedures.

Authentication. This refers to the process of confirming that a stated identity is valid. There are several methods for authentication:

Individual authentication. To establish individual accountability, a unique identifier (or logon ID) can be used every time a logon is recorded (NRC, 1997).

Network-based authentication. This method relies on the network or the host computer to authenticate the user (NRC, 1999).

Biometric authentication. These techniques rely on characteristics that are unique to each user; for example, there are iris-recognition systems, voice-print systems, and fingerprint readers. **Cryptography** can complement these authentication methods in order to prevent the interception of biometric information when it is sent across a network.

Cryptographic authentication. This form of authentication relies on encryption. Encryption is the encoding of a message to prevent unauthorized viewing and unauthorized changes to a document. Two types of encryption services are in common use. *Symmetric* (also called secret-key or shared-key) encryption uses the same key for both encryption and decryption. *Asymmetric* or *public-key* encryption is a system in which two different keys are used, one for encryption and another for decryption. The most common secret-key system is the data encryption standard (DES), which uses a fifty-six-bit key to encrypt and decrypt information; the most common public-key system is the Rivest, Shamir, Adleman (RSA) system. The public-key system serves as the basis for such encryption frameworks as Pretty Good Privacy (PGP) and is the basis of the electronic signature and related services.

Public-key systems run about one thousand times more slowly than DES systems and require longer keys (Whitfield, 1988). Therefore, secret-key and public-key cryptography are often used jointly (Computer Science and Telecommunications Board, 1996; Fiddleman, Hawthorn, & Jones, 1997; NRC, 1999; Rhodes, 1997). Health care entities should encrypt all patient-identifiable information before transmitting it over the Internet or other public networks (NRC, 1997).

It is also important to plan for eventually migrating to at least a two-factor method of authentication, using something known, such as a personal identification number (PIN), and something possessed (for example a **smart card** that electronically confirms one's identity). Eventually three-factor authentication will be practical, comprising the first two factors plus something unique to the individual, such as a biometric scan.

Passwords. Passwords can be assigned to a user and determine what information the user may access. A password is a string of characters that uniquely confirms the user's identity to the system (Marotta, 1986). Passwords can also be designed to expire at regular intervals, and a password system can be established that eliminates multiple logons for the user (Computer-Based Patient Record Institute [CPRI], 1999). It is also important that the user or the system select passwords that are difficult to guess (for example, that contain one or more special characters) and have a minimum length.

Logons and Logoffs. Once the current user is authenticated by entering a password, it is important to ensure that the same user remains the authenticated user. This can be accomplished through the use of automatic logoffs after a confirmed period of inactivity or when the authenticated user accesses the system from another computer (CPRI, 1999).

Access Controls. Access-control services protect against unauthorized access, disclosure, alteration, and destruction of any system resource (CPRI, 1999). Software tools are available to ensure that the user complies with the access privileges granted (NRC, 1997). These programs screen the contents of a medical record and allow the user to view only authorized information.

Nonrepudiation Services. **Nonrepudiation** services provide evidence that a specific action occurred (Baker & Cooper, 1995). The most commonly used instruments for documenting that an individual committed (or did not commit) a particular act are encryption (as previously described) and electronic signatures on all relevant transaction files with legally accepted time stamps and **audit trails** (CPRI, 1999).

Electronic signature. There are numerous forms of electronic signatures, ranging in complexity. To satisfy the legal requirements of a written signature, an electronic signature must typically do the following:

- Identify the signatory individual

- Ensure the integrity of a document's content

- Provide strong and substantial evidence that will make it difficult for the signer to claim that the electronic representation is not valid (that is, nonrepudiation)

Electronic signatures not only supply information about who created the file but also can be used to determine who accessed the file (Rhodes, 1998). Although an electronic record can be signed if practitioners are provided with the proper technology, this technique may not be valid in all states. It is important to note that such signatures are treated differently from state to state. For instance, Governor Gray Davis of California signed Senate Bill 820, the Uniform Electronic Transactions Act, which gave electronic signatures the same legal standing as traditional signatures on all electronic documents, including medical records.

The use of electronic signatures is also acceptable to the JCAHO, according to the *Comprehensive Accreditation Manual for Hospitals,* Standard IM.7.8 (JCAHO, 1998). However, there is no national standard for electronic signatures, and each health care entity must define its own security requirements (DHHS, 1998).

Audit trails. Health care organizations can maintain accurate access logs to all internal clinical information. They can also invest in interorganizational (global) audit trails. These newer systems will allow all patient-identifiable information to be tracked throughout multiple health care organizations (NRC, 1997). Audit trails can also be digitally signed to prove that an appropriate authority generated the audit log and to ensure that the audit log has not been intentionally altered.

Accounting methods. By tracking, auditing, and reporting remote activity, organizations can monitor usage patterns and activity. This is especially helpful when seeking to identify attempts to access confidential files. Accounting is accomplished by using audit logs within the remote access server or using a separate security audit program. These logs can highlight abnormal usage patterns, such as multiple concurrent logins by the same user or a large number of failed login requests. Another protection feature is location validation, the use of callbacks to confirm a user's location. One example of this is caller line ID, whereby the phone number of an incoming call is compared to a log of accepted phone numbers, and then access is granted if the phone number is found in the log. Another callback method is fixed dial-back, in which the system dials a preassigned number. An additional benefit of fixed dial-back is that it allows the organization to assume remote access line costs, which allows companies to better centralize and keep track of costs (Carroll, Wright, & Zakoworotny, 1998).

Universal Patient Identifiers. The use of patient identifiers has led to strong skepticism from consumers. Such identifiers are seen as necessary to deal effectively with CPRs, but consumers are very concerned about the use of patient identifiers to gain unauthorized access to their sensitive health care information (Princeton Survey Research Associates, 1999).

Standards for patient identifiers were established in 1996. A universal patient identifier may have to meet criteria in addition to those designed to protect patient privacy. For example, a report by the Institute of Medicine (1994) found that a universal patient identifier could have separate identification and authentication elements. Identification often refers to individuals' indications of who they are. Authentication allows the system to verify that the identification offered is valid. As with most transactions, security and privacy technology problems and solutions are continually being identified and regulated. HIPAA will further clarify the use of these identifiers.

System Backup and Disaster Recovery Procedures. General security procedures will be discussed in greater detail at this time. Organizations should plan for providing basic system functions, such as an alternative power supply, and for ensuring access to medical records in the event of a natural disaster or a computer failure. They also should make provisions to store backup data in secure and perhaps multiple locations.

Firewalls. A firewall can be made up of hardware and software programs that function to prevent certain Internet addresses from accessing an internal network, thus protecting the owner from potentially hostile Internet users. Several systems are available for such added security:

Intranets. An intranet is used to share company information and informational resources among employees of a particular company. It functions in many ways as a private Internet but uses techniques such as **tunneling** to send private messages through the public network. Encryption, decryption, and other security measures are used to operate within an intranet and to access the public Internet. Server-based firewalls screen both incoming and outgoing messages.

Extranets. As a private network used by companies to securely share specific information or operations with partners, suppliers, vendors, and customers, an extranet can be an extension of a company's intranet to support business between businesses. Like intranets, extranets use server-based firewalls for security and privacy. They typically also require the use of authentication and encryption of messages. They often use virtual private networks (VPNs) to tunnel through the public Internet network.

An example of a company using an extranet is Optum, a business unit of UnitedHealth Group. Optum has developed a comprehensive, interactive Web application called Health Forums that provides information and resources for members. Health Forums features a health and well-being library that includes a user-friendly medical encyclopedia and dictionary, drug information, symptom guides, feature articles, news summaries, interactive quizzes and calculators, descriptions of hundreds of prescreened national resources, and more. Members can even send most Health Forums material to friends and relatives.

Some members also have access to information about individual health plan benefits and can communicate with member services representatives through e-mail. A provider directory allows such members to search for providers by location, specialty, or language. Online maps of provider locations, including street names and landmarks, can be printed for future reference. Members can also participate in interactive chat sessions with Health Forums clinical professionals or read transcripts from past events.

Optum uses several security measures to protect confidentiality and privacy. To log into Health Forums, members must enter a member number and password known only to them. At that time, members are also asked to generate a question and answer that they use to reaccess Health Forums in the event that they forget their password. All confidential member information is contained within the company firewall and protected by secure socket layers, a state-of-the-art high-level encryption protocol.

Virtual private networks (VPNs). This term usually refers to an information network in which some of the parts are connected using the public Internet, but the data are secured via encrypted tunneling techniques, which render the entire network "virtually" private. VPNs are a relatively low cost alternative to purchasing or leasing private telephone lines.

Antivirus Software. Organizations can install antivirus software and regularly update the data files. Viruses can delete, alter, or shut down critical systems and important data. Retrieval of this information can be difficult (if possible at all) and expensive.

Continuous System Assessment. Organizations can regularly assess the security and vulnerabilities of their systems. For example, once a Web site is deployed to provide extranet services, it is important to contract with an independent third party to conduct periodic penetration testing, both scheduled and unscheduled. All users of information systems can receive a minimum level of security training. A security officer can be identified to monitor compliance with security polices and practices. He or she can run "hacker scripts" and password "crackers" against the systems monthly to determine its vulnerability. The security officer can also maintain contact with national information security organizations (NRC, 1997).

DATA INTEGRITY

Data integrity refers to the incorruptibility of the data; in other words, the data cannot be altered, whether unintentionally or for malicious purposes. Archiving and retrieval procedures are important to ensure that the integrity of data is not compromised. Written policies and procedures should be in place to ensure continuity of care at a level consistent with that taken for hard-copy imaging studies and medical records within a facility or institution. These policies and procedures can include internal redundancy systems, backup telecommunication links, and a disaster plan. Specific provisions of HIPAA also promise to address concerns with data integrity. See Chapter Eight for details.

American College of Radiology Guidelines

According to the American College of Radiology (1999), if an organization is going to employ electronic archiving, it should adhere to the following guidelines (updated versions of these guidelines can be found at <www.acr.org> by searching for keywords "PDF standards download").

• Telehealth systems should provide storage capacity capable of complying with all state and federal regulations regarding medical record transmittal and retention. To preserve data integrity, images stored at either site should meet the jurisdictional requirements of the transmitting site. Images interpreted off-site do not necessarily need to be stored at the receiving facility, so long as they are stored at the transmitting site. However, if the images are retained at the receiving site, the retention period of that jurisdiction must be met as well. The policy on record retention should also be documented in writing.

• As databases grow, database software engineers need to deal with retention and storage issues in order to maintain files while preserving data integrity. During the system development stage, organizations should establish protocols for archiving and purging old documents. A procedure should be established to back up the record's master patient index regularly, in the event of a system failure.

• Each exam data file must have an accurate corresponding patient and examination database record, which includes the patient's name and identification number, the exam date, the type of examination, and the facility at which the examination was performed. Also, space should be available for a brief clinical history.

• A clinical history of prior examinations and information about them should be retrievable from archives in a period appropriate to the clinical needs of the facility and medical staff (updated versions of these guidelines can be found at <www.acr.org>).

Standards for Document Image Capturing

The **American National Standards Institute (ANSI)** and the Association for Information and Image Management (AIIM) have jointly published standards relating to document image capture for organizations to follow to preserve data integrity. These standards include recommended practices for a number of issues, such as using image scanners, scanning roll film and microfiche, and monitoring image quality of aperture.

Other Data Integrity Considerations

A number of other considerations are important when reviewing data integrity. This list, though not exhaustive, provides an overview of issues to consider.

Prewritten Media Life Expectancy. Blank, unwritten media have limited life expectancy. Review the manufacturer's warranty and verify that the manufacture date is visible.

Postwritten Media Life Expectancy. The average life expectancy for written media ranges from ten to thirty years. The organization will need to maintain a backup copy of the written media. The backup copy can be stored on optical disc, high-capacity magnetic tape, or microfilm, and the organization needs to perform periodic monitoring of the image quality. This auditing for quality control is referred to as read-error analysis and reporting. Should a recorded image begin to deteriorate, it will be necessary to rewrite the image from the backup storage. The media manufacturer's storage guidelines should be adhered to closely.

Operating System Compatibility. Over time, hardware and software are upgraded as standards and performance levels change. Vendor maintenance contracts should be developed at the time of purchasing such technology in anticipation of future changes in hardware and software. The contract should specify how system compatibility will be ensured over time. For example, a vendor offering upgrades should also provide a formal plan for transferring the current system to upgraded technology, including a protection plan for data integrity.

Equipment Maintenance. To ensure a high-quality database, each organization should establish a routine quality-control function for health information management to audit all equipment.

Destruction of Original Documents. All applicable state and federal laws should be reviewed before destroying original documents. For example, the Uniform Photographic Copies of Business and Public Records as Evidence Act states that after the original document has been copied, it may be destroyed in the regular course of business. This holds true unless federal or state laws, or custodial or fiduciary responsibilities, require that the original document be retained.

CONCLUSION

Protecting a telehealth or e-health data system is serious business. It is easy to get excited about the power of computer and Internet databases.

Unfortunately, we all must strike a balance between this excitement and the sobering realities of our litigious society. Citizens of the United States are often quick to pursue juridical solutions if they feel their health-related rights have been violated. One of those rights concerns the protection of any information related to a patient's health. Legislators and other regulators are apparently using technology to tighten aspects of the collection, storage, and transfer of health care information that have been lax in previous years. They appear to be holding technology to a higher standard than they do traditional forms of care. Such reform may seem difficult to accommodate, but like technology itself, it is here, and in most instances, health care providers will have no choice but to adapt.

We have presented the material in this chapter to help you make better decisions regarding the care and protection of your patients' information. We encourage organizations to develop a thorough understanding of these issues, knowing that in doing so, they will be taking strides toward protecting themselves. Chapter Nine addresses many of the legal and ethical aspects of these issues as they arise in the use of telecommunication technologies.

CHAPTER 8

Legal and Ethical Issues

*A telemedicine director was frustrated with the lack of reimburse-
ment in her state for telehealth services. Her predecessor had obtained funding from Blue Cross/Blue Shield some years before, but
she felt that other third-party carriers would be more willing to fully
reimburse for such services if government agencies agreed to pay for
telehealth. The HCFA, as a federal agency, was out of her control.
Medicaid, however, which reimburses at the state level, was within
her control. Months of subtle lobbying culminated in success in 1996.
At a statewide meeting of mental health providers, the director of the
state's Medicaid office happened to be in the audience. During the
telemedicine director's speech, she challenged Medicaid to reimburse
for telehealth, and the director agreed on the spot, in front of dozens
of witnesses.*

As we have discussed, the clinical application of telehealth is in many ways still in its infancy. Although a health care professional's first mandate is to "do no harm," the use of technology brings a great many complicating issues into play. Despite these challenges, legal developments are supporting the movement toward providing responsible care via telehealth.

TELEHEALTH LAW

Laws are being enacted at the state and federal levels that will promote the rapid deployment of telemedicine and telehealth by medical and behavioral

169

health care practitioners. This section examines the underlying issues as well as specific laws that have been enacted to support this powerful movement. The issues we discuss here are relevant to the Internet as well as to a wide range of other technological advances, including interactive videoconferencing, voice response systems, and the medical support services that are enabled by store-and-forward technologies. A chronological presentation of legislation affecting patient privacy, confidentiality, security, and data integrity appears first, followed by topics related to licensure, jurisdiction, reimbursement, and credentialing.

Privacy Act of 1974

Protecting the privacy, confidentiality, and security of patients receiving telehealth services is an area of concern for consumers, providers, and the government. Playing an early role in the protection of patient privacy was the Privacy Act of 1974 (5 U.S.C. sec. 552a), which was designed to outline the responsibilities of federal agencies regarding the collection, use, and dissemination of personal health information. Section 552a(e)(10) of the act is very clear: federal systems must "establish appropriate administrative, technical, and physical safeguards to insure the security of records and to protect against any anticipated threats or hazards to their security or integrity which could result in substantial harm, embarrassment, inconvenience, or unfairness to any individual on whom information is maintained."

Copyright Act of 1976

Soon after the Privacy Act, issues related to electronic transfer of medical records surfaced in the national legislature. The Copyright Act of 1976 (17 U.S.C. secs. 101–810) affords copyright protection to all original works of authorship that are fixed in any tangible medium of expression. Copyright law protects only the expression of ideas or facts, not the implementation of ideas. So whereas the written description of a procedure cannot be duplicated without violating copyright, the procedure itself can be freely implemented (G. Alexander, personal communication, September 27, 1999).

Original works can include compilations and databases of health information, but the underlying facts in a database must be selected and arranged in an original format for copyright protection to apply. The author or "owner" of the database, once under copyright, has the right to control the creation and distribution of copies of the database and the right to control the alteration or modification of the database into a new derivative work (Office of Technology Assessment, 1995).

Medical Records Confidentiality Act of 1995

The majority of states have statutes governing the disclosure of medical records. In addition, there are federal laws that cover certain medical records. The Medical Records Confidentiality Act of 1995 sets forth standards that would govern almost all disclosures of patient-identifiable health information. It applies to electronic as well as paper medical records and requires that every reasonable effort be made to ensure the authenticity, veracity, and security of health care information.

Health Insurance Portability and Accountability Act of 1996

On August 22, 1996, Congress included provisions to address the need for transmission privacy and security in the Health Insurance Portability and Accountability Act of 1996 (HIPAA), Public Law 104-191. HIPAA, otherwise known as the Kennedy-Kassenbaum Act, called for protections of the privacy of medical information and was designed to improve the portability and continuity of health insurance coverage through administrative simplification by the Congress and the Department of Health and Human Services. Currently, health organizations and providers are working feverishly to obtain HIPAA compliance.

These provisions reduce unauthorized access to and alteration of confidential health records by creating a framework that imposes security, integrity, and authentication standards. These standards apply to all electronic health data that are transmitted by health plans, health care clearinghouses, or health care providers, whether the data reside in a practitioner's data system, are in transit, or reside in other repositories (Gilbert,

1999). HIPAA is a very large and complex act. Space limitations prohibit an exhaustive review, but we will summarize several points of direct relevance to the average health care provider or organization. Please refer to the Resources section of this book for more information.

Transaction Standards. HIPAA has a section titled "Administrative Simplification," which contains provisions intended to standardize electronic transmission of health care information and reduce associated costs and administrative burdens. These provisions call for a number of transaction requirements. They include Electronic Data Interchange (EDI) transaction standards and the establishment of unique ten-digit identification numbers for providers, payers, individuals, and employers. These unique identifiers will be assigned only after the final legislation has been passed. The EDI and unique identifiers serve to create a standard national format for all electronic transmissions. They should increase the efficiency of the existing health care system.

Clinicians will be allowed to choose whether they will complete transactions electronically or on paper. It is predicted that all health care payers will need to accept all types of transactions. Once the final rules are passed, payers reportedly will have two years to comply with HIPAA standards.

Standardizing transactions has raised concerns regarding security and privacy. Security standards and privacy legislation have therefore been proposed to ensure the protection of sensitive information (Koss, 2000a, 2000b).

Security Standards and Privacy Legislation. HIPAA standards for security will apply to all individuals who maintain or transmit health information related to the provision of health care services and supplies, regardless of the amount of the data. However, exact requirements for security techniques are not likely to be defined for each category of individual or organization. These standards will most likely attempt to focus on general security issues and require individuals and organizations to determine their own methods of compliance.

Final HIPAA rules will also address the privacy of patients. Some principles that are likely to be covered concern the limited disclosure, patient control, and authorization of one's health information. There will be no differentiation based on the sensitivity of the information. Also, use of identifiable information will not be allowed for purposes of marketing or making decisions regarding employment.

Preparing for Compliance. A person or group with senior executive reporting responsibilities should be assigned the responsibility of ensuring HIPAA compliance. These employees should be familiar with the technical operations of the organization. They should also be able to manage other personnel and interact with representatives of other companies, such as vendors. The group should review all the HIPAA literature and conduct a risk assessment to determine the organization's technological needs. Outside consultants will be available to help with these demands, but they are likely to be in high demand and expensive.

"Administrative Simplification" literature can be found at the Web site <aspe.hhs.gov/admnsimp/>, where a free download of the Implementation Guide and Data Dictionary for Transaction Standards can be found. Also at this site an organization can subscribe to a listserv to receive updates on HIPAA standards.

Once an assessment of the critical areas of your organization have been completed, a budget and timeline can be established for complete compliance. Critical areas of assessment can include considerations for the necessary types of transaction, and the security needed to protect the transmission of this information. For example, methods of information transfer to payers should be taken into account when factoring costs. The timeline should cover the design of the system, multiple testing and modifications, and the final installation of the system (Koss, 2000a, 2000b).

Failure to Comply. Failing to comply with HIPAA provisions may result in a civil and monetary penalty. Although many details of HIPAA are yet to be determined at the time of this publication, it appears that wrongful disclosure of individually identifiable health information can result in fines up to $50,000 or imprisonment up to one year (or both). In addition, if the offense is committed under false pretenses, a fine of $100,000 or imprisonment of up to five years (or both) can be imposed. A fine of up to $250,000 and imprisonment of up to ten years may be charged to individuals who use individually identifiable health information for commercial advantage, personal gain, or malicious harm (CPRI, 1999; Gilbert, 1999).

As a result of the proposed HIPAA mandate and increasing public concern about the confidentiality of personal health information, Congress and state legislatures have been considering a number of bills that address a broad range of confidentiality protections (JCAHO & National Committee for Quality Assurance [NCQA], 1998). For example, the Medical Information Protection Act (MIPA), which was introduced in Congress in early 1999, would preempt state confidentiality laws and create a single national standard for the protection of patient information.

Children's Online Privacy Protection Act of 1999

The Federal Trade Commission (FTC) in 1998 recommended to Congress legislation that resulted in the Children's Online Privacy Protection Act. This act took effect on April 21, 2000, and regulates the collection of all medical information regarding children under thirteen years of age. (For more information, visit the Web site <www.ftc.gov/ogc/>.) The FTC continues to be an advocate for general consumer privacy online and to monitor the self-regulation efforts of independent companies.

The FTC has also established <www.consumer.gov>, which links more than sixty federal agencies concerned with consumer protection and business guidance. Consumers can report any fraud complaints directly to the FTC at <www.ftc.gov>, which keeps a running record in its Consumer Sentinel and has identified over four thousand fraudulent Web sites. In addition, this site provides information for Internet businesses and online marketers on all existing consumer protection laws.

LICENSURE AND JURISDICTION

Licensure and jurisdiction issues have presented legislators and practitioners with more questions than answers. Potential solutions to various problems have been proposed or implemented, in both the local and international arenas.

Interstate Licensure

As has been evident in the United States, a state-based licensing system is a major barrier to the interstate practice of telehealth. State licensure restrictions run counter to telehealth's ability to transcend geographical boundaries. Despite this problem, many states have amended licensing requirements to include telehealth.

Practitioners are often subject to the jurisdiction of another state when they practice telehealth. How each state asserts jurisdiction depends on the "long-arm statute," which is the way a state gains jurisdiction over a nonresident. In the case of injury or malpractice, jurisdiction is questionable. When there is no signed agreement between the patient and the practitioner that delineates jurisdiction, determining which state has authority is potentially problematic in the case of a lawsuit.

Other complications arise from state licensing boards. These boards are responsible for protecting their state citizens from the actions of unqualified providers and for monitoring the credentials and performance of all the health care providers within their jurisdiction. The central point of controversy lies in whether telehealth technologies take the patient to the practitioner, or the practitioner to the patient. It is sometimes unclear which state will have jurisdiction and in which state the practitioner will need to hold a license (Schanz, 1999a).

Those involved in practicing telehealth across state lines must deal with large quantities of paperwork, the expense of obtaining a professional license, and other obligations and complications that can vary from state to state. Rural practitioners in particular may have a greater need for securing and managing multiple licenses because their lines of referral to specialists often traverse state boundaries (Nickelson, 1998).

State Decisions

Various states have already begun to regulate the practice of telemedicine and telehealth within their boundaries. Several states permit licensure by endorsement, granting a license to a professional who is licensed in another state with similar standards (Schanz, 1999a).

Moreover, the varying requirements of each state have rendered licensure by endorsement quite problematic. States differ with respect to whether they endorse licenses granted by other states (Lenoff, 2000; Sanders & Bashshur, 1995). State requirements for licensing by endorsement are also often time consuming, costly, and confusing. Practitioners are subject to numerous bureaucratic hurdles. These obstacles may involve obtaining the correct application procedures and processes from each state. Some states require that original documents be periodically submitted to licensing boards, and some states require that practitioners obtain multistate licensure (Deleon, Vanden Bos, Sammons, & Frank, 1998).

Most states also require an updated list of the licenses a provider holds, which means that the multistate provider must continually update the application. The majority of states require a physical appearance for endorsement applications. Some states also require that the provider retake licensing exams if a specific number of years have passed since the initial exam. Application fees can be yet another disincentive (Center for Telemedicine Law [CTL], 1997). Other state requirements may likewise vary, and in some cases it is more feasible for qualified professionals to obtain a license in another state by taking that state's licensing exam. Such delays and expenses can easily prohibit the clinician from practicing in states where the need for care exists (CTL, 1997).

Various possible solutions for these kinds of problems have emerged. For example, federal prisons, the military, and Indian Health Services are not restricted by state licensure laws and thus offer a model of how a future system might function through the federal government (IOM, 1996). Various professional associations are exploring guidelines for their licensing boards (Deleon, Vanden Bos, Sammons, & Frank, 1998).

E-Health, Telehealth, and Telemedicine

A proposed solution for the interstate licensing problem is the creation of a national telehealth license. Some approaches have proposed a national license because interstate commerce is involved (IOM, 1996). Others advocate the replacement of individual state licensures with a national system (Bashshur, Scott, & Silva, 1994; IOM, 1996; Sanders & Bashshur, 1995). Some nursing organizations have advocated this "driver's license" approach. Meanwhile, the National Council of State Boards of Nursing (1998) has advanced the Interstate Nurse Licensure Compact. The compact stipulates a set of articles whereby a nurse would hold a license in one state (the state of residence) and could practice in any state that signed onto the interstate compact. Nurses in compliant states must follow the laws and regulations of the state in which they practice.

The Federation of State Medical Boards (FSMB) has developed legislation allowing a state to create and administer a telehealth license. This limited type of license would allow a practitioner to "enter" a state via technology. The American Medical Association, however, has taken the position that a full and unrestricted license should be held in all states of practice (Nickelson, 1998). Ace Allen (1998) says:

> I believe that most telemedicine, as with most medicine, will continue to be practiced primarily at a local and regional (primarily intrastate) level for the next several years—and not because there are cross-state licensure issues, but because that is the way most patients will want to see their physicians.... I am also quite concerned that there are enough loopholes and uncertainties with the proposed legislation that it will be very hard to police or enforce.... Although limited cross-state licensure is a simple concept, the execution could be a nightmare—especially in this era when federalism is on the run, and states' rights are ascendant. Even "straightforward" things, such as the definitions of telemedicine, of patient records, of local standard of care, are not so obvious or universally understood as it would appear. Patient confidentiality issues, sanctions in the case of malpractice, and so on vary greatly from state to state.... My concern with cross-state telemedicine is

that the patient be afforded the same legal redress that he or she would be for an on-site encounter in the patient's state. That would mean that, in the case of a lawsuit, the case would be heard in the patient's state.

International Approaches

On the international front, similar issues and solutions have arisen with regard to licensure. For example, to practice telehealth in Malaysia, a physician requires a Malaysian medical license; in contrast, several programs from Argentina, the Middle East, and Greece are receiving consultation from professionals residing in the United States. In most of these programs, the consulting professionals from the United States are not licensed in the countries from which the consult originates (E. Saindon, personal communication, May 31, 2000).

The Committee on Medicine and Law of the International Bar Association Section on Legal Practice (1999) has proposed possible solutions for international telehealth licensure. It has proposed that each country ensure that its health and medical licensing board provides a reasonable opportunity for full and unrestricted licensure to health care practitioners from other countries. Furthermore, they suggest that health care practitioners accept the responsibility to obtain authorization for their services from the proper authorities in each country. They also suggest that if this authorization is not in place, the practitioner might be required to apply for such authorization to either the specific country or to an internationally recognized organization whose standards would be recognized by the country concerned (Schanz, 1999b). Other international initiatives are in progress. See Chapter Twelve for details concerning some of the organizations involved.

The Human Factor

Other questions and complications can arise when using technologies that easily traverse geographical boundaries. When delivering services electronically over networks such as the Internet, where distance can easily be forgotten or considered irrelevant, it can be difficult for a practitioner in the midst of a crisis to remember licensing or confidentiality restrictions mandated by state and federal legislation or by foreign countries. Many human factors may take precedence in the heat of an emergency.

For instance, in delivering consultation to a Tibetan community leader struggling with the ravages of Chinese dominance, or to an abused teenager from Utah pretending to be an adult in Florida, it could be easy for a practitioner to ignore or forget local licensing limitations (Maheu & Gordon, in press). With the rapid merging and morphing of various technologies, practitioners will find it challenging to determine which computer-based services can be provided without formal licensure.

LEGISLATION FOR TELEHEALTH REIMBURSEMENT

By developing an understanding of the history and current position of telehealth, health care professionals can learn how to make their programs profitable and sustainable. Reimbursement issues are especially important. For example, California has proven itself a leader in legislation related to telehealth by enacting the California Telemedicine Development Act of 1996, one of the first laws related to telemedicine. The proposal for this law was submitted in March 1996 and passed every committee, including the powerful Insurance Committee, without a single opposing vote. It was signed into law only eight months after its introduction. The act mandates insurance payment for telemedicine for specified providers, and defines and regulates the practice of telemedicine on a statewide level. Many other states have since followed suit with various types of laws for their particular states.

Many states already offer some telehealth coverage under their Medicaid programs. Some states (including California, Louisiana, and Oklahoma) have enacted specific legislation mandating coverage for telehealth consultation services to be provided under private insurance plans (Deleon et al., 1998). Reimbursement problems still seem to be a significant barrier to the widespread practice of telehealth, however (Cepelewicz, 1998).

Various states have placed limitations on reimbursable types of tele-health. California, for instance, in a 1997 amendment to the California Telemedicine Development Act of 1996, has removed the use of telephones and e-mail from its acceptable service category. Other delivery modes available through the Internet are not specifically mentioned in the act, making their legal status for delivery of health care unclear. An example of such a mode would be a chat room or a discussion board.

Health Care Financing Administration Reimbursement

Beginning January 1, 1999, Medicare reimbursement in rural health care began in professional shortage areas. This provision, enacted in the Balanced Budget Act of 1997, represented Medicare's first national reimbursement policy for telehealth services (Cepelewicz, 1998; Health Care Financing Administration [HCFA], 1998b, 1999; Nickelson, 1998). Payment regulations are restrictive, but they represent a significant step toward covering telehealth services. This policy also raises some important issues about how best to pay for these services.

Newer legislation promises to change some of these policies and make reimbursement less restrictive for a wide range of providers and settings. For legislative updates related to telehealth reimbursement policy, go to <http://thomas.loc.gov/> and look for S. 2505 of the Telehealth Improvement and Modernization Act of 2000.

Billing Codes

Health care services are billed for reimbursement using a variety of procedural codes, such as for initial exam, follow-up, and confirmatory consultations in hospitals, outpatient facilities, and medical offices. Furthermore, these procedures have specific codes for a number of medical specialties, such as cardiology, dermatology, gastroenterology, neurology, pulmonology, and psychiatry.

Work will be needed in the definitions of consultation and teleconsultation so that the procedural codes are universal. For example, nursing and medical specialties need to agree on what "standard practice" represents for both care and teleconsultation. The need for such agreements to be made quickly is apparent when examining impinging factors, such as the aging of our population.

Medicaid

Medicaid reimbursement for telehealth services is available at the discretion of each state. Several states allow reimbursement for services provided via telehealth. Reimbursement is subject to specific requirements or restrictions. Medicare conditions of participation (COPs) are also applicable to certain settings, such as long-term care facilities (HCFA, 1999).

Reimbursement for Medicaid-covered telehealth services must also satisfy the federal requirements of efficiency, economy, and quality of care. States are encouraged to use the flexibility inherent in federal law to create innovative payment systems for services that incorporate telehealth technology.

For example, states covering medical services that use telehealth may reimburse both the practitioner at the hub site for the consultation and the practitioner at the spoke site for an office visit. States also have the flexibility to reimburse any additional cost (for technical support, line charges, depreciation on equipment, and so on) associated with the delivery of a covered service by electronic means as long as the payment is consistent with the requirements of efficiency, economy, and quality of care. Furthermore, these add-on costs can be incorporated into the fee-for-service rates or separately reimbursed by the state. If they are separately billed and reimbursed, the costs must be linked to a covered Medicaid service (HCFA, 1999).

Some states use modifiers to the existing Physicians' Current Procedural Terminology (CPT) codes. The modifiers *TM* and *TV* are commonly used to distinguish telehealth reimbursement. Other states have developed their own local codes to distinguish telehealth services. The dust has not settled on these reimbursement issues, and more is sure to come.

FEDERAL TELEHEALTH REGULATORY BODIES

Activity at the federal level is propelled by several agencies that are working toward assessing and determining the major needs for telehealth legislation. The Food and Drug Administration (FDA) and the Joint Working

Group on Telemedicine (JWGT) have been implementing strategies for regulating telehealth. It is becoming increasingly apparent that as the regulation of telehealth changes, more regulatory bodies will eventually be needed to account for the variety of legal issues related to telehealth.

Food and Drug Administration

Many remote health care delivery systems have been inadequately evaluated and validated, and may pose a substantial risk to patients. The FDA is increasingly being called on to regulate telehealth systems and has the authority to regulate medical devices that are used in telehealth and telehealth software (Reichertz & Halpern, 1997). This situation exists because the FDA can control any telecommunications products labeled or otherwise promoted as being useful in telehealth under the federal Food, Drug, and Cosmetic Act (FDCA). This act states that telemedicine involves the use of many telecommunication technology management devices, in the form of workstations, supercomputers, satellite links, terrestrial links, and software. Each of these can be used in nonmedical contexts, but when they are used in a telehealth context, they serve to assist diagnosis or treatment. They are therefore considered medical devices in these circumstances (Reichertz & Halpern, 1997).

Thus whenever a telecommunication product with medical applications is marketed, the company or individual is subject to the requirements of the FDCA. The manufacturer or distributor is required to submit to the FDA a premarket notification (known as a 510k) that will be subject to review by six specific divisions of the FDA (Reichertz & Halpern, 1997).

As one of the first disciplines to adopt telehealth practice, radiology is continuing to set the pace for telehealth policy and standards as well as equipment. The Center for Devices and Radiological Health (CDRH) is the branch of the FDA responsible for regulating electronic medical devices and radiation-emitting electronic products. The CDRH therefore plays an important role in the development of telehealth equipment and systems in the United States (Center for Devices and Radiological Health [CDRH], 1996).

The FDA also regulates products through its Current Good Manufacturing Practices. The regulation is applicable to all medical devices, including those used in telehealth, and plays an important role in design controls for software medical devices (CDRH, 1996).

Joint Working Group on Telemedicine

The JWGT is a federal interagency group that coordinates members' telehealth activities. Several member agencies within the JWGT provide telehealth grants, and the JWGT ensures that there is no overlap in federal funding. Members bring their unique telehealth expertise to the table, creating a forum to discuss and share information, to educate its members, and to develop specific actions that reduce barriers to the effective use of telehealth technologies.

Although the average health care innovator would like to think that much is being done to advance the legitimate use of telehealth equipment, many questions related to daily practice remain unanswered. For example, in the 1999 report of a survey of state attorney's general offices regarding legal and regulatory issues related to the delivery of behavioral telehealth services, Koocher and Morray (1999) found that only 7 percent of forty-two responding states had statutes in place that address telehealth issues involving the practice of psychotherapy or counseling. Without state statutes regulating practice, professionals are left without proper direction if they wish to avail themselves and their patients of the benefits of technology, and they thus act to avoid undue risk.

CREDENTIALING

Credentialing refers to a procedure for determining whether individual practitioners possess the necessary qualifications to provide services, either generally or with certain restrictions. Credentialing is a decision often made at the organizational level. Although credentialing differs from standards used for licensing, it yields the same result: credentialing helps establish notions of appropriate training to conduct practice, and credentialing therefore defines malpractice as well.

The main credentialing authorities are individual states, the Joint Commission on Accreditation of Healthcare Organizations (JCAHO), and the **National Committee for Quality Assurance (NCQA);** there are other local credentialing bodies as well (IOM, 1996). The JCAHO evaluates and accredits over eighteen thousand health care organizations, programs, and services. The NCQA is a nonprofit watchdog organization, recognized as the leader in the effort to assess, measure, and report on the quality of care provided by managed care organizations in the United States (JCAHO & NCQA, 1998).

Issues in telehealth credentialing are so complex that some of the essential questions are still being defined. One of the many questions, for example, is whether the practitioner needs to be credentialed not only by the local organization but also by the remote institution where the consultation may be taking place. Credentialing requirements outside the practitioner's home institution will undoubtedly cause administrative obstacles for both the practitioner and the organization (IOM, 1996).

Some positions are being defined, however. For example, the JCAHO has ruled that practitioners who provide teleconsultations need privileges from an organization seeking the consultation only when the consultation involves direct patient care. If it does not involve patient care, permission is not needed (JCAHO, 1998). With regard to the jurisdiction of credentialing bodies, the requirements for maintaining telehealth records are the same as for other medical records. Regardless of the location of the patient, practitioner, or facility, JCAHO standards apply to telehealth records (Fletcher, 1999). Telehealth practitioners and organizations therefore must have adequate security measures in place to protect patient privacy. The claim of injury, either physical or emotional, caused by disclosure of a patient's confidential information is a serious one and can be followed by legal action. The patient can sue the telehealth practitioner for breach of privacy and of the implied contract of confidentiality, as well as for malpractice and infliction of emotional distress (Cepelewicz, 1998). Much more is assuredly yet to come from these credentialing bodies.

ETHICAL ISSUES

It is commonly understood that ethics are more stringent than legal codes. They are based in human values and designed to guide professional decisions in the face of many, often conflicting variables. Despite their importance, ethical guidelines for telehealth practitioners have been slow to develop, especially when compared to the rapid escalation of technology available for telehealth applications.

Key Ethical Issues

Key ethical issues in the clinical delivery of telehealth vary by profession, but generally include avoiding harm, defining the professional relationship, obtaining informed consent, discussing the limits of confidentiality, maintaining patient confidentiality, operating within one's boundaries of competence, establishing fees and financial arrangements, avoiding false or deceptive statements, providing services to patients served by other professionals, providing consultations; avoiding sexual intimacies with patients, maintaining records and data, and avoiding use of confidential material for didactic or other purposes. Professional associations generally also have other specific ethical standards for research and educational services rendered by their members.

Although most professions have delineated appropriate definitions of professional conduct for face-to-face treatment, the applicability of these definitions can easily become blurred when using technology. For example, with regard to confidentiality, most health care professionals are obligated to ensure the confidentiality of patient identity and records. In some professions, practitioners and researchers must also inform the patient or subject of the limits to confidentiality. Yet when using electronic tools, especially the Internet, professionals can easily be dazzled by the excitement of instantaneous communication with a patient halfway around the globe, and easily forget their ethical requirements.

Similarly, professionals may not be thinking of their patient records when having an office computer serviced at a neighborhood computer repair shop. Nonetheless, they may be exposing their patient files to unauthorized access and reproduction. Another area in which professionals might err in the direction of violating patient confidentiality is by using e-mail support groups for research, without obtaining the prior consent of group members.

Preliminary research with behavioral health care practitioners has shown that a significant number who offer services over the Internet are unaware of their state laws or the professional ethical requirements related to such practice (Maheu & Gordon, in press). For a detailed examination of ethical issues related to behavioral health care, see Maheu, Callan, and Nagy (1998).

Professional Associations and Ethical Standards

Professional associations typically develop and publish ethical standards for their memberships. Whereas some professional associations have led the way in developing ethical guidelines related to telehealth for their practitioners, many have not. Despite the obvious proliferation of health care technology in the last decade, including the Internet, professional associations are struggling to allocate the needed resources to developing practice standards and giving guidance to their memberships.

If professional associations want their practitioners to operate with a reverence for ethical codes, it behooves them to keep the codes timely and relevant. Even though technology may be outstripping the abilities of professional associations to "keep up," these associations have a responsibility to their practitioners to "catch up."

Practitioners attempting to operate innovative telehealth programs within the bounds of vague or outdated ethical standards and guidelines are at risk of being at a distinct disadvantage when developing a defense before a licensing board or jury (Koocher & Morray, 1999). Unclear standards and guidelines leave the innovative practitioner with many opportunities but not enough direction.

Most professional associations have provisions that admonish practitioners to work within the bounds of their competence, but they do not specify acceptable practice using telecommunication technologies. For professional associations and practitioners alike, keeping abreast of the technological demands is important, because an existing set of standards, whether outdated or updated, creates a standard of due care. This standard in turn helps establish definitions of malpractice. Similarly, if professionals of a discipline do not adhere to standards accepted by their national association, those professionals may be responsible for malpractice in tort. Therefore, it is incumbent upon the elected and staff leaders of professional associations to allocate the needed resources to develop adequate standards and guidelines to protect their practitioners in a timely manner. Some associations are making significant progress on these fronts; others have barely begun.

Exemplary Professional Associations

Some professional associations have embraced the responsibility of guiding their membership by publishing standards that address telehealth applications, including the Internet, with varying degrees of specificity. Although this is not an exhaustive list, we offer it to guide you toward some associations with existing telehealth standards.

The American College of Radiology (ACR). In 1994, the ACR (1999) adopted a standard for teleradiology mandating that "Physicians who provide the official, authenticated interpretation of images transmitted by teleradiology should maintain licensure appropriate to delivery of radiologic service at both the transmitting and receiving sites."

The American Medical Association (AMA). In June 1996, the AMA voted to adopt a policy that "states and their medical boards should require a full and unrestricted license for all physicians practicing telemedicine within a state" (National Telecommunications and Information Administration [NTIA], 1997). This policy continues the existing practice of requiring physicians to obtain endorsement of their licenses in each state in which they practice. More recently, the AMA has published guidelines for medical and health information sites on the Internet, located at <www.ama-assn.org/about/guidelines.htm>.

The College of American Pathologists (CAP). "The CAP has taken the position that a physician rendering primary diagnosis and/or treatment should have a full and unrestricted license to practice medicine in the state in which the patient presents for diagnosis" (NTIA, 1997).

The Federation of State Medical Boards (FSMB). In October 1995, the FSMB enacted a model that "would require physicians who regularly or frequently engage in the practice of medicine across state lines, by electronic or other means, to obtain a special license issued by the state medical board" (NTIA, 1997).

The National Council of State Boards of Nursing. As mentioned earlier, this organization has advanced the Interstate Nurse Licensure Compact, an innovative agreement outlining how nurses can practice in cooperative states (National Council of State Boards of Nursing, 1998). Several states have already agreed to follow this agreement, and progress is steadily being made to recruit other states.

The American Counseling Association (ACA). The ACA (1999) has approved a set of ethical standards to help guide online counselors in appropriate ways of providing care via electronic communication. These standards include considerations of confidentiality, appropriate online relationships, and legal issues involved in online counseling.

Exemplary E-Health Organizations

In an attempt at self-regulation, various Internet-based groups have evolved to help set standards and guidelines for various types of health care Web sites on the Internet. The list that follows, though not exhaustive, will help direct you to organizations that are focused on general health care Web sites, rather than specialty professional Web sites.

The Internet Healthcare Coalition (IHC). The IHC (2000) has developed an e-health code of ethics "to ensure that all people worldwide can confidently, and without risk, realize the full benefits of the Internet to improve their health." The code of ethics outlines many guiding principles to help practitioners adhere to standards for e-health. For information, go to <www.ihc.net/>.

Health Internet Ethics (Hi-Ethics). In 1999, a number of major Internet health care companies came together to discuss ethical, credibility, and integrity issues for consumer health sites. Among the topics were commerce regulations, privacy issues, content quality, and responsible advertising practices (Tschida, 1999). Subsequent meetings of these companies resulted in a formulation titled "Ethical Principles for Offering Internet Health Services to Consumers." Members agree to follow the fourteen guidelines concerning the information presented on the site and the use of information gathered by it. (For a complete listing of the guidelines, go to <www.hiethics.org/Principles/index.asp>.)

TRUSTe. This independent, nonprofit group attempts to build consumer trust and confidence in the Internet by promoting disclosure and informed consent. Approved sites display the TRUSTe icon, which signifies that the approved Web site has agreed to notify users of

Personally identifiable information collected from the user through the Web site

The organization collecting the information

How the information is used

With whom the information may be shared

What choices are available to the user regarding collection, use, and distribution of the information

The security procedures that are in place to protect against the loss, misuse, or alteration of information under the Web site's control

How consumers can correct any inaccuracies in the information collected

For more information about TRUSTe, see its Web site: <www.truste.org/>.

Health on the Net (HON). The Health on the Net Foundation Code of Conduct (HONcode) for medical and health Web sites addresses the reliability and credibility of information on the Internet. As posted on HON's Web site, "The HONcode is not an award system, nor does it intend to rate the quality of the information provided by a Web site. It only defines a set of rules to: hold Web site developers to basic ethical standards in the presentation of information; and help make sure readers always know the source and the purpose of the data they are reading." For further information, see <www.hon.ch/HONcode>.

CONCLUSION

Much has already been accomplished toward shaping the legal infrastructure for telehealth in the United States. Critical issues regarding licensure, patient protection, and reimbursement are being defined and legislated. Obviously, much more remains to be developed. Similarly, credentialing bodies are attempting to clarify their requirements for health care delivery via telehealth technologies. Ethical issues abound, and several professional associations have begun to lead the way toward elucidating practice standards and guidelines. Chapter Nine takes a closer look at issues related to malpractice and risk management for organizations and practitioners.

CHAPTER 9

Malpractice and Risk Management

Several years ago, the new director of a fledgling telehealth program devised a number of action strategies to recruit physicians in her medical center by educating them about the many benefits of telemedicine. She made a thirty-minute presentation at each department's monthly grand rounds. Every time she completed her presentation, a hand would shoot up. In each of the sixteen departmental presentations, the first question asked was, "What about malpractice liability?"

We live in a litigious society, so it is understandable that health care providers are concerned about their liability. Because e-health, telehealth, and telemedicine add a new element in the delivery of care, many providers question the level of liability when using technology. In medical practice, technology can thus add new and unforeseen factors to health care. For example, e-mail offers new ways of interacting with patients and new challenges that create new liabilities. Nevertheless, it is important to draw this distinction: telecommunication technology in health care offers a variety of new *tools* for extending existing specialties, but it does not represent a new specialty itself (Stamm & Pearce, 1995). Therefore, the discussion of ethics, standards, malpractice, and risk management related to technology ought to avoid attempts to reinvent each discipline. Rather, the goal is to examine how existing codes need to accommodate the inclusion of each telehealth tool (telephone, e-mail, chat room, fax, videoconferencing, and the like) as a

191

specific means of communication for specialized clinical care, education, or research (Maheu, Callan, & Nagy, 1998).

In this chapter, we present a review of some of the most pressing issues related to technology-based malpractice and risk management for both professionals and organizations. Although these areas are fraught with controversy, some groups have issued either preliminary or substantive papers to help make sense of the confusing landscape. We have attempted to synthesize the information from these sources in the form of suggestions to facilitate your decisions with respect to the implementation of e-health, telehealth, and telemedicine.

MALPRACTICE

Medical malpractice is generally defined as "a deviation from the accepted medical standard of care that results in injury to a patient for whom a clinician has a duty of care" (American Medical Association [AMA], 1990). For practitioners using technology, this definition presents complicated legal issues for both intrastate and interstate practice. State law generally governs malpractice liability, which defines the duty of care, the amount of damages patients may collect, and statutes of limitations.

Telehealth practice complicates issues of malpractice. One of the most difficult areas to define is the altered practitioner-patient relationships when they are mediated through technology (such as telephone or interactive videoconferencing equipment).

Altered Relationships with Patients

The area of greatest concern in the practice of telehealth is the absence of face-to-face contact between patient and practitioner. As one would expect, practitioners who traditionally perform face-to-face examinations during regular practice and have depended on physical contact for their examinations are the ones who are at the greatest risk when examining patients remotely. This risk can be reduced by having another professional present with the patient during remote consultations using technology. In many settings, a nonspecialist (the referring professional) makes a video call to the specialist (the consulting professional) and remains in the room with the patient. The nonspecialist performs the physical examination of the patient at the direction of the specialist and discusses findings throughout the procedure. This technique allows the specialist to make a diagnosis with immediate and systematic information from the nonspecialist. A nurse-practitioner, for example, is easily able to perform the needed functions for most general exams required by a wide range of physicians.

Despite the apparent effectiveness of such an arrangement, however, in some cases this practice could be regarded as delivering less than adequate care. Even with another professional present in the room, if something goes wrong, the burden of proving the effectiveness of the remote treatment falls upon the directing specialist. In addition to this problem, many practitioners do not typically operate with another professional in the room. Telehome care nurses or behavioral health practitioners, for example, typically practice without the involvement of an assisting staff. These practitioners are more vulnerable to having their actions misinterpreted and misrepresented if something goes wrong in their interaction with the patient. As much psychological literature states, transference and countertransference can easily cloud the memories of those involved when a relationship becomes heated. These misconceptions are enough of a challenge to correct when the parties are face-to-face. When one adds the dimension of geographical remoteness mediated through telecommunication technology, there can be difficulties that are not yet fully researched and for which there are no easy solutions.

Research regarding the ways in which videoconferencing technology influences existing relationships is just beginning to emerge in the medical literature. By potentially adding emotional separation as well as physical distance between practitioner and patient, technology not only changes the service delivery system but also may alter elements of the clinical relationship. For instance, when physically absent or distant from an interaction with a professional, some patients may also experience a corresponding psychological distance. Such emotional distance can result in decreased understanding and empathy between patent and physician (IOM, 1996). At the same time, researchers are beginning to study the degree to which interactive videoconferencing in particular is able to bridge emotional distance and recreate social presence (Cukor et al., 1998; Habash, 1999; O'Conaill & Whittaker, 1997; Squibb, 1999; Whittaker & O'Conaill, 1997). In fact, some researchers are reporting that in such areas as telepsychiatry, there is considerable anecdotal evidence that some patients are more comfortable relating to their caregiver in a videoconferenced encounter rather than a face-to-face one (C. Zaylor, personal communication, August 18, 1998). One can see that whereas video connections may actually be helpful for some patient populations, it is also conceivable that they will not be helpful for others. Empirical research on the impact of various technologies on various patient populations is clearly needed to determine not only the efficacy of different technologies but also the different liabilities associated with these technologies.

Although it is uncertain how such relationships will affect malpractice, it is clear that technology can alter relationships. An example of a shift caused by technology is that patients may now know more about the scientific literature related to their condition than their treating practitioner. Patients have been forming virtual communities to discuss a range of medical issues and problems as well as to gain mutual support (Bruckman, 1996; Rheingold, 1993; Shields, 1996; Turkle, 1995; Wellman & Gulia, 1995). Armed with printouts from various medical databases, libraries, conference proceedings, online support groups, and other resources from the Internet, patients are challenging the authoritarian position of many practitioners, who have traditionally been the disseminators of knowledge (Bergman, 1993; Maheu, 1997; Maheu et al., 1998).

Professionals will have no choice but to adopt a more collaborative stance with their patients and perhaps even to foster patient education. The role of the practitioner of the future may include directing patients to substantive sources of information via the Internet, rather than being the primary disseminator of such information (Ferguson, 1998). Practitioners of tomorrow may also serve as translators of information for their patients, who may not have the fundamental education for properly assimilating the information they are able to gather so easily from the Internet.

Precisely how malpractice will be affected by these changing roles is yet to be identified. Nonetheless, some predictions are possible.

Because the professional relationship as altered through technology has not been well defined, courts and ethics boards will most likely render future decisions by examining existing case law and ethics codes. They are also likely to rely on consultants and traditional perspectives to define more clearly whether a professional relationship exists in each of the new circumstances created by technology (for example, e-mail, chat rooms, and videoconferencing). The courts also may be called on to make decisions related to how responsive and collaborative practitioners have been in treating patients who have acted on knowledge they have obtained from outside resources (such as the Internet).

There are instances where practitioners and organizations could be held liable for changes in the health care relationship due to "errors in transmitting, storing, or otherwise managing information transfer" (IOM, 1996). For example, problems might arise with the use of **compressed video,** in which repetitious information is eliminated as the data are converted from analog to digital and back. The default setting on such technologies thus may be viewed as interfering with the diagnostic procedure, and the practitioner may be seen as rendering a diagnosis with incomplete information. Determining legal responsibility for misdiagnosis under these conditions is yet another area for legal debate. This same liability may apply to computer-aided diagnostic programs (IOM, 1996).

Alternatively, if delivering service through telecommunication technology becomes the standard of care, there could be instances in which liability was incurred because telehealth technology was available but *not* used, leading to delayed diagnosis and poorer outcomes. It is therefore possible to imagine a future when patients challenge practitioners and hospitals for failure to make state-of-the-art technology available (Shellens, Jones, & Lang, 1999).

Despite these possibilities, telehealth may actually decrease the threat of malpractice suits by allowing for databased informational resources and better record keeping—such as the videotaping of consultations. There are many advantages and disadvantages to having a video recording of a consultation. A videotape automatically provides proof of the encounter (IOM, 1996); however, such recordings may not be helpful if hindsight raises questions about decisions made by the reasonably cautious practitioner.

Other unforeseen complications may arise. For example, the making of audio, video, or other image records requires the written consent of the patient. The decision to make such recordings necessitates the additional steps of developing and using a thorough consent agreement. Elements to consider in such an agreement are detailed at the end of this chapter. Furthermore, although security measures are likely to be undertaken to protect confidentiality, recordings may nevertheless be vulnerable to tampering or mishandling. Practitioners and organizations ought to consider the liability risks involved with maintaining and storing such records (Brandt & Carpenter, 1999). Research and case law will undoubtedly clarify the importance of these recording and storage issues.

Altered Collegial, Mentoring, and Supervisory Relationships

Collegial relationships are increasing dramatically as technology proliferates. For example, professionals flock to the Internet not only to e-mail one another privately but also to join thousands of professional e-mail discussion groups. Although participation in these discussion groups may appear risk free, professionals need to be mindful that e-mail is not secure, and when discussing patient information, they can be exposing themselves to liability by violating a patient's confidentiality. A patient or a patient's friend may be a member of that discussion group and recognize the case being discussed. At the worst extreme, a practitioner's forwarding snippets of patient e-mail to professional e-mail discussion groups in an attempt to obtain supervision from colleagues may be cause for a malpractice suit. All patient identifiers must be removed, such as the time and date stamp of e-mail messages sent by patients.

Joint Liability. When using interactive videoconferencing equipment of any type, the respective and joint liability of referring practitioners and consulting practitioners is ambiguous. The definition of negligence and malpractice with respect to either or both types of practitioners is unclear, and varies from state to state. Courts and ethical boards are likely to examine these roles and definitions using existing case law and ethics codes (Maheu, 1999b).

Mentoring. Mentoring is another area that may be altered by technology. Given the increased readiness with which younger generations are adopting technology, the time-tested mentor model of training and decision making in health care has become more complicated. Mentors with superior expertise in ethics and practice may lack the technical expertise to make some of their mentoring as relevant as it has been in previous years, and junior administrators and clinicians with superior expertise in technology may lack the judgment in ethics and practice they need for their work to be effective.

The traditional mentoring approach in which information flows from the top down is changing with the rapid adoption of technology in health care. This sudden shift of roles for mentors and mentees may cause unexpected difficulties. Attempts at avoiding these difficulties can be complicated if the parties are invested in being "right" and are rigid in their respective positions as either mentor or mentee (Maheu, 1999b).

Supervision. The shifting of roles can be even more complicated for supervisors and supervisees, a relationship in which there is the added complication of a legal obligation and potential malpractice liability. It is wise to develop a supervisory agreement, whereby the requirements of the relationship are detailed for both parties. When developing such an agreement, be sure to delineate who has final decision-making authority. Examples of such agreements can typically be obtained from legal counsel for professional associations.

Jurisdiction for Malpractice

Jurisdiction for malpractice closely parallels that of licensure, and is equally unclear. As it stands, practitioners using telecommunication technology could be subject to the jurisdiction of the state in which they reside, every state where they practice, and the state in which the patient resides. The respective liabilities of various health care institutions (hospitals, managed care organizations, and so on) housing such services are also ambiguous.

The other issue that often arises is an effort to determine where a suit from a patient can be filed and which state laws apply. Clients will most likely sue from the jurisdiction in which they reside. With this possibility in mind, professionals and organizations need to be adequately covered by malpractice insurance in every state to which service via technology is delivered. One thing is clear, however: to initiate malpractice lawsuits, plaintiffs must substantiate that there was a patient-practitioner relationship, that the consultant somehow breached the applicable standard of care, and that this breach caused an injury (Cepelewicz, 1998).

RISK MANAGEMENT

Having reviewed the legal and ethical issues, as well as the issues of privacy, confidentiality, security, and data integrity, in Chapters Seven and Eight, you are in a good position to conduct a thorough risk assessment of each technology you or your organization intends to use. Such an assessment will guide you in reducing malpractice liability. A careful look at the literature will show a number of substantial documents outlining laws, standards, guidelines, and research comparing essential elements of responsible and reasonable practice of telehealth (American Psychiatric Association, 1998; Brandt & Carpenter, 1999; Carroll, Wright & Zakoworotny, 1998; Department of Health and Human Services, 1998; Kane & Sands, 1998; Ryboski, 1998; Spielberg, 1998).

You may also find it helpful to explore traditional elements of risk management, which can include understanding the details of applicable licensure and related liability insurance coverage for each state of practice; understanding the law in the local community and how it relates to a program; determining how courts in the relevant geographical location might determine malpractice for a program; conducting scientific research in an area prior to offering services to the public as an expert; complying with expected documentation and consultation requirements; delivering services limited to your licensure and competence; and determining which at-risk populations might be served and how to best assess and manage those populations.

Several groups, including the Physician Insurers Association of America (1998) and the American Medical Informatics Association (Kane & Sands, 1998), and some authors (Spielberg, 1998) have made specific suggestions related to minimizing liability for professional use of the Internet with patients. In general, policies that ensure privacy and confidentiality are the key to good risk management. With that in mind, the remainder of this chapter outlines potential areas of discussion. We do not offer these discussion areas as standards or guidelines, however, but rather as suggestions for your consideration or that of your health care organization. You and your organization will also need to consider state and federal law, professional ethical codes for various professional groups, and community norms in making decisions about these suggestions. Program administrators or company directors should adapt these areas of focus to the service's particular circumstance and engage in discussions with ethical, legal, and insurance counsel if questions arise. The following suggestions are no substitute for timely and thorough consultation with experienced colleagues and attorneys.

Practitioner Considerations

Practitioner considerations include boundaries of competence, licensure, malpractice insurance, standards of care, and a host of other issues. We outline a number of these issues in the next sections.

Competence. Determining boundaries of competence for telehealth and e-health practitioners is a difficult task, especially when formal education, supervision, and experience in using technology are just beginning for health care practitioners. Of greatest concern are those technologies that most severely restrict the amount of information the diagnosing and treating professional receives: e-mail and chat rooms. In the absence of clinical training, supervision, or experience in text-based diagnosis and treatment, professionals may face significant liability if a lawsuit were brought for use of such limiting technologies exclusively with unknown and unseen patients. The fact remains that professionals who have been trained exclusively to use visual, auditory, or tactile cues for rendering diagnosis and treatment may well be held accountable for practicing outside the standard of care as well as outside their boundaries of competence if a patient files a malpractice claim for services rendered in e-mail or chat rooms. As discussed in other chapters of this book, however, dozens of federally funded and private projects have shown that telehealth equipment can be used efficaciously to deliver remote treatment via interactive videoconferencing. When Internet connections are able to deliver interactive videoconferencing, new questions will arise and will need to be answered in the area of establishing professional competence for diagnosing and treating patients who have never been seen face-to-face by the treating professional. For example, an increasing number of states are passing legislation that requires initial consultation and assessment to involve at least one face-to-face encounter before the practitioner relies on remote treatment. It must be assumed, however, that the trend will be reversed if future technologies show adequate reliability and validity for diagnosis and treatment.

Another competence issue relates to the worldwide nature of the population served through networks such as the Internet. Many professionals working through the Internet are becoming keenly aware of cultural and linguistic limitations in their dealings with Web site consumers from over a hundred different countries. Cultural and linguistic competence, then, will become an area of greater concern as professionals offer increasing numbers of services to a global network of consumers through the Internet. It will become increasingly important that practitioners clearly outline areas of linguistic and cultural competence in descriptions of services rendered through telecommunication technologies.

Licensure. Although much effort is being devoted to developing a nationwide licensure for telehealth practice, such licensure does not yet exist. Practitioners would do well to obtain and maintain licensure for every state of practice. To further minimize risk, obtain copies of, read carefully,

E-Health, Telehealth, and Telemedicine

and understand the state laws regarding telehealth and e-health liability for every state encompassed in your practice. Remember that the patient's state of residence is typically considered the state within which professionals must be licensed.

Malpractice Insurance. Liability insurance for health care is not a requirement in most states, but when practicing in new areas of health care, it is highly recommended. Obtain and understand the malpractice limits of liability for the specific duties to be performed through technology. Given that malpractice policies generally cover providers only for states in which they hold a license, obtain malpractice insurance for each state of licensure. Obtain a written agreement from the malpractice carrier regarding its coverage of specific services to be delivered. Do not settle for written agreements or form letters that do not specify the services or technologies to be used.

Standard of Care. Be fully informed of the accepted standard of care. This can differ from community to community as well as from state to state. For example, delivering care electronically may incur an obligation to be aware of the norms and customs of the people treated. You should be informed regarding the expectations of the populations served, as well as local events, including floods, wars, or other natural disasters and catastrophes. Your use of the Internet could result in allegations related to a slow rate of transmission or allegations that information you suggest for the patient's consideration online is unreliable. The best sources for such definitions of expectation are the state licensing board of your state and that of your patients, ethics boards of local chapters of professional organizations, and peers in your community whom you can consult. Be aware of emergency backup services in each community served. Obtain the name of at least one practitioner on call within the patient's geographical location, or other emergency referral services.

Know and adhere to the relevant practice guidelines and critical care pathways. If you are performing work for an organization, provide evidence of service in accordance with the organization's practice guidelines related to the use of telecommunication technology (National Committee for Quality Assurance [NCQA], 1999).

Keep current all online statements that are related to your training, hospital affiliations, managed care contracts, or licensure. Maintain an appropriate balance between professional and personal disclosure in the development of Web sites. Review any Web sites recommended to patients.

Prescriptions. Be cautious when discussing prescription medication. The AMA stipulates that a doctor should write new prescriptions without an in-person physical exam only if that doctor, who has the patient's history and written medical records, recently saw the patient in person. In addition, the physician should have a medical history available, inform the patient of the benefits and risks of the medication, perform a medical examination of the patient, and initiate follow-up care to check for side effects (AMA, 1999).

Peer Review and Approval. Write to the ethics and licensing boards of your local, state, and national professional association for peer review and approval of services to be rendered. Provide as much detail as possible in your descriptions of referral recruitment strategies; consent agreements for patients and their families; services delivered, including assessment protocols; medical records, including the procedures for storage and retrieval; and protocols for termination and case disposition. Ask for specific recommendations regarding how to properly identify your credentials and training in documentation related to communications with participants via specific modalities such as e-mail, Web sites, chat rooms, telephones, audio bridges, or interactive videoconferencing. Furthermore, clearly define the service you intend to deliver, such as assessment, diagnosis, medication consults, psychotherapy, or education. Even if the ethical boards respond by saying they cannot render a decision at this point in time, the documentation you will have obtained from the boards could be valuable in any subsequent lawsuit.

Obtain specific consultation from leaders in the telehealth community, and document details of such consultation, including dates, the topics you discussed, the suggestions the leaders made, and your rationale for your decisions regarding whether or not to follow the suggestions. If another professional requests a consultation from you, make a complete notation in the medical record (NCQA, 1999).

Patient Considerations

A number of risk management issues relate directly to the treatment of patients. Some key suggestions for limiting liability related to patients will be detailed in the following discussion.

Professionals are expected to guide patients with respect to safety and due precautions related to health care. Patients do not know what they do not know. It is therefore important to establish a working relationship with patients in the form of verbal and written agreements. These often take the form of consent agreements.

Consent Agreements. The consent agreement can be the single most important document for protecting an organization and provider in a malpractice suit from a patient. Many states require that professionals obtain a consent form and discuss it verbally as well as have it signed by the patient before the patient receives treatment. A patient consent agreement for treatment via telecommunication technology might include the following basic elements (check with your state licensing board and legal counsel for specific requirements):

- If a community's standard of care does not cover telecommunication technology, fully inform all clients (both verbally and in writing) of such practice as being "outside the professional standard of care, and in an area not yet validated by research."
- Describe how electronic service delivery differs from face-to-face service delivery.
- Discuss positive and negative consequences of engaging or not engaging in telehealth consultation. Detail the risks and benefits of working electronically.

- Discuss the limits of confidentiality. Be sure to mention that technology-based consultation may lead to breaches of confidentiality that may be difficult to remedy.

- Describe inherent deficiencies in the electronic equipment that can possibly interfere with diagnosis or treatment. Discuss issues related to equipment failure, describe how to resolve issues of jurisdiction, give a brief description of the equipment and the services to be delivered, and explain the purpose of remote contact.

- Describe the specific roles of any consultant or local referring practitioner. Explain who will have ultimate authority over patients' treatment, and state whether the information will be stored in a computerized database.

- Give the details of your licensure.

- Describe procedures for practitioner follow-up when patients do not appear for remote consultation.

- Provide patients with written lists of alternatives and behavioral suggestions in the case of equipment failure, accident, catastrophe, or natural disaster.

- State whether at any time e-mail will be forwarded to third parties for consultation.

- Inform patients of who will have access to their e-mail address, phone number, or any other contact information and who else might contact patients on your behalf.

- Document vacation arrangements, intended patient e-mail addresses, average response time, and topics not appropriate for discussion via technology.

- Make provisions for nonreceipt or delayed receipt of e-mail, problems with servers, or unannounced changes in the schedule of e-mail communications. Discuss how easily human error can lead to incorrectly delivered messages.

- Inform patients that cellular and cordless telephones are a confidentiality risk.

- Allow patients the opportunity to prohibit identifiable medical-related communication from appearing in any electronic medium. E-mail is particularly vulnerable because the Supreme Court has held that there is no reasonable expectation of privacy in e-mail.

- Give patients the choice to prohibit identifiable images or information derived from the telehealth interaction to be transmitted or used by researchers or other, unidentified entities (Schanz, 1999c).

Documentation. When working with the newer technologies, there is an increased need for documentation. Document the following: the identity of the patient in the medical record (using the name or an ID number), the participating family members, the treating professional, and the attending support staff, both medical and technical; the location of all health care providers; the date of the encounter; and the beginning and ending time of the encounter. Personal biographical information should also include the address, employer, home and work telephone numbers, and marital status of each patient. For patients fourteen years and older, you need to make appropriate notation concerning their use of nicotine, alcohol, and other substances (NCQA, 1999).

Basic Health Care Practice. Remember the basics of practice, regardless of the technology you are using. Ensure that the history and physical exam identify appropriate subjective and objective information pertinent to the patient's presenting complaints. Also ensure that any necessary laboratory and or other studies are ordered or obtained. When working with children, review the patient's immunization record (available through the medical record) (NCQA, 1999).

Release of Information. Follow appropriate procedures regarding the release of information before sharing patient information electronically. Arrange for proper scanning and sharing of release forms signed by patients so that local practitioners, remote consultants, and patients can have copies for their files. If you are treating a minor, it is often necessary to obtain appropriate written authorization from a parent or caregiver. Before undertaking actual treatment of a minor, you may need further evidence of the authenticity of the individual presenting himself or herself as the caregiver; this may be a situation requiring initial face-to-face contact before delivering service.

Videotaping. Securely store videotapes of procedures and consultations, and limit the number of copies. In addition, document every video recording in the medical record. It is important to note that audio- or videotapes can be used to prove innocence as well as guilt, and both parties may be entitled to complete, unedited copies if copies are kept (Brandt & Carpenter, 1999). When dealing with children, understand that videotaped and photographic records are more sensitive and can be highly controversial. For these reasons, some providers choose to keep only minimal electronic video and photographic records for children.

Security of Medical Records. Patients should have access to documented security measures for your institution, group, or practice. For patients seeking to protect their medical privacy, you might encourage them to obtain a copy of their medical records. You can also inform them that they can request a copy of their personal medical file from the Medical Information Bureau <www.mib.com>. Urge patients to read authorization forms before signing and to protest disclosures that they find inappropriate. Inform patients that they have a right to protest if their medical information is being shared without their explicit permission. Patients in many states also have the right to examine and correct their health records (California Healthline, 1999).

Patient Feedback. Seek active input from patients regarding policies and their implementation. This is particularly important when discussing the consent agreement, as described previously. Regularly collect patient satisfaction measures with regard to both technology and health care service.

Research. Obtain approval from a university human subjects committee before conducting research. Be sure to obtain proper release forms from all subjects. Debrief all patients who have participated in research, and document your debriefing.

Fees. Patients may not know what to expect when using technology for consultation. Potential patients ought to know in advance if they will be charged regular office fees or any extra fees for equipment rental. You may also need to mention hidden costs to patients, such as Internet access or long-distance telephone charges to teleconferencing services. Some states prohibit charging patients for the use of equipment or for transmission fees. Check with your state licensing board and other legislative bodies for specifics regarding these fee-setting and reimbursement issues.

Supervision. Inform patients if sessions are being supervised and if (and how) the supervisor is preserving session transcripts. Give patients the credentials of the supervisor.

Multilingual and Multicultural Competence. Working remotely places an extra duty of care on you as a professional. Determine whether patients are using English as a primary or secondary language. Depending on your practice specialty, you may need to determine your patients' level of language comprehension before you can deliver diagnosis or treatment. Obtain training in multicultural issues in general, and training in the cultural mores of the patient populations you will be treating. The professional relationship brings with it a duty to protect patients from harm, regardless of citizenship.

The absence of contextual cues and background information can also be a significant impairment. You must therefore use caution when recommending any specific course of action before gaining an understanding of the individual's full familial, sociopolitical, and cultural situation. Cultural norms and traditions unknown to you may render some treatments ineffective or perhaps even dangerous.

Staff Training and Documentation Considerations

You can be held accountable for the policies and procedures followed by your employees. It is therefore essential that staff be trained to use technology properly, that their skills be updated regularly, and that such training be documented. Although the following information is not exhaustive, it comprises some of the factors to consider when developing staff policy manuals.

Standards of Care. Be certain that staff members are informed of and following whatever standards of care might exist for using technology. Adhere to the basic standard of care for all services delivered to patients; in other words, use encryption for e-mail exchanges to protect confidentiality during transmission, learn about other possible causes of breaches of confidentiality and security, learn about storage and retrieval procedures for audio and video records, and understand and adhere to appropriate supervision protocols. Check professional associations for their statements regarding e-health and telehealth practice, research, or education.

Continuing Education. Provide staff training regarding the importance of patient confidentiality, backup procedures in the event of equipment failure, and security measures for medical record keeping. For example, consider devices that make use of **biometrics** to control access to records. These devices analyze fingerprints, voice patterns, or retinal patterns of blood vessels in the eye. Biometric measures are often combined with electronic signatures, identification codes, and passwords. Encourage staff to attend continuing education classes in e-health and telehealth, including legal and ethical practice workshops; be sure they document their attendance.

Confidentiality. Take measures to ensure that staff members are dealing with the person with whom they think they are dealing—using code words, passwords, or both. When working with minors, verify the identity of their parents, and develop procedures for contacting the parents in an emergency. Determine the level of security most appropriate when obtaining parental consent. For example, under the requirements of your state licensure, may you obtain valid permission from parents via e-mail, fax, or surface mail?

Separation of Duties. Develop staff procedures that involve a separation of duties. Assign checks and balances within a system to limit the impact of a single user. Give staff members the least amount of access to information needed for them to accomplish their duties. For example, use read-only access to data files so that files cannot be manipulated. Define documentation procedures clearly; in other words, include intake forms, releases, case notes, e-mail exchanges, and selected audio and video footage in the patient's medical records.

Organizational Considerations

If you are working for an organization, obtain and understand the statement of the organization's requirements regarding use and misuse of confidential information in computer systems. Pay particular attention to regulations regarding videotaping of patient sessions if you are using videoconferencing services. If possible, work for organizations offering immunity from suit. This immunity could take the form of a monetary cap on economic damages or include provisions that would protect against litigation based on claims of negligent use of technology (Office of Technology Assessment, 1995).

General Technological Considerations

As a first order of business, develop a solid project management system. Whether technical support staff are employees or outsourced from vendors, require that they provide information regarding the technology they use. Set the same requirement for clinical staff. Each form of technology presents its own considerations, and much risk management hinges on proper documentation of how each technology is used and by whom. We discuss some general points in this section, then look at the specifics of e-mail technologies in the next.

Use of Technology. Require that the technical staff document the following, along with all other related technical issues:

- Who uses which equipment
- Who owns each piece of equipment
- Schedules for equipment maintenance

- Who is responsible for equipment maintenance
- Format for transmitting medical information
- Arrangements for record storage
- Hours of technical staff availability
- Procedures for repairs
- Quality assurance mechanisms, such as the issue tracking system and resolution process
- User requirements
- Frequency and format of technical reports

Clinical staff can be required to document schedules of equipment use and purposes for accessing equipment.

Transmission Verification Procedures. Develop transmission verification procedures for both local and remote transmission sites. All entries in the medical record should contain the author's identification in the form of a handwritten signature, unique electronic signature, or initials (NCQA, 1999). In transmitting patient records, for example, you will need procedures for confirming the receipt of the data, checking for errors, and certifying that test scores or values are appropriate for rendering diagnoses. For each technology used—e-mail, chat rooms, electronic medical record transmissions, or videoconferencing—be aware of the opportunities for security leaks.

Security. Document and regularly update all security measures. These measures ought to include file addition and deletion security, electronic audit trails, and immediate deactivation of passwords for departed personnel.

Invest in well-designed systems that offer the greatest security with respect to cost and to prevention and deterrence of privacy abuses. As we have mentioned elsewhere, security measures that go beyond needed levels can be unduly expensive, delay the access of information, and make access inconvenient. Computers can be built and programmed from the

E-Health, Telehealth, and Telemedicine

beginning to offer greater security, only disclosing necessary information to authorized users.

Specific E-Mail Considerations

Because e-mail is the lowest common denominator, aside from the telephone, for most users of technology, e-mail procedures and precautions have been more widely developed than for other, more advanced forms of technology. Therefore, this section contains suggestions derived from lessons learned by professionals using e-mail and from several professional associations that have documented guidelines for the use of e-mail by providers.

Policies. Discuss policies and limits for contact when offline. Explain exactly how often e-mail messages will be checked. Establish a turnaround time for messages, given a realistic estimate of your availability. Explain to patients how to deal with time delays related to the sending and receiving of e-mail messages. Establish policies regarding preferences for labeling mail. Instruct patients to put the category of the transaction in the subject line of the message, to facilitate filtering: for example, "processing," "appointment," "referral," or "billing question."

Patients may also benefit from advance knowledge of any limitations you will be placing on e-mail or chat room communications. This knowledge will help them set reasonable expectations regarding e-mail exchanges. For example, you could inform patients that if e-mail exchanges become cumbersome for them or for you, telephone, video, or face-to-face meetings might be required. Specify the limits of e-mail or chat room interventions with each patient, basing those limits on the type of relationship with that patient. Establish acceptable types of transactions for e-mail messages, such as appointment scheduling; inform patients of whether or not medication overdoses, suicide threats, homicide threats, domestic violence, rape, HIV, or other sensitive subjects will be discussed in e-mail. Instruct them to avoid anger, sarcasm, harsh criticism, and derogatory references to third parties in e-mail or chat messages.

Explain the possibility of technology failures, and inform patients of what to do when an e-mail message is lost in cyberspace, when they haven't received a response in the expected time frame, or when they are in crisis and the technology malfunctions. Include all such information in the patient consent agreement.

If responding to e-mail received from a Web site, be sure to include a disclaimer stating that the response is not intended to establish a professional relationship with the sender. Be aware that even if you make such a disclaimer, it is possible that responding to specific questions with advice in private e-mail may be interpreted as having formed a practitioner-patient relationship. As the practitioner in such a case, you may be held liable for poor or incomplete advice.

Emotional Reactions. Inform patients that e-mail interactions can generate unexpected emotional reactions. Given the overall lack of training, supervision, and experience provided for practitioners in using text-based media for treatment, it is reasonable to assume that strong emotional reactions may require added time and energy to clarify, especially with highly medicated, elderly, mentally ill, or gravely distressed patients. Encourage patients to set up a telephone, videoconference, or face-to-face appointment to discuss emotionally charged or critical issues.

Alternative Resources. If consulting only in e-mail, provide hypertext links or Web addresses or telephone numbers of emergency telephone services, and give patients contact numbers for appropriate certification bodies and licensing boards to facilitate consumer protection.

Record Keeping. Encourage patients who wish to maintain records of e-mail or chat sessions to do so in a confidential manner. Explain that e-mail is easy for family members, visiting friends, and employers to find. If you give any specific advice in an e-mail or chat room, make a hard copy of the exchange and keep it in a paper file for future reference if needed.

Limits of Confidentiality. Inform patients of the limits of confidentiality when using electronic communication tools. In cases where limits of confidentiality are unknown, disclosure of such ambiguity is appropriate. Inform patients about which parts of messages are to be included in the medical record; also inform them that staff members may process messages if this is true. Establish policies before discussing personal information with patients in e-mail. Be aware that e-mail programs operate in numerous ways; for example, depending on the manufacturer, the "reply" function may or may not include the original message. Consider if including original messages from either the patient or the practitioner is appropriate, how much is beneficial, and how much of this will not violate the patient's confidentiality if intercepted by a child, spouse, friend, or roommate. Discuss whether it would be appropriate to send a confirmation of receipt of e-mail before responding more fully.

E-Mail Security. Always use the highest possible level of security, such as encryption and electronic signatures, when discussing patient issues with colleagues or with patients directly. Do not send group mailings in which patients' names can be visible to other recipients. Be cautious about using "blind mailing" features in e-mail. Specialized settings can allow some readers to see an entire list of names supposedly "blind copied" to a group of recipients. If using e-mail accounts for patient contact, document each one, and limit access to your e-mail account by other individuals. Take precautions against unauthorized access to files by computer repair staff, clerical assistants, or others who may ordinarily have access.

Vendor Considerations

Regardless of the requirements for vendor accountability imposed by the HIPAA, working with a reputable and reliable vendor is important to avoid potential problems and diminish risks. Determine whether the vendor has product liability insurance to cover suits from disgruntled patients seeking recourse for faulty hardware, software, or support services. You should be indemnified in the event of a breach of obligation.

With particular respect to the HIPAA, the vendor must at minimum agree to keep all patient information in strict confidence and to use it only for the purposes mutually agreed on. Sensitive information should be disclosed only to vendor employees who have signed confidentiality agreements. For further information regarding full HIPAA requirements, see the Resources at the back of this book for updated HIPAA regulation sites.

In addition to meeting HIPAA requirements, the vendor should have disaster recovery protocols and instructions for accessing emergency information during scheduled and unscheduled downtimes. The American Medical Association's Web site <www.ama-assn.org> provides a list of considerations for establishing e-commerce relationships. More information about vendor considerations is given in Chapter Three and in Appendix B. To adequately protect yourself and your organization from risks associated with working with vendors, please refer to these sections as well.

CONCLUSION

Malpractice and risk management policies in telehealth and e-health are just beginning to take shape. Nonetheless, core elements of existing treatment and practice standards are not likely to change. Refinement of these standards will necessarily extend their application to the use of telehealth and e-health. These processes are under way and are already shedding light on the new practice arenas being developed. Chapter Ten details how you and your organization can get started by writing and following through on a business plan.

CHAPTER 10

A Beginner's Blueprint: How to Get Started

The administrators of a large mental health facility decided that they wanted to deliver telepsychiatry. The Department of Defense offered hundreds of thousands of dollars in funding, so the facility hired an executive director to simultaneously secure this funding and start a telemedicine program. Many months passed, much money was spent, and a change in directors occurred before the funding was eventually obtained. After three years, the facility conducted only a handful of telemedicine consultations. What went wrong?

There had been no planning. Rather than applying a rigorous and methodical plan to the creation of a telehealth program, the facility tried to start in the middle. Unfortunately, this mistake is all too common.

A reasonable summary of advice from developers of technology-based services would be this: plan, plan, and then plan some more. One of the most common mistakes people make in developing remote health care services is underestimating the number of issues needing attention. Health care has always been a complex industry, and the effort to begin delivering services through technology is forcing a reassessment of existing strategies. This reassessment is leading to much innovation directed toward the elimination of duplicated effort and the streamlining of services. The introduction of automation and telecommunication technologies will ultimately improve health care, but for now there are significant challenges in the design

215

and implementation of profit-making programs. Depending on the nature and complexity of a project, we recommend allowing six to twelve months for planning and implementation.

Nearly every guide to program development stresses the importance of creating a business plan. Because each business plan requires a specific and individual focus, this chapter serves only as a general outline, a blueprint describing the most important issues in launching a telehealth program or creating an e-health business. Each business will need to modify this outline to fit its requirements. Please also note that although these components are presented in linear order, you will need to address many of these topics simultaneously when actually developing a service.

Table 10.1 summarizes the basic steps needed to develop a business plan. This chapter discusses these general steps, and we invite you to modify them to fit your setting, be it a telehealth project or an e-health company.

Table 10.1. The Business Plan

Step	Activity
1. Understand the overall organizational mission and goals	Make sure the service is in line with the overall values and strategies of the organization
2. Identify needs and the specific services to be delivered	Conduct a needs assessment to determine which services are in demand
3. Identify the target audience	Identify an audience that needs (and will pay for) the service
4. Identify the resources you need	Delineate everything required, including personnel, equipment, transmission channels, and consultation

5. Design an effective organizational structure	Situate the program within the organization. Staff it appropriately to maximize flexibility
6. Identify accountability	Clearly delineate lines of responsibility as soon as possible
7. Forecast costs and identify funding sources	Develop a budget detailing start-up and operating costs, a break-even analysis, a profit-and-loss statement, and cash flow projections or detailing capital and angel financing
8. Establish clear and measurable goals	Set benchmarks and goals that can be measured quantitatively
9. Create project timeline	Set specific target dates for meeting the objectives and goals
10. Develop feedback mechanisms	Create systems to provide information regarding successes and failures of the business plan
11. Evaluate the program annually	Formally measure successes and failures; use this data to improve the program

1. UNDERSTAND THE OVERALL ORGANIZATIONAL MISSION AND GOALS

It is vital that the service(s) you develop are in line with the overall values and goals of your organization. For example, if an organization is strategically placing itself to provide more health-related services for chronically ill patients, it would make sense to launch home-based telehealth services. In short, unless your organization exists solely to provide telemedicine or e-health services, these services must exist within an extant organization. Although some businesses may be developed solely to deliver a particular service, most operate within the framework of an overarching organization or parent business. Keeping those parameters at the forefront of planning is essential to avoid costly fundamental errors.

2. IDENTIFY NEEDS AND THE SPECIFIC SERVICES TO BE DELIVERED

Each project or business should clearly identify the existing demand for the product or service in question. Conduct a market assessment to determine community needs and likely services to meet those needs. Service developers all too often focus on obtaining equipment or technology. Because consumers compose the most critical half of the business interaction, it is essential to keep their preferences and spending patterns in mind.

The ultimate effectiveness of health care services can be determined only by a thorough needs analysis that considers consumer and professional preferences as well as technical options. For example, practitioners seem to prefer high-bandwidth technologies, but patients consistently report satisfaction with lower-bandwidth technologies if they can be spared the trouble of traveling to obtain health care.

Lessons Learned from Telehealth and Telemedicine Pilot Projects

Given the number of telemedicine and telehealth pilot projects developed internationally in the past decade, you will probably find it helpful when undergoing your needs assessment to interview developers of such projects and to conduct a thorough review of the literature in your specific health care area.

Another crucial aspect of needs assessment is the early identification of revenue sources. Keep focused on the most promising of these revenue sources during the start-up phase, and allocate those resources wisely. Dazzled by technological possibilities, health care service providers may misallocate limited funding if they have failed to properly assess basic patient needs. For example, although high-bandwidth technologies are preferred by professionals, access to them is often limited by budgetary constraints. When a program is facing such constraints, a thorough analysis of patient needs may uncover that less sophisticated and less expensive technologies may be equally effective. More specifically, for applications that have not demonstrated increased efficacy with a video link, it might be wiser to first evaluate the relative value of video and audio links to determine whether video links are a significant improvement over telephone connections (Squibb, 1999).

A good example of the lengths to which thoughtful program developers will go to conduct needs assessments is found in the work of B. Hudnall Stamm, who is employed at the Institute of Rural Health Studies at Idaho State University. Dr. Stamm works closely with rural communities to plan health care services, at times even flying to the area via bush plane. She draws from a variety of information sources, including Western medicine and technology, and the community's history, stories, material culture, and traditional medicine. She works with community members across the life span, including leaders and elders, to understand the community and their health care goals (for example, to provide better access to a particular specialty, to provide health care without transporting people away from their families, to enable more expedient access to care, or to allow more local or tribal control in decision making).

These communities use Stamm's knowledge to help them examine how, or even if, technology might be used to meet their goals. Incorporating a community's specific culture can be very difficult in communities where previous infusions of Western culture and technology have caused cultural trauma. Developing services or purchasing equipment without respecting the primacy of the community's authority can be a form of colonialism. Aside from issues of cultural fit, there may be such challenges as limited bandwidth and high cost of access from remote areas; overcoming the digital divide requires flexibility and ingenuity. In an extreme case, specialists in an urban hospital may be accessed by having a runner take data back and forth from a rural community to an intermediate town with an Internet connection. Going forward on a project without humility and a clear assessment of the recipient community's culture, goals, and resources is a recipe for program and cultural disaster (B. H. Stamm, personal communication, April 24, 2000; see also Stamm, 1998, 2000; Stamm & Friedman, 2000; Stamm & Perednia, 2000).

Literature reviews may uncover findings that are relevant to patients, their communities, providers, and the overall project or business. The care network clinical needs assessment team of the Hôpital Sainte-Justine in Montreal (Poitras, 1999) conducted a literature review and concluded that the network needed a vast territory with a high rate of medical needs and a low number of subspecialists; specifically, it needed a desire on the part of local professionals to work with specialists, clearly outlined procedures, clear lines of responsibility, and reliable and easily upgraded equipment.

As reviewed in Chapter One, federally funded telehealth projects tested many ideas and found many dead ends. One large program in the southeastern part of the United States opened a multipurpose telehealth program that promised to do everything for everyone. The program managers soon realized they lacked the specialists to deliver the services they promised. This oversight led to an overexpenditure of funds to quickly identify and train clinicians to provide a wide range of services. Yet 75 percent of the trained physicians were never called on to provide care because there was no demand for their services, and consequently the business lost thousands of dollars. The program managers also lost credibility with the medical staff by preparing them to provide services that were never used.

Challenges in Starting a Telehealth Program

We conducted interviews with several telehealth company executives to get a firsthand look at telehealth start-up processes. We felt it was important to provide input throughout this chapter from people who have launched telehealth programs. The comments in this first section are a distillation of responses to questions related to the greatest challenges faced by telehealth start-ups.

Robert Cox, M.D., Hays Medical Center, Kansas

- Communicating needs of recipients of telemedicine services to the providing institution.
- Obtaining physician buy-in.
- Obtaining administrative buy-in (personal communication, November 16, 1999).

Michelle Gailiun, Director of Telemedicine, Ohio State University

- Figuring out who is going to pay for everything.
- Figuring out who your clinical and administrative champions are and how to use them.
- Figuring out how to change human behavior in general. This perception usually presents itself in inverse proportion to the amount of change you are actually needing (personal communication, September 28, 1999).

Warren B. Karp, Ph.D., D.M.D., Coordinator of Telemedicine and Distance Learning Activities, Department of Pediatrics, Medical College of Georgia

- Figuring how to set the appropriate level of expectations for the technology in the mind of the users. If you set expectations too high, users may be disappointed. If you set expectations too low, users might not thoroughly explore the capabilities of the technology.
- Training all the necessary people (providers, families, clients) in using the technology. One important part of training is using the technology in the actual application environment.
- Facilitating the understanding of the value brought by technology. Some services provided by telehealth may be reimbursable by contracts. In most states, telehealth is not reimbursable by third-party payers or Medicaid insurance. You can say your program is

cost-effective when you are able to provide a contracted service in a more cost- and time-effective manner or when more patients or clients are referred to you because of your ability to use tele-health (personal communication, November 15, 1999).

Steven W. Strode, M.D., University of Arkansas for Medical Sciences
- Securing the needed funds.
- Reducing the initial suspicion of the physicians in remote sites.
- Dealing with hostility from our local newspaper (personal communication, November 12, 1999).

Rosa Ana Tang, M.D., M.P.H., Professor of Ophthalmology, University of Texas Medical Branch, Galveston
- Finding committed and qualified personnel.
- Finding commitment from superiors.
- Finding resources to enable upgrading (personal communication, November 11, 1999).

Peter Yellowlees, M.D., Department of Psychiatry, Royal Brisbane Hospital, Australia
- Convincing one's own colleagues to use telemedicine systems.
- Finding the time to devote to program development while juggling other work priorities.
- Finding good people to work with you and, in particular, people who can support clinicians, train them, and develop the appropriate policy background, as well as perform evaluation studies (personal communication, February 10, 1999).

To aid in "determining the nature and extent of the problems that a program is designed to address" (Siden, 1998), developers should meet with focus groups. These small discussion sessions are designed to obtain in-depth information from individuals who are knowledgeable in specific areas. Participants are selected not at random but through nonprobabilistic sampling in order to find subjects who are most likely to represent the group or experience being studied (Krueger, 1988; Siden, 1998).

So as best to serve the needs of the community, the strategic planning process should involve four main focus groups, as follows:

1. *Health care institutions.* They will be directly affected by technology-based services because of the increased information sharing (that is, sharing of medical records) and service distribution between the institutions.

2. *Key individuals within the health care provider organization.* They are needed to identify the organization's goals and to evaluate the existing level of technological and human support.

3. *Key individuals in each community.* Community leaders can identify common needs and the potential for shared resources, including funding, facilities, equipment, personnel, and so on (California Tele-health/Telemedicine Coordination Project, 1997).

4. *Strategic partners.* When developing an e-health company, early alignment with other companies or enterprises with compatible services is recommended. Partnering with other companies can help address shared needs.

Selecting Strategic Partners

John Bringenberg, President, <Lifescape.com>

- With strategic partners, the most important thing is a commonality of mission and culture. Of course capital, market positioning, competitive edge, and market penetration are also important. But having a strategic partner who is culturally compatible will be a great asset in reaching your goals. In the case where your relationship with a strategic partner is more an alliance or a cooperative extension of your business, you need to find a win-win scenario in which the alliance helps both parties (personal communication, May 30, 2000).

Richard Flanagan, CEO, <Epotec.com>

- When working with strategic partners, you must have incredibly clear agreements, because everyone assumes you are thinking the same way, and there are so many ways to be thinking differently. You can't assume they know what you are talking about (personal communication, May 30, 2000).

Mitchell H. Gold, M.D., CEO, <Elixis.com>

- Two goals of partnerships ought to be to achieve rapid distribution and have long-term revenue opportunities that might include technology improvements and enhancements.
- Partnerships give you credibility, but each partnership uses resources, so you want to maximize them.
- Leverage partners to project and manage your growth. The challenge lies in aggressively driving growth yet maintaining the standardization that needs to occur (personal communication, May 30, 2000).

G. Ed Kriese, CEO and Founder, <Medicalrecord.com>

- Pick strategic partners that have a solid, traditional, bricks-and-mortar business model and add an e-health component, making it a "bricks and clicks" model. Make sure they are large enough and have a good management team. Look for people who have had some experience in business development with Web companies (personal communication, May 30, 2000).

Michael Weiss, CEO, <CancerEducation.com>

- It is important to be persistent with potential partners. Expect a minimum lead of six months to have substantial conversations and a year lead time to ink a deal (personal communication, May 30, 2000).

Carl Tsukahara, Vice President for Marketing and Alliances, <Confer.com>

- Acquire leverage for yourself—look hard to build proper alliances to fan out and scale at a rapid pace. Partners can help growth enormously, but more is not better. Sometimes fewer is better. The worst thing is having lots of partners who produce nothing; they can use up lots of time and energy. Young companies are always starving for resources. Invest in the partners that are important (personal communication, May 30, 2000).

Sources of Further Information

Most state governments have a department of community health or an office of rural health (or both) that can aid in conducting research on the existing health care market. (Please note that some related state offices do not go by this name.) These departments often keep statistics on areas in the state that may have a shortage of providers, or they track physicians (and often nurses and allied health providers) through censuses on a county-by-county basis. In addition, state medical schools may track rural health shortage areas as part of their mandate to provide care to all citizens.

Other good resources are the National Rural Health Association <www.nrharural.org/> and the federal Office of Rural Health Policy <www.nal.usda.gov/orhp/>, which maintain a list of state offices of rural health and a list of medically underserved populations. The Office for the Advancement of Telehealth can also be a valuable resource.

Larger medical institutions often apply a "mutual fund" approach to the creation of a telehealth program. They attempt to minimize their risk (or maximize their investment) by using a single network for several types of services. To find information related to these types of services, inquire at local city hospitals. Almost all large hospitals today, and certainly most integrated delivery networks, have a central resource to help outside clinicians navigate through and refer into their system. Access points usually consist of a Web site and an individual assigned to these duties within the hospital system.

3. IDENTIFY THE TARGET AUDIENCE

After identifying a specific need to be served, businesses must next identify the audience they will serve. This can be accomplished in two ways: by payer population or geographically. Looking at the payer population re-quires targeting a group that is either within a single paying network (as was done by Ohio State University's prison telehealth program) or that provides a single point of service for patients with various benefit plans (as was done by Appal-Link in Virginia). While directing the telehealth program at the University of Kansas, Pamela Whitten commonly applied the latter approach by seeking formal contracts with providers in the state. One example was a fee-for-service contract for adult and child psychia-trists with the Crawford County Mental Health Center. Another example was a capitated contract with Hays Medical Center for rheumatology serv-ices. By negotiating specific contractual arrangements, the University of Kansas successfully identified clients who needed, and could pay for, its services. All too often, telehealth programs fail because they establish themselves without ensuring a client body.

With respect to identifying underserved populations by geographical area, a new business should analyze the target area geographically. The di-mensions of the geographical area must be matched to the individual business, depending on the service it intends to provide. For example, if the goal is to bring care to children in elementary schools, the target area could be the eastern part of a state (as was done by Eastern Carolina Uni-versity) or a neighborhood in the inner city (as was done by the University of Kansas).

Because e-health companies that work over the Internet serve a world-wide audience, geography becomes secondary to language. For example, an English-language Web site can serve many different geographic locations around the world.

Retaining Consumers

Retaining e-health consumers poses a number of new challenges. This sec-tion will outline some of these challenges and some possible solutions.

For years, patients' health care information and options have been limited to local providers, books and magazines, and television—all of which operate on their own timetable or are located away from home.

With the emergence of e-health, patients now have many options and an enormous amount of information that can be accessed easily and instantly. These patients, or "cyberchondriacs" (Goldstein, 2000), are often busy and well educated. They are taking their health care into their own hands (Haugh, 1999). The e-health sites that can locate, attract, and maintain a consumer mass will survive—all others will fade away. What follows are some important tips to help your business keep pace in this highly competitive market.

Advertising. There are millions of products and services available over the Internet. Consumers must be able to find your site or know about your service in order to take advantage of it. It has been estimated that only 13 percent of the consumers interested in buying online health care know what sites to visit and therefore do not use the Internet to the extent they might (Bard, 2000). This shows that potential consumers need strong advertising campaigns to direct them to a site; for lack of guidance, many will simply revert to familiar methods of purchasing services. Traditional e-commerce methods, such as commercials or banners, are ideal but often too expensive for smaller companies. Some start-up companies offer an incentive to physicians in exchange for referrals to their service.

To maximize the effectiveness of advertisements, it is important to direct them to the target audience. Many start-ups buy personal information to accomplish this. Companies can track individuals' buying patterns, personal information, preferences, interests, and so on by gathering bits of information found on the Web. They then sell this information to other companies, which use it to target consumers for advertising. As discussed in Chapter Seven, there is controversy over the methods used to acquire this information, and some laws are being formulated to regulate this practice.

Brand Name Image. Branding, or developing a brand name image, establishes the general identity of a product or company. Companies can use audio or visual cues that associate their brand with quality and value superior to that of the competition. A recognizable image or song promises to attract browsers and establish customer loyalty. Eye-catching colors, ear-tingling jingles, cute animals, and so on are all techniques used to implant a memory into consumers' heads to help them remember a product or service. Every communication with the potential consumer, be it image, text, or sound, should produce only sentiments that the company wishes to engender. (For example, a company would be unwise to develop a logo that resembles a Nazi symbol.) The goal of advertising is to strengthen a company's image and promote instant recognition of its product(s).

Virtual Communities. Consumers who frequently visit a Web site are more likely to purchase the products or services offered. Building a virtual community can create an incentive for the consumer to repeatedly return. These communities can be developed along three lines: geographical location, demographic characteristics, or topical issues.

Geographical communities can provide information about specific issues and events affecting the location in which all the members reside. Demographic communities focus on groups of people who share a characteristic—age, gender, ethnic origin, life circumstance, or any other characteristic that makes a person feel like part of a group. Topical communities focus on a common interest or issue. For example, weightlifters may visit a site to pick up the latest tips; people who enjoy simulation games come together to play. The majority of communities are topically based.

At any type of virtual community site, your company can develop discussion boards, offer site registration and membership (with incentives for joining), make articles available, or present testimonials—all of which entice the consumer to return. Continually updating and revising the content on the site will pull the consumer in to find out the latest information (Hagel & Armstrong, 1997).

Consumer Trust and Loyalty. Building and maintaining consumers' trust promotes return customers. A conspicuously displayed list of members of a medical advisory board informs the consumer on product and service reliability. Visibly displaying your privacy policies regarding the handling of personal information can assuage the reluctance of many consumers to use online services (Reents, 1999b).

Patients often feel loyal to their personal physician. Developing a personalized and sensitive site that simulates the role of the trusted provider is another way to strengthen customer loyalty. Customers who feel a link or kinship with a site are more likely to use it.

4. IDENTIFY THE RESOURCES YOU NEED

Given that delivering traditional health services is a complex endeavor, it is easy to underestimate just how many resources are required to deliver remote consultation. These resources include personnel, equipment, telecommunication options, and consultation services. The next sections look at these and other resources.

Personnel

Think carefully about the expertise needed to start *and* maintain a telecommunications health care service. Because e-health companies are an outgrowth of telemedicine and telehealth, it is only reasonable to assume that e-health companies will generally require many of the same personnel positions as telehealth programs. Common examples from the business world include such positions as the chief executive officer (CEO) and the chief operations officer (COO). At a minimum, your company or program will require the following positions and skills (where different roles exist for personnel in e-health companies versus telehealth or telemedicine programs, the job titles for telehealth programs are in italics):

• Founder, *visionary director*. This is a person with vision, thick skin, good business instincts, and an entrepreneurial spirit to launch and lead a program. In a study examining active telepsychiatry programs (Whitten, Zaylor, & Kingsley, 1999), the researchers found that the individuals leading a telehealth program and their personal style were among the biggest predictors of success.

• Chief executive officer (CEO). This individual is responsible to the board of directors for the overall functioning of the company, revenue, staffing, products, and services. In start-up companies, the CEO is often responsible for developing a business plan and obtaining one or more rounds of funding based on that business plan, as well as developing the company for an initial public offering (IPO), whereby stock is made available to consumers on the open stock market. Overseeing major corporate collaborations and strategic alliances also falls within the function of the CEO.

• Chief operations officer (COO). This employee attends to the overall business functioning of the organization and performs organizational tasks for the CEO.

• Chief medical officer (CMO), *medical director.* This employee sets the professional tone in accordance with professional guidelines for patient services, medical record keeping, professional training, and other record keeping.

• Chief technical officer (CTO), *technical expert.* This individual must be well versed in telecommunications and networking. Telehealth is a broad area with an ever-increasing range of telephony and other technical options. Hiring a CTO with both hardware and software skills is desirable. Often one expert in each area will be necessary, but for dot-com companies with lean start-up budgets, finding one person who can fulfill both needs is a wise investment of early funding dollars. It is a mistake to assume that the telecommunications company and equipment vendor can fulfill this need.

• Security director. Given the increasing need to be compliant with various pieces of legislation related to the security, privacy, confidentiality, and data integrity of health care information, it is wise to have a management team member who is devoted specifically to keeping abreast of these issues and forming policies.

• Marketing director. This individual must be well aware of the research on the target audience, the services to be delivered, and the overall direction of the company. Moreover, because branding is essential for e-health companies, this employee ought to have expertise in branding for dot-com companies.

• Program director. Someone must oversee scheduling, the recruiting of clinical providers, event planning, and so on, to ensure that the company delivers services correctly and in a timely manner.

• Business manager. This individual is typically responsible for managing the company's day-to-day business functions, such as tracking revenue and expenses, ensuring timely billing and collections for provider services, supervising staff, and so on. Someone with organizational and motivational skills would optimally handle these tasks.

• Training director. Nearly every employee will require some type of training. Clinicians will need to be taught how to perform a consult and possibly how to operate equipment. Marketing personnel must understand overall business operations and strategies to help identify potential markets. The entire staff will need to be cross-trained in how to run equipment, in the capabilities and limitations of the equipment, or in how to schedule a consult. Training requirements vary with each company. A dedicated training director can also help orient new employees and direct work flow to them, thereby harnessing the enthusiasm of new employees and shortening the time period (usually several weeks) typically required for new employees to learn the ropes and become maximally productive.

• Ergonomics director. Offices and treatment rooms require proper lighting and acoustics, and furniture and equipment need to be designed for the comfort of patients and providers. An ergonomics director selects or designs rooms with an optimal location and size, accessibility to phone and power systems, accessibility for patients or for provider flow (or both), and proper lighting and acoustics. Although smaller health care services typically cannot afford a full-time salary for such a person, it is worth considering hiring a professional who is knowledgeable in both this area and another key specialty.

• Clinical personnel. Licensed and reputable physicians, nurses, therapists, psychologists, and so on, are crucial for attracting potential clients and delivering responsible service.

• Consultants. Start-ups need assistance in many areas, including raising funds, leveraging assets, forming partnerships, negotiating, contracting, making management decisions, and managing day-to-day operations. You may choose to have an official advisory board or to employ specialized consultants. Advisory board members to e-health companies are typically paid a salary in the form of cash or equity for their time and expertise.

Lessons Learned from E-Health Start-Ups

Thousands of e-health start-up companies in 1999 and 2000 had similar learning experiences as they improved on telemedicine and telehealth approaches and tried to incorporate successful revenue models. A lesson that has become most evident during these years of experimentation is that a new business must start with a clearly articulated revenue model and be able to shift rapidly as the market demands different services. Microsoft was not built in a day. Another lesson learned by many companies is that to avoid unnecessary expenses, e-health businesses ought to hire Web-savvy officers and start with services that are clearly in demand. If a company can remain financially steadfast long enough, it may indulge in its temptation to expand into new areas. Once it has established a clear revenue source, a hospital system or e-health company is ready to expand.

One way to expedite growth is to find other companies who can serve as strategic partners to offer complementary and not competing services. These partners ought to be equally well established in their own areas of specialty. If they are start-up services or companies, the agreement you develop with them ought to be such that the potential demise of the start-up will not substantially detract from your program's revenue stream.

Challenges in Starting an E-Health Company

We conducted interviews with several e-health company executives to get a firsthand look at e-health start-up processes. These comments are a distillation of responses to questions related to the greatest challenges faced by e-health start-ups.

John Bringenberg, President, <Lifescape.com>

- Market timing. Lifescape took several years from concept to operations because, as a health niche service, we felt it made sense to build and launch in 1998–1999, when several high-profile health Web businesses hit the market.
- Maintaining focus. Focus is critical. Let's face it, the Web is so vast, and entrepreneurs are so inventive. It is easy to want to do many related things. Keeping focused on building a core service and doing it better than anyone else is a critical success factor (personal communication, May 30, 2000).

Richard Flanagan, CEO, <Epotec.com>

- You need to know what people want, what's functional. It is essential to have riveted focus not only on what you are doing but also on the landscape, which changes so rapidly that it is breathtaking.
- Producing high-quality scalable products (that is, used efficiently by thousands and thousands of people) in a very short time frame is a significant challenge. Windows for production are very short. Technology is constantly changing and improving (personal communication, May 30, 2000).

Mitchell H. Gold, M.D., CEO, <Elixis.com>

- Refining and focusing the vision and seeing what the marketplace will accept.
- Creating the buzz behind the company, creating brand recognition, defining what your company stands for and leveraging mainstream media (newspapers and TV) and industry, and then leveraging that

recognition for further funding for second- and third-round funding for an IPO (personal communication, May 30, 2000).

Ann Garnier, Senior Vice President, <Healinx.com>

- One of the biggest challenges to start-ups is getting the physicians to adopt technology. That means you must educate physicians through trade shows, lectures, and advertising, and by developing relationships with organizations, medical associations, hospitals, or physician groups (personal communication, March 13, 2000).

Vince Kuraitis, principal, <bhtinfo.com>

- Struggling with competing themes in business plans when seeking investors.
- Lack of clarity regarding successful applications of new technology.
- Unpredictability in cash flow (personal communication, May 30, 2000).

Carl Tsukahara, Vice President for Marketing and Alliances, <Confer.com>

- Customers have a difficult time telling all the e-health companies apart—a company has to have a fairly concise positioning for itself. A company can have a compelling solution, but it makes the mistake of trying to apply it to all the world's evil. Many companies make the mistake of "trying to boil the ocean." You need to clearly articulate the service.
- Choose your investors wisely. Money is not just money. There is sometimes the danger that you start believing your own story too much; trusted adviser-investors can help give you a better perspective (personal communication, May 30, 2000).

Greg Tullman, CEO, <Allscripts.com>

- Competitors. One of the biggest challenges we must face is that competitors lie better than we tell the truth. Competitors lie about the capabilities of their products. The solution is to build strong reference sites and have customers talk with customers as opposed to accepting the Internet hype. We provide real product, but we also have to be selling a vision of the future. You need to strategically position your company against competitors; some of that is what you do, some is what you will do.

- Execution. Just after we arrived at the company, a very substantial competitor announced that it would be entering our market space with a directly competitive product. We were a million; it was a billion. Our answer was, "Well, we're here, and we don't have any choice, so we'll still go out and execute." The lesson was that we executed, and the other company did not. We are now the industry leader (personal communication, May 22, 2000).

Equipment

The cost of equipment varies depending on the technology needed and the network configuration. Technology has evolved rapidly and decreased in price in the past few years. Space considerations make it impossible to discuss each individual piece of equipment; see Chapter Three for a detailed discussion of interactive videoconferencing equipment. For regularly updated information, refer to the *Telemedicine Today Annual Buyer's Guide and Directory*, which provides a comprehensive listing of equipment, specifications, prices, and services.

Equipment Considerations for Telehealth Programs

Warren B. Karp, Ph.D., D.M.D.,
Coordinator of Telemedicine and Distance Learning Activities,
Department of Pediatrics, Medical College of Georgia

- We have found that even the simplest technology requires a support system for users.

- Even "plug-and-play" equipment does not address the need to integrate the technology into an existing health care system, where factors related to human behavior, billing, and scheduling can inhibit the efficient use of technology.
- If you buy equipment without providing a specific framework for using it, your project will fail.
- The framework that you provide must allow users, not technologists or administrators, to be the enablers.
- You should perform a needs assessment prior to purchasing any equipment. Seek input from users during the process of deciding which technologies will be appropriate. There is nothing worse than one person making decisions about technology to be used by another person (personal communication, November 15, 1999).

Transmission Channels

Traditionally analysts have looked at telehealth services in relation to the level of interactivity inherent in the service. Previously, this had often been constrained by the available bandwidth. Regardless of the modality (traditional interactive videoconferencing, Internet, and so on), the quality of the telehealth event is determined by the quality of the chosen telecommunications option. See Chapter Three for information to help you make an informed choice about such transmission channels.

Consultation Services

Organizations with technical and applications expertise in-house may find outside input unnecessary. However, as mentioned previously, many organizations will need a consultant to develop links among the technology, administration, and specific medical disciplines. Consultants are available to provide a wide range of services: creating a business plan, conducting a needs assessment, recommending technical solutions, providing training, doing ongoing audits and evaluation, and more (Allen, 1995b). Good consultants can help telehealth projects and e-health companies run smoothly and help save money by bringing their experience from past projects. Buyers beware, however: a business that hires an inexperienced consultant will be paying for his or her on-the-job training.

Miscellaneous Requirements

The need for other resources varies, depending on the goals and nature of each telehealth program. For example, if a program covers a large geographical area, it will need appropriate resources to travel throughout this area. Telehealth technologies do not eliminate the need for travel; it is often necessary for project directors or company principals to meet in person at least initially to establish a business relationship. Furthermore, when creating a telehealth system, it is often wise to invest early in many services that will be needed. For example, because teleradiology is important for acute care triage, critical care support, and follow-up care in many programs, early implementation of a teleradiology system makes sense. Early implementation will also help alleviate scheduling problems.

5. DESIGN AN EFFECTIVE ORGANIZATIONAL STRUCTURE

A study conducted in the mid-1990s (Whitten & Allen, 1995) documented the importance of setting up telehealth programs within an effective organizational structure. Established organizations must determine where new technology-based services will optimally fit into their existing structures. Some telehealth programs have created freestanding telehealth centers, which operate autonomously within the health system (for example, the Medical College of Georgia); other programs create departments that operate within a division (for example, the University of Kansas Medical Center's program, which is housed with the Information Technology Division); still others simply situate the program within the clinical department (for example, the University of Brisbane in Australia operates its telepsychiatry program out of the psychiatry department). Visibility, flexibility, and support from key administrators are factors that require consideration when making these decisions.

It is also important to develop an effective structure within your telehealth program. As discussed in the section on resources, make sure you have the appropriate personnel and that the division of labor and the hierarchy are clearly established. Structure your program to maintain flexibility. In telehealth, you must be able to turn on a dime. With small staff sizes, everyone must be able to cover for everyone else. Programs must aim to reduce error and increase efficiency and satisfaction. Protocols need to be established that define functional policies and procedures. Clinical protocols must deal with the lack of direct contact between the patient at the remote site and the practitioner at the consulting site.

Challenges to an Effective Organizational Structure

**Peter Yellowlees, M.D., Department of Psychiatry,
Royal Brisbane Hospital, Australia**

Convincing major tertiary hospitals to use videoconferencing in the public (HMO) sector is a challenge to our telemedicine program. There is relatively little for these hospitals to gain from providing extra services to rural or remote areas. The doctors, in particular, have an extra level of work that they are required to perform in the major hospitals, without any extra remuneration or support beyond the feel-good factor of helping their rural colleagues manage patients more appropriately. In comparison, the rural hospitals have taken up telemedicine very quickly, and have generally driven the use of telemedicine from that remote end (personal communication, February 10, 1999).

Staffing Challenges

A telehealth project creates a new environment with new types of clinical experiences that allow health care practitioners to cooperate with people outside their field. Although merging several disciplines can bring new opportunities, it also can bring competing agendas that surface in projects, communities, or health care reimbursement plans. These conflicting agendas can also lead to staffing conflicts that will disrupt the overall integrity of the program.

Challenges to Obtaining Multidisciplinary Staffing in Telehealth and E-Health

Steven W. Strode, M.D., University of Arkansas for Medical Sciences
Accept the challenges related to overcoming the suspicion of the physicians in the remote areas, and the lack of interest of physicians at the consulting site (personal communication, November 12, 1999).

One way to address multidisciplinary needs and potential staffing conflicts is to organize focus groups to achieve internal homogeneity based on the type of technology needed by each professional. For example, focus groups can be organized around requirements for content and timeliness of user information. Linking practitioners from different departments who share similar bandwidth requirements for images will result in internally homogeneous groups that can actively cooperate with each other (Siden, 1998).

When the scope of a telehealth project involves many different professionals, each working with specific applications, careful strategic planning is required to ensure success. Large organizations should consolidate services to maximize their bandwidth use. By acquiring equipment that is compatible and usable throughout an organization, the program may be able to share telecommunications cost among disciplines. The same system that is used for patient care can also be used for continuing education and communication within the organization. The main problem that arises with shared use is scheduling. The program needs to establish rules so that emergency telehealth services can be performed when needed (Puskin, Morris, Hassol, Gaumer, & Mintzer, 1997).

E-Health Staffing Challenges

E-health company principals had several key comments related to staffing.

John Bringenberg, President, <Lifescape.com>

- Putting together the best team. Building a team that has the combination of expertise, shared vision, and culture in place to lead the company is tough. Furthermore, as we begin to see the public markets for dot-coms wobble, stock options are losing their tensile strength, making middle and senior management more available for hire (personal communication, May 30, 2000).

Richard Flanagan, CEO, <Epotec.com>

- Hiring and training is another challenge—finding really good people and getting them up to speed with the Internet world. We focus on finding incredibly well trained technology folks (personal communication, May 30, 2000).

Mitchell H. Gold, M.D., CEO, <Elixis.com>

- Bringing on the personnel and capital to grow the company. You have to be willing to exchange ideas with a number of people and bring on consultants to poke holes in models (personal communication, May 30, 2000).

Greg Tullman, CEO, <Allscripts.com>

- Burnout. This is a twenty-four-hour business. There are no such things as weekends or time off. We are always connected, always in touch. The situation doesn't give some people downtime, and it can lead to burnout. We have tried to create a management team that is somewhat interchangeable, so some people can step in for others (personal communication, May 22, 2000).

Michael Weiss, CEO, <CancerEducation.com>

- If you are coming from a health background, managing and coordinating information through the technical staff in a meaningful way is one of the biggest challenges. It is not easy to communicate with programmers.
- Sometimes it is best not to know what can and can't be done. Tell your staff what you want and be willing to pay for it to get done, and they just might surprise you.
- Develop a working advisory board and establish relationships with patient advocacy groups to give you direction (personal communication, May 30, 2000).

Scheduling

Scheduling is often one of the biggest problems faced by telehealth programs. The University of Kansas Medical Center (KUMC) grapples every day with the telemedicine scheduling issue. Until the summer of 1995, clinicians requesting a telemedicine consultation had to set up their own telemedicine events. They had to find their own consultant, book line time, make room arrangements, and coordinate patient record transfers. On average, they were making more than twelve calls to set up a single consultation—and they were not happy about it. In July 1995, KUMC launched "one stop telemedicine": the telemedicine coordinator takes all incoming requests and makes the twelve-odd calls to schedule telemedical events (clinical, educational, and administrative). A survey showed that its clients were quite pleased with the service. Several start-up companies are currently developing and marketing scheduling software; however, its effectiveness remains unproven.

Referral Patterns

Multidisciplinary telehealth projects should consider the effects of changing existing referral patterns. Many practitioners report that protecting preexisting referral patterns is a primary concern to ensure that patients receive the highest quality of care.

Whitten and Franken (1995) conducted an investigation to determine the knowledge of, attitudes toward, and use of interactive telemedicine for specialist consultations among rural practitioners in Kansas. The important role played by relationships and extant referral patterns emerged as a major finding in this study. Another interesting finding was that use of telemedicine services was dependent on programmatic efforts to accommodate existing referral patterns. The data analysis also showed widespread but superficial knowledge of telemedicine services. It showed that professionals had a high appreciation of the value of technology but demonstrated relatively low usage of the available services. Physicians did not appear to be afraid of the technology or the change introduced by telemedicine. Use of technology was also not predicted by any characteristics of the physician.

Reimbursement

Reimbursement of telehealth services presents several further complications. Reimbursement of services cannot only finance operational costs but also increase use of a system. The opposite is true as well: for example, the use of telehealth services has been slow to develop among psychologists and their patients, due at least in part to the initial reimbursement policies of the Health Care Finance Administration (HCFA), which did not allow reimbursement for psychology services (Klein, 1999; Rabasca, 1999).

Another barrier to technology use is payer systems that reimburse providers directly rather than reimburse the facilities that incur the bulk of operating costs. One possible solution to this impediment is to seek support from managed care companies for system setup and operating costs, rather than seek selective reimbursement for practitioners. Another way to provide adequate funding is to have the different users of the system cross-subsidize the cost of the system. Cross-subsidization occurs, for example, when a telehealth system is designed and sustained with funds designated for clinical care to patients but is also used to provide continuing education to professionals in the organization. This model works when the project goal is to provide a service to the community, so that a department does not pay for the bulk of operation costs.

Legislation promises to change some of these practices, opening reimbursement to a much wider group of providers and settings. For legislative updates related to an expansion of telehealth reimbursement policy, go to <http://thomas.loc.gov/> and look for S. 2505 of the Telehealth Improvement and Modernization Act of 2000.

6. IDENTIFY ACCOUNTABILITY

A telehealth service needs a champion who will fight to make it survive and thrive. In creating a telehealth project, the organization must identify who is in charge (and who will get the credit or the blame). If it doesn't, the organization will find it too easy to get rid of its telehealth project at the first sign of trouble.

Politics rule organizations, so you must identify and recruit centers of political power in the early phases of program development. You must also identify specific tasks within the telehealth service and assign accountability for the fulfillment of those tasks. Marketing, scheduling, billing—each task must be assigned to a specific individual or department, and that person or department must issue regular reports and updates.

In e-health companies, accountability is often delegated to specific executives. In the early phases of company start-up, multiple tasks are often assigned to these overworked executives while the company awaits additional staff funding. These key executives need to be chosen wisely. Executives who have proven themselves in nontechnical health care industries may not be the best choice for an Internet-based company. For example, hiring executives who are not Internet savvy or who have never developed Web sites can be a significant detriment to the effective launch of a Web business. Holding people accountable makes sense only if they were chosen for the needed abilities in the first place. Holding nontechnical staff responsible for giving direction to a technical staff is going to slow a business launch significantly. It is wisest to choose e-health company executives who have both administrative and technical expertise, to make goals very clear from the onset, and to allow those executives to initiate projects as they see market demand for them. Accountability can take the form of weekly reports and updates from everyone during the first critical months of business launch.

7. FORECAST COSTS AND IDENTIFY FUNDING SOURCES: TELEHEALTH PROJECTS

For systems based in hospitals, clinics, or universities, the first step to gaining organizational support for any telehealth development program is to secure a written commitment from the director of the organization. Once such a commitment is obtained, you can develop a formal business plan. Such business plans typically include start-up and operating budgets for the project, a break-even analysis, income projections (a profit and loss statement), and cash flow projections for the entire life of the project. These details will vary depending on whether the program is operating within a nonprofit organization and on who is sponsoring it. Regardless of the type of organization and which patients are to be served, the start-up budget should include sufficient funds to support operations for the first six to twelve months of operation (IOM, 1996).

A common error is to underestimate the start-up costs of a telehealth program, so do not make the budget conservative. Next, determine how the program will receive funding for the start-up and how funding will be maintained once the program is established. There are two general categories of funding: internal and external.

An organization can fund internally and consider the program to be an investment. Ten years ago this approach was almost impossible due to the high cost of technology. Now more organizations, such as Kaiser Permanente and the Michigan Department of Corrections, are adopting internal funding strategies thanks to tremendous changes in hardware and telecommunication options. Technology can often cost less than $20,000.

E-Health, Telehealth, and Telemedicine

Just ten years ago, similar services would require technology that ranged in price from $150,000 to $200,000. (Unfortunately, nontechnical resources such as rent and personnel have not enjoyed a similar decrease in cost.)

External funding is available through many government and private foundations. Although the competition for it has become increasingly stiff, this funding is worth pursuing if you have developed a strong project (or if someone in the organization has befriended a congressional representative with influence). Current federal telehealth granting agencies include the following:

Rural Utilities Services

USDA Distance Learning and Telemedicine Grant Program

Office for the Advancement of Telehealth

Office of Rural Health Policy

National Telecommunications and Information Administration

National Library of Medicine

Technology Opportunities Program (Department of Commerce)

In addition, a number of federal agencies (including the National Institutes of Health) provide grants for telehealth projects that meet the goals of their overall health-related agendas. In these cases, telehealth services are secondary to the actual clinical services being provided. The Telemedicine Information Exchange Web site <http://tie.telemed.org/> and the previously mentioned federal agencies and foundations are the best resources for identifying sources of funding.

One of the advantages of external funding is that programs receiving such funding typically have the luxury of a "grace period" before they need to become sustainable. On the negative side, it is of interest to note that in a 1997 survey of telehealth program administrators (Wachter & Grigsby, 1997), researchers found an inherent problem with the continued financial viability of externally funded programs upon the withdrawal of funding. A majority of these administrators believed that specific requirements of their granting agencies placed limits on operational decisions that could have promoted the long-term sustainability of the program. The perception was of being "locked in" with regard to fundamental decisions, such as those related to the purchase of equipment or the type of services to be offered.

External funding may be the only option for some telehealth projects, but internal funding can have distinct advantages. One of the most important benefits of internal funding is its flexibility. Flexibility is critical to maintaining a sustainable telehealth program. A difficulty with external funding is that it often hampers a program's ability to adapt quickly to newly identified needs within the community or to changes in those needs, or to advancements in technology. Such inflexibility inhibits the program's ability to invest in and offer only the services for which there is a demand. Internally funded programs operate from a needs-driven approach that allows them to be better positioned to become sustainable once they have established themselves. These programs only purchase and use equipment when necessary, and are not burdened, for example, with the cost of supporting costly rural sites.

Internal funding has its disadvantages as well. One is the pressure to generate adequate revenue for a hospital, clinic, or university system. Another is the expenditure of time and energy required to seek new sources for funding, which reduces resources available for optimizing the telehealth program within such organizations. The search for alternative sources of revenue can cause other problems, too. For example, when telehealth equipment is rented to outside users to generate additional revenue, that equipment is not available to the primary organization for which the system was originally intended (Wachter & Grigsby, 1997).

Whichever funding strategy you will apply for your program, it is critical to clearly identify projected reimbursement for ongoing services before incurring expenses. Important considerations include whether reimbursement for telehealth services in the designated service region is available from third-party carriers, such as Blue Cross/Blue Shield or

Medicaid. Some negotiating may be necessary with certain providers; you may need several months of lead time for such negotiations.

The bottom line is that the steps needed to gather funds, whether internal or external, will vary greatly depending on whether you are working with private foundations, federal or state governments, or internal budget decision makers. However, there are a few universal principles, which transcend the funding source.

The first step to obtaining funding for a telehealth project is to develop an effective proposal that addresses the type of funding required. Be sure to clearly identify whether funding will be needed only to support start-up costs or whether it will be needed to sustain long-term operations as well. This distinction is important because some projects are forced to end operation when funding ceases.

View each proposal from the perspective of those who will grant the funds. In other words, it is important to design the proposal so as to meet the requirements of a project and be in keeping with the mission of the funding organization. Certain agencies focus on funding technology infrastructure, others focus on software, still others focus on staffing.

By applying to potential sources of funding whose organizational goals are most similar to those of your program, you significantly improve your program's odds of being funded. Grant providers are looking to maximize their dollar by investing in programs that are fiscally sound. They also seek ambitious projects that make cost-effective use of financial resources, have long-lasting educational effects, and have a record of fulfilling and completing grant requirements.

Suggestions for Funding Telehealth Projects

Michelle Gailiun, Director of Telemedicine, Ohio State University
- When purchasing your system, consider your future needs with respect to financial feasibility and the security constraints of your network configuration.

- Understand and accept the fact that the greatest economic benefits to telemedicine fall to the health system and not to individual players.
- Find the funding to foot the initial bill (personal communication, September 28, 1999).

FORECAST COSTS AND IDENTIFY FUNDING SOURCES: E-HEALTH COMPANIES

Although forecasting revenues and costs has been one of the keys to obtaining traditional funding for start-up companies, e-health companies have set new standards for approaching funding sources. Financial projections for dot-com companies have proven to be remarkably unrealistic, despite the predictability of sources for funding such companies. Founders often begin with their own (generally modest) capital and then raise initial capital through their own resources, including borrowing "seed money" from family and friends. Other founders obtain "angel" financing after developing a business plan with clearly defined financial statements that outline future revenue streams and projections.

Most start-up companies seek the advice and direction of an advisory board, consisting of six to eight senior executives with experience in business start-up and development. These board members are typically paid $5,000 to $15,000 per year. Some of this fee is often offset by offering advisory board members shares in the company being built, otherwise known as equity. These early advisers often not only help guide the company during its early months but also occasionally become early investors as angels or first-round venture capital investors.

An initial round of angel funding typically raises $50,000 to $200,000 to launch a company. This money may be adequate, for example, to pay part-time salaries for key personnel, such as a founder (typically taking a title such as chairman of the board or CEO), lawyers, accountants, and so on, who will help further define the business plan and prepare it for future funding. Angel capital typically provides for the first product prototype and customer relationships, and moves the enterprise to a level at which it appears that the firm has the initial evidence of a viable business model and the people and processes to execute the business plan.

Venture capital funding is often then sought to hire other key corporate officers, purchase needed equipment, rent office space, establish or solidify product and customer relationships, and document the next-phase business plan. Venture capital investors become investment partners in the company and often are given from 25 to 35 percent of the company's equity in exchange for taking the risk of infusing the company with working capital. These investors often make their influence felt at the decision-making level by contributing executive personnel to the staff or by occupying seats on the company's board of directors.

The next round of funding is often much larger and should allow a company to begin generating significant revenue. Once a company generates revenues, it can become self-funding or can support debt and additional stock sales to provide the capital needed for growth. At some point, a company may have sufficient intrinsic value or growth prospects to hope to attract many investors. When it does, the company may contemplate selling stock on a public stock exchange through an IPO.

E-health start-ups have displaced some of these time-honored traditions, generating unprecedented amounts of angel and venture capital funding and greatly accelerating funding cycles. Companies have been valued at inflated ratios and have obtained IPO status before proving their financial viability. With the stock market fluctuations in the early part of the year 2000, it is more difficult than ever before to predict the successful raising of capital of e-health companies in the decade to come. In fact, considering the thousands of new e-companies and initiatives within existing companies, it is certain that many lessons will be learned (as was the case with pilot telemedicine projects), and many companies will not be able to sustain themselves financially.

8. ESTABLISH CLEAR AND MEASURABLE GOALS

Be concrete in setting goals. No goal should be stated in a way that cannot be quantitatively measured. For example, one goal could be to provide the first consult by a certain date. Another goal could be to obtain five service contracts in the first six months. Another goal could be to perform so many consults in a twelve-month period.

In addition, establish an acceptable level of revenue returns. Do not be afraid to establish clear benchmarks, even if they require employees to stretch themselves to meet the stated goals. Employees often are able to meet goals if those goals are clearly identified.

9. CREATE A PROJECT TIMELINE

Once you have set concrete goals, you need to establish specific target dates for all the phases of starting and maintaining the project. Businesses can get discouraged when they encounter roadblocks and challenges. A key employee may resign, or some unreliable vendors may be six weeks late delivering equipment (as discussed in Appendix B, vendor contracts should specify installation timelines whenever possible). Unexpected happenings are the nature of business, but a clear and specific timeline should allow for some wiggle room and keep organizational goals in perspective.

10. DEVELOP FEEDBACK MECHANISMS

Unless there is adequate feedback among all levels of the program, decisions made at higher levels may inadvertently cause a program or business to lose direction and subsequently miss critical opportunities. For example, some health care operations can be performed sequentially or simultaneously. Gantt charts are often helpful in providing both guidance and feedback. These charts help organize tasks sequentially and are a basic tool of most program managers. There is also project management software designed to automatically develop such charts (for example, Microsoft's

Project). Such software can help create a spreadsheet of tasks accomplished and keep all relevant information readily available. If adjustments need to be made, for example, with respect to equipment installation or staffing changes, the software will help pinpoint optimal parameters.

Obtaining feedback on completed steps is also essential. While directing the KUMC program we described earlier, Pamela Whitten did a number of things to obtain feedback through the course of the project. For example, after launching a new scheduling process, she conducted a market survey among the telehealth sites in Kansas to see how they liked the new system and what could still be improved. Another goal was to catch potential problems before they got too serious, so Dr. Whitten set acceptable ranges for activities. Whenever an activity fell outside the accepted range, she would be notified. For example, she set a range of 1 percent as the acceptable maximum amount of time the system could not be brought up for a consult. When this was exceeded, she was quickly able to determine the cause, such as a miscommunication between the scheduler and technician. She could then adjust the intraoffice processes to prevent such occurrences in the future.

Obstacles to Maintaining a Telehealth Program

Warren B. Karp, Ph.D., D.M.D., Coordinator of Telemedicine and Distance Learning Activities, Department of Pediatrics, Medical College of Georgia

- Turnover of personnel means that we are constantly retraining.
- Updating equipment is a challenge because of added expense and potential incompatibility of software and hardware.
- Complacency can be a detriment. It is important to motivate people to constantly explore new uses for the technology. As users become more and more comfortable with the technology, they should also "push the envelope" by experimenting with new applications (personal communication, November 15, 1999).

Sally Davis, Program Director of Telehealth and Management Development, Marquette General Hospital, Marquette, Michigan

- A continual struggle lies in promoting clinical services to practitioners and getting them to adopt those services.
- Even with all the current telehealth programs around, models that we can replicate in our area are still minimal.
- The politics (the referral patterns; the administrative, practitioner, and community politics) involved in the start-up and maintenance of various clinical initiatives present a significant barrier. So often, something can be done technologically, but politically it is difficult (personal communication, May 30, 2000).

Rosa Ana Tang, M.D., M.P.H., Professor of Ophthalmology, University of Texas Medical Branch, Galveston

- It is important to train patients to know what to expect when seeing you on a TV instead of face to face.
- Not having adequate personnel and the necessary patient records at the remote site can severely limit the success of patient services (personal communication, November 11, 1999).

Steven W. Strode, M.D., University of Arkansas for Medical Sciences

- One ongoing challenge is balancing the need to repair the technical infrastructure while trying to "sell" the increasing dependability of the services, with little interest and poor service from state telephone companies.
- It is tough to cope with campus administration and college deans with ambiguous lines of authority who flip-flop from wanting to call all the shots to expressing frank disinterest.
- It is difficult to recover from the loss of program champions when they change roles or relocate (personal communication, November 12, 1999).

Robert Cox, M.D., Hays Medical Center, Kansas

- Our three biggest challenges are obtaining reimbursement for clinical services, dealing with maintenance and transmission costs, and maintaining physician interest (personal communication, November 16, 1999).

Peter Yellowlees, M.D., Department of Psychiatry, Royal Brisbane Hospital, Australia

- Continuous staff training must be available, requiring both formal sessions and the production of videos, protocols and papers, CD-ROMs, and Internet programs.
- Operating in a setting where there are numerous doubters and other barriers thrown in one's way is very challenging. It is hard to maintain personal morale and to continue to be a driver. It is clearly essential to develop a core of supportive colleagues (personal communication, February 10, 1999).

11. EVALUATE THE PROGRAM ANNUALLY

For sustained growth and clarity of direction with all staff, prepare an annual report that addresses the goals of the program, use of the budget, feedback obtained, personnel decisions, adherence to the timeline, and serendipitous accomplishments. In developing such a report, it is important to be comfortable with identifying missed achievements and the underlying reasons for any weak areas. Even if the report isn't all good news, the review of achievements from the previous year can serve to boost employee morale. Therefore, all employees should review this annual report. An added benefit of such a report is that the subsequent discussion can generate good ideas from the people who are actually implementing the day-to-day operation of the program.

CONCLUSION

There is a tendency to rush through the planning and strategizing phase of a telehealth or e-health program. Yet proper planning is the key to success.

Begin by identifying the services to be delivered, the target audience, and needed resources. Design an effective organizational structure, and identify who is accountable for which tasks. Then forecast costs and funding sources. Establish clear and measurable goals, as well as clear project timelines. Develop feedback mechanisms and evaluate your program on an annual basis. Follow these guidelines, and you will find the success you are seeking.

Chapter Eleven explains how to conduct research to evaluate a program and outlines solid research techniques that will be needed by grant-funded projects.

Research: Issues, Methods, and Outcomes

A telehealth program in the southeast received a large grant for telemedicine. One stipulation of the grant was that the recipient must conduct a "telemedicine evaluation." The principle investigator (PI) for the grant was well suited to launch a demonstration project. However, he was not formally trained in conducting research. The PI decided to design a satisfaction survey for patients and providers. After collecting a year's worth of data, the PI learned that most of the data from his survey were useless. For example, he had written questions with multiple constructs, so there was no way to clearly identify which embedded concept the respondents were addressing. Having never clearly defined the meaning of some of his questions, he was unable to derive any meaning from his results when later probed by administrators. Moreover, he did not properly delineate experimental and control groups, so no valid comparisons could be drawn. Unfortunately, weak research design appears to be the norm in telemedicine evaluation.

Evaluation should be planned up front; it should not be an afterthought. It is important for a study to have a question to answer, but too many telehealth research publications report on studies that instead were completed merely for the sake of conducting some type of evaluation. Your program can avoid this trap.

Applications of telecommunication technology in health care are fertile ground for valuable research questions. At a minimum, a program can evaluate its progress and success. The evaluation process includes identifying clear objectives for the project; determining what results would suggest that the project has met its objectives; and stipulating the steps for data collection, analysis, and interpretation concerning the project's operations and effects (IOM, 1996).

This chapter gives you the background necessary to decide which type of research is appropriate for evaluating your telemedicine, telehealth, or e-health project. We begin with a general definition and discussion of research; next is an overview of how to structure an evaluation suitable for technology-based health care. The third section outlines the types of research preferred by federal agencies, and we conclude with a discussion of the types of research specifically needed by e-health start-ups.

GENERAL PRINCIPLES OF RESEARCH DESIGN

Research is commonly divided into two major categories: basic and applied. Basic research usually uses a theoretical or scholarly approach. The purpose of this research is to understand a phenomenon and its effects. Applied research is commonly conducted by private sector evaluators and seeks to generate data that will be used for decision making. Both basic and applied research require that the evaluator rigorously conduct the study according to scientific method, have a clear understanding of how the phenomenon being studied can be measured or observed, and apply appropriate procedures to test the observations or measurements.

Whether you are doing basic or applied research, there are four major types:

1. Laboratory experiments. Research studies in which the variance of almost all the independent variables not pertinent to the immediate problem is kept at a minimum by isolating the research in a physical situation apart from the routine of ordinary living.

2. Field experiments. Research studies in a realistic situation in which the investigator manipulates one or more independent variables under as carefully controlled conditions as permissible.

256

3. Field studies. Nonexperimental scientific inquiries that attempt to discover the relations and interactions among sociological, psychological, and educational variables in real social structures.

4. Survey studies. Studies that examine large or small populations by selecting and studying samples chosen from the population to discover relative incidence, distribution, and interrelations of variables.

Regardless of the type of research undertaken, there are universal steps for conducting research. The typical research process consists of these nine steps:

1. Select a problem.
2. Review the existing research and theory.
3. Develop hypotheses (research questions).
4. Determine an appropriate methodology and research design.
5. Select the appropriate subjects.
6. Collect data.
7. Analyze and interpret the results.
8. Present the results in an appropriate form.
9. Replicate the study when necessary.

These steps are based on a common understanding of the relationships among theories, hypotheses, concepts, constructs, variables, selection of subjects, data collection, data analysis, and interpretation. We briefly review these terms and processes in the next sections to give you a sense of their importance to the success and meaningfulness of your efforts at research.

Hypotheses, Concepts, Constructs, and Variables

Research is traditionally conducted to evaluate one or more hypotheses (questions) derived from a theory (an unproven assumption). This is done by identifying and testing the theory's underlying concepts (abstract ideas formed by generalizing from particulars and summarizing related observation) and constructs (combinations of concepts that cannot be directly observed). (It is of note that most research in technology-based health care has been conducted at the observational level and has not followed this approach. The body of early telehealth and telemedicine research, then, has serious theoretical flaws.) The goal of conducting research, then, is to answer questions.

The testable counterpart of a concept or construct is called a variable. Variables are understood by their relationship with one another. The researcher systematically changes the independent variables (the experimental conditions); he or she then observes the dependent variables (the subjects' responses that the researcher seeks to explain). The subjects' responses are presumed to depend on the effects of the independent variable or variables. There may be more than one independent variable in each experiment, though the researcher must be careful to attribute the correct effects of each one to the subjects.

For example, suppose that a researcher is attempting to examine the effectiveness of teleconsultations as opposed to face-to-face sessions in relation to the overall behavior of mentally ill patients. The independent variables are the different therapeutic techniques used and the mode of service delivery: teleconsultations or face-to-face sessions. The dependent variables are the behaviors of the patients. The researcher, in a very controlled manner, varies the types of therapy used and the modes of service delivery, and records the changes in the patients' behaviors.

Selection of Subjects

Selection of appropriate subjects is critical to the success of any study. Develop protocols for selecting research participants with input from experts in the clinical areas to be investigated. Chapters Eight and Nine discussed important ethical and risk management issues that also need to be taken into account. Ethical standards for working with research participants (regarding informed consent, safety, confidentiality, and so on) have been clearly defined by the American Psychological Association (1992) in "Ethical Principles of Psychologists and Code of Conduct."

Data Collection

There is a wide range of data collection methodologies and analytic strategies for each of the four types of research mentioned earlier. These are often broken down into two categories: qualitative and quantitative. Qualitative research refers to several methods of data collection, including field observation, focus groups, in-depth interviews, and case studies. Even though there are major differences between these techniques, their ability to enable the researcher to get "close to the data" unifies them under this category. Quantitative research requires that the variables under consideration be measured numerically and uses such data collection strategies as close-ended surveys or interviews to collect data that can be reported numerically.

The boundary between these two categories is not rigid. For example, many qualitative methodologies lend themselves to reporting data in numerical form as well. A researcher should select qualitative or quantitative strategies (or both) in accordance with the goal of the research. A qualitative approach is a good choice when investigators need (1) to view behavior in a natural setting, (2) to increase their depth of understanding of a phenomenon under study, particularly for a phenomenon that has not previously been studied, and (3) to be flexible and to allow them to gather data not anticipated during the design of the study.

A quantitative approach should be considered when researchers wish (1) to use numbers for greater precision in reporting results or (2) to take advantage of powerful methods of statistical analyses. Many researchers have realized that the validity and reliability of a study are often enhanced when they use both methods to study a phenomenon, a strategy commonly called triangulation.

Other characteristics to consider in data collection include reliability, validity, responsiveness, interpretability, and flexibility. An evaluation instrument or criterion is *reliable* if repeated use under identical circumstances by the same or different users produces the same results. It is *valid* if it measures the properties, qualities, or characteristics it is intended to measure. Validity is essential in health care outcome research, so we will give this element additional attention here.

A study is useful only if the results are valid and reproducible; that is, it is useful to the degree to which it actually measures what it purports to measure and can be replicated by all independent parties who follow the guidelines of the original experiment. Control over research conditions is important because it enables researchers to rule out plausible but incorrect explanations of results. Validity provides a check on how well a study fulfills its function. The study must be internally and externally valid, as will be discussed here.

Internal validity is determined by the processes used to collect data in the experiment. Incorrect findings, or artifacts, can arise from a variety of sources, such as the maturation or mortality of subjects, instrument decay over the course of a study, experimenter bias, or problems with sample selection. To maximize the internal validity of a study, it is important to evaluate a variety of potential experimental designs and try to keep strict control over the research process so that subjects and researchers do not intentionally or unintentionally influence the result.

Researchers should also be striving to maximize external validity. External validity refers to how well the results of a study can be generalized across populations, settings, and time. Common procedures used to guard against problems with external invalidity include (1) using random samples, (2) using heterogeneous samples, (3) selecting a sample that is representative of the group to which the results will be generalized, and (4) conducting the research over a long period of time (Cook & Campbell, 1979).

An evaluation instrument or criterion is considered *responsive* if it can detect important differences in outcomes across evaluation groups or periods. It is *interpretable* if users find the results of its application understandable. An evaluation instrument or criterion is *feasible*, another important characteristic, when researchers can accomplish the required activities, collect the necessary information, and analyze the resulting data within available evaluation resources and without imposing excessive burdens on those whose cooperation is required for the evaluation. If it is adaptable to a variety of evaluation problems or circumstances, it is considered *flexible*.

Data Analysis

Once researchers have collected data, their next step is to perform an analysis, or the categorizing, ordering, manipulating, and summarizing of data to answer the research questions. There are many types of analytic strategies—for example, content analysis for qualitative methods, or statistical tools for quantitative methods (such as frequency distributions, measures of central tendency and variability, measures of relations, and analysis of variance). The choice of type of analysis generally depends on the overall research design and the questions to be answered.

Interpretation and Generalizability

Once they have analyzed the data, investigators must interpret the data by drawing conclusions. If the research has been conducted properly, its findings are generalizable to other programs. As discussed, generalizability is dependent on how well the study has met requirements for reliability, validity, responsiveness, interpretability, feasibility, and flexibility (IOM, 1996). When research is well conducted, then, its interpretations are generalizable and can help decision makers guide the further expansion of services and expenditure of resources.

PROGRAM EVALUATION

There are many ways to combine the elements of research described in the first section to evaluate a technology-based health care service. The following discussion provides some criteria to facilitate these decisions.

The type of evaluation to conduct varies somewhat depending on the program's funding structure (see Chapter Ten). If a technology-based health care program is internally funded, it is free to choose to evaluate any aspect of its program. At a minimum, a program should conduct a market analysis to track the success of the program and services. This analysis includes benchmarked levels of activity, client and provider satisfaction with various aspects of the service, issues related to quality assurance and utilization review, and cost-benefit analyses. For programs with an academic bent, research avenues are unlimited and typically range from efficacy to provider-patient communication.

When funding comes from external sources, such as federal offices or foundations, the granting institution often requires specific research. Unfortunately, many telehealth programs to date have been short staffed and unable to hire experts trained in research design. As a result, much of the telehealth research to date is methodologically flawed.

Many pilot telemedicine and telehealth programs have conducted poorly designed evaluations. An area particularly fraught with inconsistencies and poor research design is that of patient and provider satisfaction, as revealed in Mair and Whitten's systematic review of telehealth satisfaction research (1999). More specifically, this research failed to contribute substantially to the field's understanding of how patients and providers feel about telehealth and the subsequent effects on the consultation. Mair and Whitten found that much of the published satisfaction literature to date has presented a rather superficial examination of satisfaction.

Mair and Whitten (2000) posit a number of potential explanations for these deficits. One reason is that although the granting agencies require evaluations, they have not funded the required level of evaluation. Another has to do with the methodology employed to perform satisfaction research. Most telehealth researchers have used only Likert-style surveying techniques. Although this technique is inexpensive and easy, employing only this method has clear limitations. In addition to providing a limited scope of data, problems with specific surveys are confounded when used as the sole source of data. Poor design of questionnaires and administration protocols often create biased and unreliable results, according to Mair and Whitten. Without well-designed and standardized questionnaires and administration protocols, interpretation is difficult, as is generalizability across studies. Another confounding problem within satisfaction research is the construct of satisfaction. Few studies clearly defined what satisfaction meant, so when participants indicated they were "satisfied," the researchers were unable to determine whether participants meant "Telehealth didn't kill me," "Telehealth was OK," or "Telehealth was a great experience."

Structuring the Evaluation Plan

The following section outlines the general steps for creating an evaluation plan. Researchers go to graduate school to get the full level of training needed to conduct most clinical research, so we present only a brief outline here. However, there are basic attributes of any solid evaluation plan; they should be taken into account when you hire a trained researcher.

Getting Started. Regardless of the type of research selected, the first step is to establish clear objectives for an evaluation. An evaluation committee should be established to determine the types of decisions to be affected by the results, and who will use the evaluation results. The committee should identify the key elements of the service to be delivered and evaluated.

If a project is funded to answer specific research questions, definition of the questions should precede development of the program. Given the nature of funding cycles, it is often the case that many programs and activities evolve gradually, without regard to previously established rationales. This practice is often inappropriate.

The lessons learned from the analysis of satisfaction research to date are important and can be applied to almost any research theme. First, the research question or questions should be both relevant and specific. What exactly needs to be better understood? The more specific a question is, the better the research will be. Hypotheses and theory should drive the research. Drawing hypotheses from theoretical underpinnings ensures that the research focuses on specific measurement objectives. This also helps ensure that the researcher has thought through all the potentially confounding issues.

The second step is to hire a trained researcher to conduct the evaluation. This does not mean that project coordinators should turn to a high-priced consultant. Many university professors are willing to conduct research as an academic challenge and do not charge high fees. Many junior faculty are interested in conducting research so as to increase their number of publications for eventual tenure. This group will be professionally trained and are usually not focused on financial gain. Academic appointments at major research institutions are extremely competitive, so the quality of researchers tends to be quite high.

Early inclusion of this professional evaluator is essential to developing a relevant and pragmatic research plan. A researcher who is brought aboard at a late stage may be ill positioned to create the type of data needed. When brought in at a late stage, researchers are often forced to work with poorly designed data sets and often can do very little to salvage a study, despite their best attempts.

Categories of Evaluation. The next step is to determine the level and perspective of the evaluation. There are three overlapping categories: clinical, institutional, and societal (IOM, 1996). The clinical perspective analyzes the potential benefits, risks, and costs of alternative strategies to health care. For example, does telepsychiatry provide the clinical information necessary for diagnosis (Cukor et al., 1998)? The institutional perspective focuses on the organizational context of the telehealth application, which includes clinical protocols, administrative structures and practices, patient and practitioner satisfaction, and other clinical personnel (IOM, 1996). For example, does the use of technology reduce the number of medical evacuations (Stoloff, Garcia, Thomason, & Shia, 1998) or affect referral patterns (Whitten & Franken, 1995)? At the societal or system level, evaluation examines the overall health care delivery and financial issues, mainly involving the distribution of public resources (IOM, 1996).

Elements of the Evaluation Plan. The Institute of Medicine's publication on telehealth research (1996) states that an evaluation plan should contain eight key elements.

1. The *project description* identifies the distinct characteristics of the application being assessed and the alternative modes of health care delivery or control groups to which it may be contrasted. It also details the specific research question, the length of the study, the key personnel, the equipment involved, the type of service delivery, and the clinical population to be studied.

2. *Strategic objectives* explain how the design and evaluation of the technology-based health care service will affect the supporting organiza-

tion's objectives (IOM, 1996). These general objectives may be, for example, to reduce casualties on the battlefield (Blakeslee & Satava, 1998) or to improve a community health network (Puskin, Mintzer, & Wasem, 1997).

3. *Clinical objectives* "state how the service is intended to affect the individual or health population by changing the quality, accessibility, or cost of care" (IOM, 1996, p. 146). For example, a correctional telehealth project might be designed to provide cost-effective health care to HIV-positive inmates (Mazmanian et al., 1996; McCue, Hampton, Marks, Fisher, & Parpart, 1997). An e-health company's objective might be to automate back-office record keeping and payer reimbursements through secured transmissions via the Internet.

4. As discussed in Chapter Ten, a *business plan* sets out the framework for how the implementation and evaluation of the service will provide decision makers the proper information related to financial sustainability. A business plan can range from a simple project management plan that outlines the health care service's management and leadership personnel and its work plan and budget, to a highly detailed functional analysis of how the service fits within the organization's overall strategic plan (IOM, 1996).

5. Once the research questions and objectives have been determined, *evaluation level and perspective* can be established at three broad levels: clinical, institutional, and societal (IOM, 1996).

6. The *research design* "describes the strategy and steps for developing valid comparative information, including the sources and techniques for collecting data" (IOM, 1996, p. 144). It specifies whether the strategy is experimental or quasi-experimental.

7. The *analysis plan* "outlines the methods for analyzing and interpreting the resulting information" (IOM, 1996, p. 149). These methods may range from relatively simple statistical comparisons to more sophisticated multivariate regression analyses. Overall, the basic task in research design is to balance the validity of the research findings with the relevance, feasibility, and affordability of the evaluation. Measurable outcomes "identify the variables and the data to be collected to determine whether the project is meeting its clinical and strategic objectives" (IOM, 1996, p.152).

8. *Documentation* is perhaps the most important step in the evaluation process. The publications *Telemedicine Journal* and the *Journal of Telemedicine and Telecare* are examples of specific media that demonstrate the proper way of documenting technology-based health care evaluations. (At the time of this writing, both journals are considering a name change to reflect e-health research, which they also publish.) The main point is to follow a formal procedure to produce credible and usable results (IOM, 1996).

Challenges to Performing a Solid Evaluation. Organizations may be faced with several problems when developing an evaluation plan. One problem is that resources dedicated to evaluating technology-based health care applications seem to be limited. This is often the case because funding for an evaluation may compete with funding for the services that are to be evaluated (IOM, 1996). Setting priorities for the use of limited resources is difficult. One goal of this chapter is to suggest that outcome research ought to be a high priority if a program hopes to achieve fiscal sustainability over time.

Another problem that often arises with outcome research is that information necessary for the evaluation is not easily available. This is particularly true when a researcher has not been hired from the inception of a service. Inadvertent problems can become apparent after data collection has already begun. For example, consent forms may be inadequately designed, thereby prohibiting the full use of collected data; essential demographic data may be missing because computerized medical record fields were improperly developed; and questionnaires may use inappropriate scales for response sets.

Another common problem is that data collection timelines are often underestimated. Time demands for information collection should be relative to the specific project and allow enough time to permit data collection to be reliable. Many evaluations look for effects within a relatively short period and therefore may neglect unexpected longitudinal results (IOM, 1996).

Although the first part of this chapter has aimed to give you a general overview of research and outcome evaluation, there is no one-size-fits-all evaluation plan. Evaluations differ because they are intended for different purposes. In the early to mid-1990s, most telehealth evaluations simply looked at the feasibility of using a telehealth system. Many granting agencies have moved beyond funding yet another "telemedicine demonstration project." Millions of dollars have been spent on these demonstration projects with almost universal findings of feasibility. As a result, the current focus is more on conducting empirical research to answer specific outcomes questions.

The remainder of this chapter will first outline research agendas established by federal and cooperative telemedicine ventures, then look at e-health research agendas and their complications.

FEDERAL AGENDAS

Several federal agencies and private organizations have recognized recent advances in telehealth and are developing improved evaluation strategies and frameworks (IOM, 1996). These organizations are also funding evaluation research and are requiring demonstration projects to conduct their own separate internal evaluations. For example, the Office for the Advancement of Telehealth focuses on quality, accessibility, and health care costs primarily in rural areas. The Health Care Financing Administration (HCFA) is also interested in quality and access, but the projects it sponsors are primarily intended to provide information to formulate payment policies for Medicare. Other organizations include the National Library of Medicine, the Agency for Health Care Policy and Research, the Department of Veterans Affairs, and the Department of Defense (IOM, 1996).

The federal Joint Working Group on Telemedicine (JWGT) has made an effort to develop a broad evaluation framework for all applications of telehealth (Puskin, Brink, Mintzer, & Wasem, 1995). The JWGT identified three operative goals for evaluations. The first was to accentuate data collected from civilian and military projects by determining reliable ways to combine similar results. The next goal was to minimize the repetition of resources by developing and maintaining a centralized inventory of all available data collection protocols. The third objective was to facilitate data collection at individual sites by centralizing information common to multiple areas (IOM, 1996).

The Agency for Health Care Policy and Research (AHCPR) has also addressed the need for telehealth evaluations (Fitzmaurice, 1998). It suggests that there are currently several barriers to good telehealth evaluation, such as multiple objectives, proof of concept, the variety of specialty services, lack of a "normal" patient flow, a small number of patients, and a wide variety of patients' conditions. The AHCPR also sees several threats to the validity of telehealth evaluations that include a relatively small number of patients and a subsequent low statistical yield: there may be selection bias; there may be changes in the telehealth system during the evaluation that affect outcome measures; and it may be impossible to assign practitioners and patients arbitrarily to experimental or control groups.

Despite these various concerns, the AHCPR has developed the following telehealth evaluation variables:

Clinical outcomes

Technical acceptability

Health systems interface

Costs and benefits

Patient and provider acceptability

Access to care

No program can or should try to incorporate all these evaluation components in a single project. Instead, the purpose of the project as well as the expertise of the individual evaluators will drive the selection of the category or categories to measure. Although the federal government suggests these content areas, each organization may have different agendas regarding their goals in learning about telehealth.

ISSUES THAT TRANSCEND FUNDING SOURCES

It is important to acknowledge that not all research is conducted to comply with federal funding. Unfortunately, telehealth literature to date focuses primarily on the technology itself (Fisk et al., 1995; Ong, Chia, Ng, & Choo,

E-Health, Telehealth, and Telemedicine

1995; Caramella, Lencioni, Mazzeo, & Bartolozzi, 1994; Cook, Insana, Mc-Fadden, Hall, & Cox, 1994). However, if one accepts the literal definition of telemedicine as "medicine at a distance," then it becomes evident that the focus should be placed on the service or program, not the technology. Unfortunately, very little existing research in this field recognizes that organizational issues serve to make or break telemedicine programs.

Even with increasing evidence that managerial and administrative issues play a vital role in the effectiveness and utilization of such services, few studies have attempted to document the influence and role of structure, leadership, job roles, or training factors (Perednia & Allen, 1995). Research has demonstrated that organizational factors are critical determinants of the success or failure of a telemedicine program (Whitten & Allen, 1995). This research suggests, for example, that telemedicine programs may benefit particularly from redefining the roles and responsibilities of certain personnel, increasing the efficiency and decreasing the complexity of the consultation scheduling process, and clarifying and formalizing leadership and decision making. Other research of organizational factors has documented how telehealth is organized for delivery to unique contexts (Zaylor, Whitten, & Kingsley, 1999); charted successful and unsuccessful strategic approaches toward operationalizing telemedicine (Whitten, Sypher, & Patterson, 2000); and charted the protocol and steps for providing telehealth services (Whitten, Cook, Swirczynski, Kingsley, & Doolittle, 1999). Innovations in telemedicine technology need to be matched by innovations in organizational communication and structure.

E-HEALTH RESEARCH ISSUES

Although e-health is an outgrowth of telehealth and telemedicine, its measures of success are not limited to satisfaction surveys, feasibility studies, or empirical research. Consumers decide if a business is satisfactory and feasible. The type of evaluation conducted by writers of e-health business plans is focused more intensely on the nature of consumers' behavior, with ever-increasing consumer choices related to technology. Such behavior is often measured by opinion polls or surveys, as well as by the speed of IPOs and by stock market prices.

Despite its seemingly unique features, research conducted through the Internet is particularly vulnerable to some of the traditional errors in measurement. This is especially true because of the global nature of the population being measured and the wide variety of linguistic, cultural, and economic factors that can influence a consumer's choice of telecommunication technologies. Research with an online population is vulnerable to the following errors in measurement:

Coverage error. Occurs when all units of a population do not have a known probability of inclusion greater than zero in the sample drawn to represent the population.

Sampling error. Occurs when researchers sample only a portion of the survey population rather than all members.

Measurement error. Occurs when respondents give inaccurate answers to questions due to poor wording or interviewing; survey, administration, and effects; or the answering behavior of the respondent. This kind of error is particularly relevant in e-health because Internet users might have limited reading skills or might not use English as a primary language.

Nonresponse error. Occurs when responses are not obtained from people who, had they given responses, would have provided a different distribution of answers.

Greenberg (1999) identifies problems related to the reliability and validity of testing instruments online, despite their relative ease of construction. Data security and individual anonymity are also confounding variables when conducting research on the Web. As mentioned in previous chapters, it is becoming commonplace for Web sites to collect information about visitors without their knowledge, which raises ethical as well as legal issues for researchers. Moreover, with regard to anonymity, it is currently impossible to ensure the anonymity of a person completing an assessment instrument on the Web when using common desktop technology. Test security is also an issue. There is no guarantee that an outcomes instrument won't be printed off and distributed to other study participants.

Inklings of these complications occur regularly to Web site owners who receive mail from readers from around the world and who analyze log files of their Web site traffic. For example, <www.SelfhelpMagazine.com> traffic statistics regularly report visitors from over 106 different countries. Although mail received from readers is written in English, it is only reasonable to assume that not all these readers are using English as a primary language. Occasional mail in very broken English is merely a glimmer of the range of people accessing an average American informational health care Web site. Developing assessment tools to measure health-related values for these readers is fraught with problems that have as yet been unaddressed by the majority of researchers.

Although existing research strategies can be useful in measuring some aspects of dot-com activity, additional strategies will most certainly be needed. It has already been documented that the complications of conducting research through technology to assess technology-related behavior are particularly complex (Barak, 1999; Mehta & Sivadas, 1998; Smith & Leigh, 1997; Stanton, 1998; Swoboda, Muhlberger, Weitkunat, & Schneeweib, 1997). For example, the tradition of collecting information via telephone survey has now been complicated by consumers with multiple phone lines, with each phone line being used for a variety of services. It is possible for people to have a telephone line at work, another one at home, a cell phone, and a fax line located at their home or office (or both). If a researcher wants to assess a particular consumer's behavior, the choice of which telephone line to call is now significantly complicated.

Nonetheless, the polling industry is making strides, learning lessons, and studying the survey-taking literature (Coy, 2000; Groves, 1989; Krosnick, 1999; Mitofsky, 1999; Rogelberg & Luong, 1998). Other research approaches are based on visitor profiling studies, which record the user's movements on Web sites and the time spent at each page of the site, and usability studies evaluating the user-friendliness of Web sites (Hollenbeck,

1999). As researchers collaborate to develop research designs across disciplines, the future of Internet-based outcome research is bright. How these new tools will be applied to evaluating the success of e-health companies will nonetheless be tempered by the ultimate determinant of commercial success: consumer behavior.

CONCLUSION

Research methods and outcomes are the backbone of any solid project or business. Although the focus on technology in health care is relatively new for many professionals seeking to expand their range of services, research and outcomes techniques and protocols have existed for decades. With a well-defined question, it is possible to develop the proper research methods to test ideas and obtain valuable information for telehealth and e-health. By understanding the type of research sought by various funding sources, project planners can increase their chances of winning the funding needed for the project, and corporate decision makers can maximize the bottom line. Telehealth program developers must allocate enough funding to hire qualified staff to conduct empirical research if they wish to draw valid and reliable conclusions from their work. Program evaluators must think beyond simple satisfaction and decide on the specific questions that need answering and how best to address these questions. Such an approach is vital to improve the knowledge base related to the effects of telecommunication technologies. This knowledge is vital to improving services based on these technologies and to defining their possible limitations in clinical practice. More important, this knowledge is needed to shape the growth of future programs and put an end to the needless expenditure of research funding and start-up investments.

Chapter Twelve peers into the future and gives you a brief look at what is likely to be commonplace in health care within the next decade.

Visions into the Future of Health Care

You hear the sound of a motor and know the Park Ranger saw your flare. You feel relieved that you do not have to try to make it back to the Ranger station on your broken ankle. The transport back is painful and bumpy, but you know that medical attention is near. At the Ranger station, a pleasant Dr. Miller asks you for your Guardian Angel. You pull the small device out of your pocket and type in your access code.

Dr. Miller thoroughly examines your ankle, then sits at a desk and researches your medical history on the Guardian Angel. "Looks like you've had problems with this ankle before. Normally, I'd tell you to go home and put ice on your ankle for the next forty-eight hours. But I'm concerned that the ligaments never fully healed from the soccer accident. The two injuries seem to have affected the same area of the ankle, so I'm recommending an MRI to see if surgery is necessary," he says with a compassionate smile.

You are disheartened at the news, but at least your examination was thorough, unlike the last doctor, who didn't even access your past records. "Well, that won't happen to anyone else," you think to yourself, "since I reported that guy to my insurance company after checking my Guardian Angel and finding out what he did—and didn't do."

The Ranger station offers you a cot to rest on while your friends come to get you. With a little help from the medication Dr. Miller gave you, you fall fast asleep. You are not concerned about missing the time to take your next pill: your Guardian Angel will wake you when it's time. And as you sleep, the Guardian Angel is taking care of scheduling your MRI, paying for your medication, and ordering your custom ankle brace.

The device known as the Guardian Angel already exists at the Massachusetts Institute of Technology (MIT). It is being tested as a prototype for a lifelong health adviser. Developed by Peter Szolvits and his research group at MIT Laboratory for Computer Science, the Guardian Angel software module is designed to store an individual's medical record throughout his or her life span, instead of that record's being held in separate pieces at various doctors' offices, hospitals, and pharmacies. Different components of this record are being designed for housing in an individual's portable device, home computer, and personal physician's or insurance carrier's computer. The individual would have sole control over the personal files by setting a password on the portable device. The Guardian Angel will also be able to track conditions over time, perform accountability tests, issue reminders to both the patient and the treating professional, and send alerts concerning inconsistencies in body chemistry, medications, and behavioral decisions, such as exercise, food, or alcohol choices that may lead to illness (Dertouzos, 1997).

This chapter peers more deeply into the future of telecommunications technology. The first section discusses three areas that will be central to the future of health care: issues concerning wireless communications (including broadband satellite systems), globalization of health care and international policymaking, and overall digitization through e-health and the Internet. In the second section, we discuss specific technologies that will give you a sense of what is to come: biosensors, smart cards, **virtual reality,** and telesurgery.

FUTURE HEALTH CARE TRENDS

In the future, health care will combine changes in the telecommunications marketplace and changes in the health care industry, leading to improved diagnosis and treatment and reduced costs of patient care throughout the world.

The efficient management of time, resources, and information will continue to be the top priority for the health care industry. Moreover, information technology will be more critical to the quality and economic viability of health care as we move further into the twenty-first century. The growth rate of the telecommunications market in the United States is expected to be 30 percent per year until 2003 ("New Technologies," 1998).

The main forces driving the current and future development of telehealth technology are the notions that caring for sick and injured people is expensive and that optimizing the health of the chronically ill saves money. Telehealth can be applied to a disease management model whereby phone- or video-based interactions between patients and practitioners lower health care costs. This model is already contributing to decreased service utilization by chronically ill patients and those at risk for acute episodes. The result is that the role of communications in health care, whether based on videoconferencing, computers, or telephones, will increase dramatically when that use translates into monetary savings (Holt, 1997).

Wireless Technology

Wireless technology in health care has been most commonly used for telemetry, emergency medical services, and transport. For example, paramedics already use wireless telemetry and wireless interactive video for communicating with emergency physicians to permit assessment before the patient arrives at the hospital. In the hospital setting, wireless technology is also useful in allowing emergency room physicians to remain with their current patients while consulting other staff members via portable wireless devices.

These systems also facilitate general patient care in hospital systems, where doctors no longer need to swing by the clerk's desk to check for the arrival of their next patient or to obtain a medical record. With a few pen taps on their lightweight, wireless laptops, they can quickly retrieve and update medical records as they move from patient to patient. These systems will undoubtedly become smaller and more commonplace as physicians realize how much time and energy they can save.

Wireless Application Protocol. Companies in the United States have already introduced wireless handheld computers, such as the Palm series and its competitors. More recently, mobile phone providers, such as Sprint PCS, have introduced products with the ability to access limited Web pages for text information. Direct access to the Web and its graphics is not yet possible without appropriate technical standards. However, a standard called the wireless application protocol (WAP) is already under development. WAP is a way of converting information on Internet Web sites into a form that can be displayed on a mobile handheld phone device. Once mobile systems are able to offer the capacity to support high-speed connections to the Internet, so-called microbrowsers will also soon be available; WAP proponents believe that consumers will be able to get message notification and call management, electronic mail, mapping and location services, weather and traffic alerts, sports and financial services, address book and directory services, and corporate intranet applications on their handheld devices.

International Developments. In countries that have adapted to digital wireless phone systems faster than the United States, a wide range of wireless technology is already available. For example, in Japan, Nippon Telephone & Telegraph provides Internet e-mail access to one million customers via its wireless phone services. With this wireless technology, practitioners may eventually be able to consult through e-mail with their patients from remote sites.

Japanese companies have also introduced a mobile videophone that can transmit live video at 32 Kbps. In the Netherlands, Nokia has already introduced the Nokia 9110 Communicator, which can link to a digital camera, store images, and then e-mail them. Nokia's Communicator should be available in the United States by now, and mobile videophones will soon follow. All these products will greatly enhance medical and behavioral health care in the United States. Counselors will be able to visually communicate with their patients in times of crisis via mobile videophones. In addition, clinicians will be able to consult with staff in emergencies.

Broadband Satellite Systems. Mobile satellite communications also promise to extend the global reach of voice, data, and other services. In a cooperative effort known as Internet in the Sky, the FCC has proposed affordable worldwide access to high-quality telecommunications services, including videoconferencing. The FCC has granted orbital locations and Ka-band licenses to thirteen companies, including the following: EchoStar, Hughes, Loral, Motorola, Ka-Star, NetSat 28, and PanAmSat. Motorola and Boeing have invested in an ambitious plan to put up an Internet in the sky.

Unlike terrestrial mobile phone systems, satellite technology may be several years away from offering affordable services. Once they are fully functional, however, these systems will provide several advantages. Larger satellite systems can reach a global audience and at the same time offer data transmission rates three times faster than an ISDN connection; they all aim to transmit information at speeds up to 155 Mbps. It is projected that purchasing broadband satellite service will be akin to purchasing Internet service from an ISP (Montgomery, 1997). An antenna attached to a satellite-to-computer gateway intercepts signals, much as antennas attached to a radio intercept radio waves.

According to the FCC, these satellite systems will be used for the same sort of applications as a terrestrial telecommunication line: desktop-to-desktop videoconferencing, Internet access, electronic messaging, faxing, telehealth, direct-to-home video, electronic transaction processing, distance learning, and even news gathering. The broadband satellite system is designed to support millions of simultaneous users and provides not only high bandwidth but also shorter latency periods, that is, the amount of time required for data to get from point A to point B. The system consists of two earth orbit levels, low earth orbit (LEO) and geostationary earth orbit (GEO).

LEOs will aim to serve two-way high-speed networking, teleconferencing, telehealth, and other interactive applications. LEOs already are used as tracking services to monitor the location of trucks or other vehicles. Several more satellite systems are becoming operational, including Lockheed Martin's Astrolink, scheduled to begin operations in 2001, and Hughes Network System's Spaceway.

GEOs will serve one-way information downloading and video distribution, such as broadcasting and multicasting (Montgomery, 1997). Users reportedly will have two-way connections that provide up to 64 Mbps on the downlink and up to 2 Mbps on the uplink. Broadband terminals will offer 64 Mbps of two-way capacity. This represents access speeds up to two thousand times faster than today's standard analog modems. For example, transmitting a set of x-rays may take four hours over one of today's standard modems, whereas the same images can be sent over the Teledesic network in seven seconds (*Teledesic Overview,* 1999).

In the United States, satellite technology promises to provide increased access to high-speed telecommunications systems for those living in rural areas. In other areas throughout the world, it will allow isolated communities, where terrestrial lines were previously not available, to have access to high-speed communication networks.

For example, NASA has developed the Advanced Communication Technology Satellite (ACTS). This is the world's first processing Ka-band satellite for remote patient monitoring and care of astronauts and other telehealth applications. ACTS allows the use of small, low-cost portable antennas attached to equipment, providing affordable high data transmission rates (up to T-1, 1.544 Mbps) for medical records, images, and live video. For example, ACTS is developing applications in telemammography. This will improve access to care for underserved communities by providing fast, low-cost, high-quality communication with centralized mammography specialists. New image compression techniques and faster data transmission will lead to significantly lower communication and digital storage costs and will increase productivity.

Satellite technology in general will not only facilitate data transmission important for telehealth images but will also enable access to e-mail, telephone, and the Internet from anywhere in the world. Inexpensive pocket-sized, battery-powered wireless communicators will give patients and practitioners the ability to consult with colleagues or specialists, access medical records, or obtain medical advice, regardless of location.

Satellite technology has led some to refer to it as "unwiring the world." It will directly address the problems of inadequate health access and educational, economic, and cultural opportunity. Moreover, "unwiring" tends to level differences between rich and poor, because it works as well in remote regions as in modern cities and will be economical enough to be spread everywhere.

One example of this concept is the Costa Rican Foundation for Sustainable Development (1999), which has developed a program called LINCOS (Little Intelligent Communities). LINCOS envisions immediate access to a wide array of information technologies from a number of small villages and communities. Each village is to have a digital satellite link and integrated local wireless telephone connection, analytical laboratories, telehealth services, a computer lab, electronic commerce and banking services, and a multipurpose information center.

The developers of this system plan an image-and-text database that can be customized and built on by the local health worker, permitting other health workers in a region to share experiences and data. These databases are to include sophisticated image analysis capabilities to help with faster, more accurate identification of problems. Other public health facilities, such as laboratory analysis for environmental, agricultural, and public health analysis, would ideally be housed within the network.

Barriers to Wireless Technology. Wireless technology still faces numerous barriers to its widespread use. The FCC, for example, has proposed that a new spectrum be developed for wireless medical telemetry service, because of occasional interference from digital television broadcasts. These occurrences highlight the dangers of electromagnetic interference with the operation of critical medical equipment.

Security concerns over the transmission of sensitive data will need to be addressed before this technology can be fully realized in health care. Wireless signals can be easily intercepted, as they are during cellular telephone conversations. Therefore, failure to safeguard the confidentiality of information exchanged between the patient and provider using any form of wireless technology increases risk and could result in legal recourse.

Globalization of Health Care Delivery

Opportunities for international telehealth applications are great. The need for such services is particularly apparent in countries where the demand for high-quality health care outstrips supply. However, opportunity does not come without significant challenges. Just because a country needs or is receptive to telehealth does not mean it is properly positioned to receive it.

Barriers to international growth exist at ethical, political, social, and economic levels. These barriers can involve differences in cultural environments, legal and regulatory requirements, payment policies and structures for practitioners, hardware standards, and software availability.

With regard to technical standards, the need for international technical standards will become more critical as global services and communications expand in reach. Despite the many obstacles, advances are being made toward telecommunications standards by such groups as the International Telecommunications Union (ITU). More specifically, the ITU has developed the "H" standard series for videoconferencing, which is gaining wide acceptance.

With regard to economic factors, countries under consideration for investment by U.S. health care providers must meet two criteria: health care must be considered poor in the region seeking assistance, or a substantial portion of the country's population must be wealthy enough to afford services from U.S. health care deliverers (Jones, 1997). Nonetheless, the self-sustaining push of the Internet offers an ever-growing potential to overcome these and other obstacles.

Many international groups are focused on telemedicine and telehealth. As discussed in Chapter Five, the G8 nations are also involved in the deployment of telemedicine to developing countries as a primary vehicle for introducing new health care services. Similarly, the World Trade Organization (WTO) is engaging in health services negotiations, after successfully negotiating both financial and telecommunications basic services. The new global trade discussions by the WTO will include important decisions related to telehealth and distance education (OAT, 1999a).

E-Health and the Internet

Digitization of health care information is ubiquitous. In the international arena, it is obvious that the area with the most promise for rapid growth is the Internet. The demand for health information through the Internet is increasing at an astonishing pace. The continued growth of the Internet is inevitable, due to its global span, its ability to merge and surpass the power of television and telephone, and its stimulus to innovation (Cairncross, 1997).

As we discussed in Chapter Two, with increased access to e-health through the Internet, patients have the ability to contact many more people than ever before. Although it is too early to predict with complete accuracy the specific role the Internet will play, it does appear to be developing as a potential universal pathway for telecommunications of all kinds. With the development of inexpensive higher-bandwidth access, such as cable modems and digital subscriber lines, videoconferencing will soon be available to the desktop via Internet connections.

It is already obvious that health care consumers of the future will be more actively involved in decisions that affect their health care. They will expect high levels of choice, control, customer service, interaction with their health care practitioners, and access to information (Mittman & Cain, 1999). The health care industry will need to meet those expectations with increased availability and reliability of online information services.

Strong market forces—managed care organizations, employer purchasing coalitions, assertive government agencies, and patient organizations—are at work in health care. Internet technologies, intranets, and extranets will serve as low-cost, rapidly deployable stages for distributing information. As discussed in Chapter Two, competitive health care organizations will be pressured to use the Internet to promote a wide range of products and services (Mittman & Cain, 1999).

The Next Generation Internet (NGI), otherwise known as Internet2, is a joint venture by academia, the federal government, and industry to resolve problems with bandwidth constraints, quality, and security issues. This group is using a backbone with a core subnetwork consisting of a 2.4 gigabits per second (Gbps), thirteen-thousand-mile research network to test Internet applications requiring greater capacities to quickly transmit large amounts of information.

When Internet2 debuted in February 1999, project leaders chose a surgical procedure to demonstrate its telehealth potential. Doctors in Ohio and Washington, D.C., were involved in a simultaneous transmission of data at 2.4 Gbps in real time. The event marked the beginning of a communications network that connects thirty-seven universities. It demonstrated two important characteristics of NGI: real-time interaction on the Internet without delays, and the ability to use applications that require a large amount of bandwidth (Carrington, 1999b).

In addition, NGI promises to deliver much higher quality of service than the relatively unregulated "old" Internet. More specifically, it is being developed to provide the following (Next Generation Internet Initiative, 1999):

An increased ability to handle real-time, multimedia applications such as videoconferencing and streams of audio and video—very important for telemedicine and distance education. The ordinary Internet cannot make any guarantees about the rate at which it will deliver data to a given destination, making many real-time applications difficult or impossible.

Sufficient bandwidth to transfer and manipulate huge volumes of data. Satellites and scientific instruments will soon generate a terabyte (a trillion bytes) of information in a single day. For instance, the printed collection of the Library of Congress is equivalent to ten terabytes.

The ability to access remote supercomputers, construct a "virtual" supercomputer from multiple networked workstations, and interact in real time with simulations of tornadoes, ecosystems, new drugs, and so on.

The ability to collaborate with other scientists and engineers in shared virtual environments.

The Promise of E-Health

Given the unprecedented and unpredictable changes of the last decade, the promise of digitized, wireless, globalized e-health is difficult to imag-

E-Health, Telehealth, and Telemedicine

ine, let alone describe. Nonetheless, three groups are sure to benefit: patients and their caregivers, practitioners, and health care organizations.

Patients. Patients in the future will be guided by high-speed search engines using **intelligent agent** software systems to sort through health information. These systems will include personalized navigation tools that store information derived from previous interactions with the patient so as to enhance future searches. Increasingly sophisticated medical services and products will be accessible and available for purchase online.

Patients will be able to avail themselves of a wide variety of electronic health care devices that perform routine home health exams, such as thermometers, EKGs, and blood pressure cuffs. Their results will then be transmitted over secured Internet channels to their physician's office computer. In fact, home health care was the fastest-growing segment of the medical device industry in the 1990s, and this rate is likely to continue as medical equipment becomes less expensive and more specialized (OAT, 1999b).

Health Care Professionals. Health care professionals are already using the Internet in many ways: for professional supervision, consultation and discussion through e-mail discussion lists and Web site forums, and research through Web sites and targeted e-mail newsletters (Kikuchi, 1999).

The transition of many academic journals to online versions and their being augmented by advanced search engines that enable quick screening of information are two important online contributions to health care. Medical education will also be increasingly delivered through distance learning programs housed on the Internet. As we have seen, medical records will become further integrated with Internet technology. Speedy access for practitioners to these types of informational resources will serve to improve the reliability and quality of health care services.

Increased pressure from patients will drive practitioners to use e-mail more widely for clinical purposes. With pressure from patients and health care organizations, practitioners will be forced to overcome their fears of being overwhelmed with electronic messages, liability problems, and breaches in security (Carrington, 1999a; Eysenbach & Diepgen, 1998;

Spielberg, 1998). In time, despite the lack of reimbursement for e-mail communications, practitioners will come to accept and use e-mail as they have the telephone and fax machine (Mittman & Cain, 1999). Some professional associations are already developing practice guidelines for health care professionals using e-mail (Kane & Sands, 1998).

Health Care Organizations. Health care organizations, from insurance to hospital to pharmaceutical companies, are increasingly replacing more expensive communication channels with access to the Internet. Electronic insurance claims and data from clinical trials or for FDA filings are already being transmitted cost-effectively. Once security regulations are clarified, large claims clearinghouses will also use the capabilities of the Internet.

Challenges to the Future of E-Health

In its ability to combine transactions, information, education, and online communities, the Internet holds great potential for health care. The potential future of health care on the Internet (e-health) is that of maximizing care management remotely and automating it to involve a minimum of human intervention (Dertouzos, 1997). The most significant challenge is to develop incentives and practice solutions for professionals to encourage them to adopt such technologies into their workday routines.

Although there are characteristics of the Internet that will fuel its use in health care, several characteristics will damper its use as well. Whereas patients' use of the Internet for health information is likely to continue growing at a very rapid rate, use of e-mail by health care professionals is likely to proceed more slowly due to the time required by professional associations to develop practice standards for electronic contact with patients.

There will inevitably be increased strain between patients who become increasingly empowered with their newfound information resources and some practitioners who feel a loss of control over their patients' care (Ferguson, 1998; Mittman & Cain, 1999). As practitioners grow accustomed to their lost dominance over patients, they will most likely form collaborative teams with patients and their support systems.

The rapid pace of change in the Internet might outpace the ability of many health care and professional organizations to develop up-to-date practice standards (Cepelewicz, 1998). Practitioners who venture forth and offer services on the Internet through e-mail alone are in danger of being used as fodder for the development of case law regarding e-mail practice, which does not yet exist in many states. For example, the proper use of disclaimers, screening tools, encryption programs, consent forms, and credentialing has not yet been challenged in civil court. Proper use of these devices and agreements is the responsibility of the professional, and case law will develop to clarify the exact lines of responsibility related to each.

Professionals are expressing increasing concern for public safety and protection regarding the Internet related to the variable quality of information, the lack of credentialing and accountability from unlicensed or unqualified practitioners, and the lack of alternatives with respect to consumer protection (Maheu, 1997; Maheu & Gordon, in press; Rusovick & Warner, 1998). Moreover, individuals are showing serious signs of physical and cognitive dysfunction due to the stress imposed by daily use of technology (Murray, 1998; Weil & Rosen, 1997).

Successful development of e-health in the future will force developers of health care applications to acquire a comprehensive understanding of the essential elements of the doctor-patient relationship (Sampson, Kolodinsky, & Greeno, 1997), the role of adjunctive professionals, the proper ownership and handling of the medical record (Waller & Alcantara, 1998), and the roles of health care institutions and third-party carriers. Until these essential elements are identified, the digitization and automation of interactions between these central parties will lag.

Furthermore, health care analysts will need to prove that digitized and electronically transmitted health care lowers utilization and leads to better outcomes. The health care environment, with its focus on cost containment and risk avoidance rather than on long-term patient outcomes, will limit e-health's impact in this regard. New incentives will need to be developed for the health care industry to shift its focus to patient-centered care (Holt, 1997).

Technology fueled by legislation may soon provide such incentives. Channeled by federal legislation such as the Healthcare Information Portability and Accountability Act, as discussed in Chapter Seven, software and hardware developers are envisioning a world in which patients will be protected by such devices as electronic signatures and secured high-speed transmission. The Internet will become a centralized office for many professionals within a few short years. As discussed in Chapter Two, products are already being deployed toward this end both on and off the Internet.

For example, in September 1999, Bill Gates announced the Microsoft product known as Windows Distributed interNet Architecture for Healthcare (Windows DNA for Healthcare), which he described as "an industry architectural 'blueprint' that enables corporate developers and independent software vendors to build and rapidly deploy high-performance applications that support integration, analysis and delivery of information between disparate health-care information systems" (*Microsoft Announces,* 1999).

Many other companies are also in competitive pursuit of the health care market. For example, several companies are developing digital certificates to create the necessary infrastructure that enables organizations to securely exchange patient information. Digital certificates and digital signatures are electronic forms of identification that cannot be forged or altered. When used with the other pieces of an e-commerce system (browsers, servers, and Web applications), digital certificates support digital signatures and the security services—data confidentiality, authentication, authorization, data integrity, and nonrepudiation—needed for functions such as secure exchange of patient records, online scheduling, and secure messaging. The future is likely to bring many improvements in this remarkable technology.

Reimbursement is also an issue. In a recent survey of 249 telemedicine and teleradiology program managers conducted by *Telehealth Magazine* (Dakins, 1999), delays in Medicare reimbursement reform were reported to be one of the main obstacles to telehealth growth. For a small percentage of telehealth programs, legal and regulatory obstacles pose substantial problems and may lead to the discontinuation of their services. The study also found that future growth of telehealth projects is highly dependent on

E-Health, Telehealth, and Telemedicine

whether the program is funded internally or externally. Among managers of internally funded video-based programs, 80 percent stated that they anticipate expansion in the next five years.

Another problem is that health care record-keeping and billing practices have too much overlap and waste and too many standards for electronic communications and transactions. A universal system, though still far in the future, would be one solution for consolidating practices and standards (Mittman & Cain, 1999).

SPECIFIC TECHNOLOGICAL TRENDS

Although predicting the future growth of specific technologies is akin to investing in the stock market, we nevertheless offer you an outline of some of the most promising technologies. As is true of the stock market, the perceived value of these new technologies may easily shift as the global marketplace experiences unexpected twists and turns. Today's predictions of winners can easily become tomorrow's losers. Nevertheless, considering how much each of these areas has developed, their future growth in some form is assured.

Biosensors

Remote care and disease management in the future may utilize biosensors that will be temporarily attached to—or even permanently implanted in—patients to monitor and record vital signs, provide medication reminders and monitor dosages, and alert health care practitioners via a network (typically the Internet) when there is an abnormality. These sensors will lead to better outcomes, with fewer hospital days and increased patient and payer satisfaction (Holt, 1997). One organization paving the way in biosensor development is the U.S. military.

Military Applications. The military is concentrating heavily on developing biosensors for monitoring the position and health status of soldiers (Satava, 1997). They have developed a prototype device that is worn on the wrist.

Called the personal status monitor (PSM), it has a vital sign monitor that includes pulse rate and oxygen saturation and has an EKG attachment. The PSM also can provide the location of the soldier via a geoposition satellite locator. This feature can be of particular benefit if a soldier encounters a health problem, because the PSM transmits an alert signal that includes the soldier's location and vital signs to the closest medic. Ensuring that this information remains in the proper hands is an issue that will obviously need close attention from those who choose to use such technology.

Developments from NASA. Like the U.S. military, the National Aeronautics and Space Administration (NASA) is also leading the way toward developing advanced devices. To accommodate the needs of astronauts in the future, NASA is adapting and developing technology in application-specific biosensors, biotelemetry and noninvasive monitoring, medical informatics, smart medical and environmental sensors, decision support systems, image compression, new teaching aides, holography, and virtual reality ("NASA's Telemedicine Future," 1997). These innovations can provide cost-effective remote, continuous biomedical monitoring of outpatient data to support the range of specialists needed in space. NASA has also expanded the use of these sensors in a telehome care project (*Biomedical Sensors,* 1999).

For example, NASA is involved in a project that provides continuous ambulatory monitoring of the condition of the mother and fetus following in utero surgical repair of life-threatening congenital birth defects. (The surgery is conducted at the Fetal Treatment Center at the University of California, San Francisco.) NASA is helping develop a miniaturized, implantable, fetal health monitoring system (FHMS) to reduce postnatal health care costs (by a factor of ten) and to significantly improve the immediate and long-term health of these infants.

The FHMS can provide continuous data for ambulatory patients during postsurgical recovery lasting two to four weeks. Because the transmission of the data for the FHMS does not require high bandwidth, there are many potential applications of these technologies to telehealth, ranging from fetal surgery to emergency trauma care (*Biomedical Sensors,* 1999).

E-Health, Telehealth, and Telemedicine

Another example of NASA's contributions to telehealth is the focus on measuring physiological status without using invasive procedures. The ability to analyze blood without obtaining a blood sample has tremendous benefit both in space flight and on Earth. It reduces the consumables that need to be taken into orbit and eliminates the need to return samples to Earth for postflight analysis. Similar technology has already begun to benefit environmental sampling ("NASA's Telemedicine Future," 1997).

From Mars to Main Street. As we look out into the future, it is safe to say that many new discoveries in the area of telehealth and telemedicine will be made because of increased planetary exploration in the twenty-first century. For example, humans traveling to Mars will require systems that provide autonomous operation to support the astronauts' every need, including health care.

In one of the most innovative and comprehensive programs launched to date, Sanders and colleagues are working with NASA to develop a self-contained health care delivery system for the Mars probe. With transmission times of up to twenty-two minutes from Mars to the Johnson Space Center, it is impractical to conduct emergency telemedicine. Classic telemedicine, then, is useless for health care delivery in deep space. Sanders and colleagues are therefore developing a computer-driven, multicomponent branched logic and artificial intelligence system to diagnose and treat a wide variety of health conditions aboard spacecraft. The computer system will be able to compare an astronaut's history and symptoms to a large databank of similar histories and signs and symptoms of illness or disease. The physical exam will probably be conducted by a handheld color Doppler ultrasound unit connected to a probe for wired or wireless scanning of the astronaut's body. The computer will compare the scan to a databank of images. The computerized history and physical exam will give a differential diagnosis and identify a therapeutic plan, and medication will be on board to treat the illness.

Surgery will be performed by astronauts trained in surgical simulation procedures; they will work with holographic images of the operative sites as guides. The system will incorporate safety measures, so that any body part incorrectly approached with a scalpel will trigger a warning. The most exciting part of this project is that "everything on that spacecraft will be in doctors' offices within five years. These systems will help set standards for health care where they did not previously exist. For example, we have no hearing standards for physicians who use a stethoscope. This project will help set those standards" (J. Sanders, personal communication, May 29, 2000).

Smart Cards

Smart cards containing an embedded silicon chip that provides medical information in the form of an implantable or wearable device will be perfected in the near future. They hold at least one to eight kilobytes of memory and include a microprocessor, which contains an operating system permanently written to ROM (read-only memory). The card is referred to as "smart" because its silicon chip is able to securely store and process various types of information, from images to personal data. Compared to magnetic stripe cards, smart cards are more reliable, can store up to a hundred or more times the information, and are more secure due to advanced encryption and biometrics.

Smart cards are enhancing security in many different areas by providing digital authentication for access control, both physical (facilities, hardware) and logical (networks, intranets), and by making verification protocols faster, more rigorous, and more convenient. Digital certificates stored on a card support public-key cryptography, making digital signing and encryption of electronic documents and mail a simple operation. Smart card systems with multiple applications may have several layers of security, secret passwords, and data encryption keys. Each data area on the card can also be protected with independent security passwords and encryption processes.

Smart cards can serve many different functions and contain important medical and other data on one card—for example, one's name, date of birth, social security number, as well as immunization record, drug allergies, current medications, or dental history. The health care industry will be able to utilize smart cards to speed and improve medical services, expedite insurance claims, and provide medical histories in emergencies.

The military is beginning to use smart cards to record training certification and replace dog tags.

Virtual Reality

The application of virtual reality (VR) in medicine has the potential to refine many different areas of telehealth, including telepresence surgery, three-dimensional (3-D) visualization of anatomy for medical education, surgical simulators, complex medical database visualization, rehabilitation, and virtual prototyping of surgical equipment and operating rooms.

Rehabilitation medicine made possible through VR allows individuals with impairments to experience lost sensations, facilitates accurate assessment and therapy, and helps specialists plan personal living space for easier access. The operating room and hospital of the future can be initially designed and tested in VR before physical construction (Satava, 1995a, 1995b).

Advanced technology such as VR will help better manage rehabilitation projects that involve telemonitoring. For example, the Rehabilitation Engineering Research Center is evaluating the use of passive data sensors placed throughout a patient's home to monitor daily activities such as how many times he or she opens the refrigerator or uses a closet. The information is then fed back into a computer database that analyzes the results so that the therapist can better manage the rehabilitation process (Kincade, 1999).

In the future, VR will have a great impact on the teaching and training of surgeons. It can teach surgeons complicated medical procedures and determine their level of surgical competence before they operate on real patients (Ota, Loftin, Saito, Lea, & Keller, 1995). VR also allows an intern or medical student to repeat the same procedure several times, which reduces the need for expensive animal training models. It should be noted, however, that the use of VR in the future may lead to a reduction in Medicare reimbursement to teaching hospitals (Akay, 1996).

VR psychotherapy is also proving to be useful for such psychological disorders as panic disorder, agoraphobia, and a wide range of phobias, including the fear of flying. At the California School of Professional Psychology in San Diego, Brenda Wiederhold combines real-time physiological monitoring with VR graded exposure therapy at one of the five VR sites operating in the United States. The equipment includes a head-mounted display that immerses the patient in a simulated situation on a commercial aircraft. Patients are guided through a variety of flying situations from takeoff to landing, all in a controlled environment. In the future, the application of VR systems will offer new opportunities for practitioners and patients to simulate real-life situations in a controlled and safe environment.

Other VR applications include plastic surgery, allowing medical students to practice procedures on virtual cadavers ("Plastic Surgery," 1997). The "virtual embryo" and 3-D visualization of the fetus are also possible with the use of VR technology (Akay, 1996).

A good example of a VR system that may become standard in the future is the Green Telepresence Surgery System. It consists of two components: the surgical workstation (a 3-D monitor that handles with haptic, or force, feedback) and the remote work site (a 3-D camera system and responsive manipulators with sensory input). Practitioners use this system to get a different perspective on anatomy by using a helmet-mounted display and DataGlove to "fly" inside and around different organs, using 3-D visualization (Satava, 1995a, 1995b).

Telesurgery

In the field of surgery, telehealth is used for medical education, diagnostic or therapeutic assistance, and consultations with remote patients (Sezeur, 1998). Telesurgery can also include a scenario in which a surgeon at a primary operating site consults with a colleague when he or she encounters complex or unexpected problems during surgery (Cheriff, Schulam, Docimo, Moore, & Kavoussi, 1996). Future possibilities for this area of telehealth include the use of remote robotic arms that are able to perform precise surgical procedures directed by a practitioner from a distant site.

Telesurgery data and information requirements are much higher than other applications of telehealth. Telesurgery requires a network with high reliability, an acceptable transmission delay, the ability to transfer vast amounts of data, and low data error rates (Smithwick, 1995). Fortunately, telecommunication technology is advancing at an exponential rate, and with the development of both satellite and inexpensive land-based broadband capabilities, the future of telesurgery is very promising.

The military is also experimenting with telesurgery to intervene quickly on the battlefield to reduce the morbidity that occurs when there are delays in operative intervention. An intuitive telemanipulator system that would allow surgeons to remotely treat injured patients could improve the outcome of soldiers suffering from severe injuries.

Bowersox, Cordts, and La Porta (1998) evaluated a prototype of a four-degrees-of-freedom telesurgery system that gives a surgeon a stereoscopic video display of a remote operative field. Using robotic manipulators, the surgeon can precisely control surgical instruments at the remote site. Surgeons were able to use the system to perform successful organ excision, hemorrhage control, and knot tying on anesthetized swine, thus demonstrating the feasibility of performing standard surgical procedures remotely. Because the times required for complex manipulations were often long, the system would not be capable of supporting resuscitative surgery or of playing a role in early trauma management; the researchers concluded that the system may be a unique research tool for acquiring basic knowledge of operative surgery.

An important limiting factor for telesurgery is the vestibulo-ocular disruption known as simulator sickness. This results from the lag time in transmission between the sending and receiving sites, and occurs when the receiving operator is wearing a head-mounted VR display. Over 50 percent of VR system users experience dizziness, nausea, or headaches within twenty minutes of donning VR headgear. Simulator sickness is minimized when images are sent over high bandwidths with little compression (Allen, Bowersox, & Jones, 1997).

The future of telesurgery may involve the use of robotic assistants to replace human assistants. The main motivator behind the idea is that robotic assistants can be cost-effective and can deliver telesurgery services over distance. Turner (1996) evaluated twelve patients undergoing laparoscopic bladder neck suspension. Six of the procedures used a human assistant, another six used a robot arm to hold and maneuver the laparoscope and camera. In each case, use of the robot arm improved steadiness and the clarity of the picture compared to use of a human arm.

Overall, the cost of the robotic arm was less than that of human assistants, but this depends on the volume of surgery and may vary between institutions. Other findings confirm these results and mention further benefits, such as reduced time for surgeries.

CONCLUSION

Computers and communications technologies are changing the nature of American life as we know it. They will soon make specialty expertise available whenever and wherever needed. Patient information will be available not only for patients when they are assessed but also as part of electronic records that are available immediately and at any time.

Technology influences behavior. As technologies become more powerful, accessible, and affordable, their impact on patients and practitioners must be assessed. Much further study is needed to examine the relationship between people and technology before the health care industry can confidently assert its place in the world of telehealth.

As we glimpse the future, we can only hope that professionals worldwide will actively and responsibly embrace the potential of this technology. Professionals need to be involved in its evolution, with patient care in the forefront of all decision making. Despite the planning and funding issues, the legal and regulatory challenges, the ethical entanglements, and the reimbursement struggles, telehealth is becoming part of the way health care is delivered.

E-health, telemedicine, and telehealth are here to stay. Just as every physician must know about x-rays and what they can contribute to health care, it is time now that every clinician learn about the contribution that telecommunication technologies can make to their care of patients, to their education, and to patient self-care. To do less will deny them and their patients the benefits of higher efficiency and faster, better access to care and information.

Tips from the Experts

I n the course of conducting research, we spoke with dozens of telemedicine professionals to discuss the information they felt should be included in this book. They universally commented that telemedicine books rarely provide any space for input from the other professionals in the field. In response to these comments, we posed several questions to top managers working in e-health, telehealth, and telemedicine. Their responses have been interspersed throughout the book as case extracts, but some comments remained. This appendix serves as a forum for the remainder of their unique insight and expertise.

Robert Cox, M.D., Hays Medical Center, Kansas

Vice President Gore, in a Washington, D.C., hotel, was visiting over POTS with an eighty-year-old woman in her home in our community. They were connected by both audio and video. The vice president said, "It would be nice to have this type of technology for people like my parents on the family ranch in Tennessee." My response was, "Expansion of this technology will be difficult since Medicare doesn't pay for it." As he left the demonstration, the vice president responded, "That's wrong. . . . We'll fix it" (personal communication, November 16, 1999).

Sally Davis, Program Director of Telehealth and Management Development, Marquette General Hospital, Marquette, Michigan

- For us it has been the specialists at the regional referral center, not the end-site rural practitioners, who have initiated the clinical consults.

- Telehealth does not exist in a vacuum. Successful telehealth programming requires a meld of various services within the organization: information technology, education, community relations, program directors, practitioners, and, of course, a supportive administration.
- The connectivity of independent hospitals and other health care partners has greatly improved in our region. This area of Michigan has worked hard to build cooperative health care networks, and these networks have used videoconferencing extensively. We began with a focus on professional education but soon realized the benefits of the system for administrative purposes. The image of our regional referral hospital and of the smaller health care organizations in our network has benefited. Because the technology is present within our organizations, and because we make it available to community groups, we are seen as being current with technology.
- Telehealth has a global effect on organizations. Every department and every service has the potential to use the technology to improve some component of business or patient care. It's up to the leaders of the department to maximize its use.
- When I have a chance to sit in on a clinical application and see that it really works and that the patient is getting better care because of something I influenced, all the work has definitely been worth it.
- The other thing that has been fun is watching the paradigm shift in our organization. When we started, it was something that people were afraid of or hesitant to use. At that time we had only one system at our main campus. Now when I walk down the halls of our conference center, I can pass one room where a videoconferenced in-service is going on, the next room has a videoconference meeting going, and I know there's a patient telemedicine consult happening in another area of the hospital later that day; then the room scheduler comes up to me and says she's getting heat from three different groups because there isn't a system available when they want one. Videoconferencing has become the norm for our health

care system and the other health care systems in our network. This paradigm shift also strikes me when I'm at a meeting and one of the participants will correct someone else on their video etiquette or will pick up the keypad, dial in, and start moving the camera around. They don't need a telehealth staff person around anymore. That's when I like to think back to the early days and compare them to where we are now (personal communication, May 30, 2000).

Warren B. Karp, Ph.D., D.M.D., Coordinator of Telemedicine and Distance Learning Activities, Department of Pediatrics, Medical College of Georgia

Facilitating change in people can be frustrating, unless you take a long-range view. I would say that, overall, telehealth has been very rewarding. It has allowed us to create windows into people's natural environments to observe functional outcomes, so that we are not limited to observing clinical outcomes in a hospital. If you view telehealth as an evolving behavior, you can cut down frustration levels. Although there are "early enablers" of technology, most people require time and behavior modeling to adopt new technology. Allow individuals to adapt to the technology at the pace that is comfortable for them. If one steps back and takes an overall view of the process, it is more rewarding (personal communication, November 15, 1999).

Steven W. Strode, M.D., University of Arkansas for Medical Sciences

Although the interactive television network serves credit course education, continuing education, education for the public on health matters, and teleconferencing, the campus has stressed the potential and actual value of clinical telemedicine services. The single surviving statewide newspaper sent their health reporter, who spent half a day on campus and traveled two hours each way to visit a remote site to discuss the clinical uses. This was very early in our use of the network for actual cases (although we had run a few simulated cases to "shake down the system").

When the story appeared on the front page of the newspaper, the reporter or her editor had creatively taken the entire cost of the network and divided it by the (incorrectly calculated) number of true clinical cases we had performed. The headline screamed that the network was costing the taxpayers one-eighth of a million dollars per case. My picture appeared on the back page of the first section in the article's continuation.

The next day there was a flurry of crisis meetings with the chancellor and dean. The campus PR experts said that contact with the media was always a gamble, that about four times out of ten they distort the story to sensationalize it, but that you are likely to "win" the other six times.

I decided that the best test was what people said in church three days later. There were at least two to three times as many who complimented me on the picture and story compared to those who understood that this was a slam against the program and me personally. I decided that the influence of the press was greatly overrated (at least by me), although I would love to run whenever the local media snoops around again.

When I think of satisfying telemedicine moments, these come to mind:

- Early in the program, an elderly cancer patient was able to cancel a painful three-hour drive to the medical center for wound care because the cancer specialists looked at him over interactive television.
- Within a week after Dr. Waner, one of our ENT faculty, was on the cover of *U.S. News and World Report* with a story on his use of lasers to treat birthmarks, we got a request from Israel for him to evaluate a child there for treatment. Dr. Waner had never seen our equipment before (although this is becoming more rare on our campus). The equipment worked, and the child was set up for treatment when Dr. Waner traveled to Israel for a meeting a month later.

E-Health, Telehealth, and Telemedicine

- A chest x-ray of a newborn with suspected pneumothorax was evaluated by a pediatric radiologist and neonatologist, and the baby did not need to be airlifted here.
- Any time I am working with our picture phones, I just remind myself that although these are primitive, the future will likely use regular telephone lines and special phones or PCs. Someday, the technology will be reliable, cheap, widespread, and not dependent on the whims of the telephone companies.
- It is always satisfying whenever I hear that another insurance company has paid the first telemedicine claim our campus submitted to it (personal communication, November 12, 1999).

Rosa Ana Tang, M.D., M.P.H., Professor of Ophthalmology, University of Texas Medical Branch, Galveston

I was asked to see a lady who had a brain tumor that had been radiated several years back when she was in Arequipa, Peru. She was ready to be sent to Miami to be treated with a new modality of radiation called the gamma knife.

Her church had taken several months to raise the $30,000 necessary for her trip and treatment at a discounted rate. Using a 384 Kbps ISDN connection, I examined the patient online and reviewed all of her x-rays from Lima, Peru, where I was visiting. I immediately called in my neurosurgery professor and a neurologist colleague, and the three of us agreed that the patient's problems were related to having had excessive radiation; there was no need to give her more radiation, but also there was no tumor left. We spared her the trip and its costs and sent her for physical therapy instead.

Two years later when I connected with her physicians, they told me she was learning to walk again, and the x-rays had not shown any progression for two years. This event made me feel I had made a difference, thanks to the availability of telemedicine (personal communication, November 11, 1999).

**James Reid, P.A.-C., Director, Midwest Rural
Telemedicine Consortium, Des Moines, Iowa**

Years ago, early in my telemedicine career, I remember being totally enthralled by telemedicine technology. Even as a clinician who had spent ten years focused on caring for patients, I found it easy to become distracted by all the cool capabilities of the technology and to forget what we were really trying to accomplish. One day, an encounter with a patient and her family quickly brought me back to reality and left me with an indelible memory that reminds me why I became involved in telemedicine.

A mother of two, in her late twenties and residing in a rural community in eastern Montana, developed a severe case of depression that required hospitalization. She was transferred to the nearest inpatient psychiatric unit, 150 miles away in Billings. Because the father was not a part of the family, her two children, a girl age six and a boy age four, were placed in a foster home. After about a week the children began to ask questions about the whereabouts and well-being of their mother. The foster father was also the director of the local mental health center, which had just joined our telemedicine network. Inspired by the desire to help these children understand their situation, he recognized that a videoconference between the children and their mother could potentially benefit them all. He scheduled the videoconference between his rural mental health center and our urban hospital telemedicine studio for the next day.

At the appointed hour, the mother and the children were brought to their respective telemedicine rooms, the connection was established, and the magic began to happen. First the children told their mother they loved her and that they missed her. Then, as they all grew more comfortable with seeing each other on the TV, the children began to play hide and seek, encouraging the mother to remotely search the room with the camera to find them. They played games, teased, and showed obvious love for each other. When it was time to close the session, the children again told their mother of their love for her and asked her to "come home soon."

I watched their interaction through our observation window and heard their conversation on our monitor. It was then, as tears traced a tortuous path down my cheeks, that I realized beyond any previous doubt why I was so enthralled by telemedicine. The allure of telemedicine for me was not then, and is not now, because it is glitzy—although it is. It is not because telemedicine uses cool, leading-edge technologies to expand the boundaries of your imagination—although it does. It is the potential of telemedicine to touch people's lives in meaningful ways that grabs me. That interaction was not just about a mother visiting with her children, although that would have been enough. Given the circumstances, nothing could have better motivated the mother to follow her treatment regimen and the path to recovery. The gentle reminder of her responsibility to her children afforded by that videoconference was therapeutic. It was perhaps as therapeutic as anything else we could do for her in the hospital.

I saw the impact then, and I still see it today. When periodically bogged down in the day-to-day challenges of implementing telemedicine, I take myself back to that early experience, remind myself that we are doing this for the patients, and then carry on with passion (personal communication, October 5, 1999).

Peter Yellowlees, M.D., Department of Psychiatry
Royal Brisbane Hospital, Australia

My main reward from telemedicine has been the knowledge that patients can be treated effectively now who were not treated effectively in the past. When I talk about telemedicine, I include all forms of electronic technology, particularly the Internet; I know that patients find the Internet especially important to them. I was on a national radio program with a talkback component, and it was extraordinarily rewarding to hear of the very positive experiences that patients have had through being *information empowered,* via the use of these technologies.

The other reason I am pleased to have been involved in telemedicine is that I feel now that these systems are truly on the verge of being integrated into the normal health care environment and will no longer be "special" in the future. All these technologies are simply tools to assist clinicians like me provide the highest possible care, and access to care, for our patients, and it is great that they are being fully integrated and increasingly used as such nowadays (personal communication, February 10, 2000).

Vendor Agreements: A Primer

Many health care professionals enter into contracts with vendors, only to learn that they needed to have their agreements reviewed by an attorney or, at the very least, needed to consider some basic principles in the negotiation process. This appendix is intended to help you make better choices when negotiating contracts for products and services.

Suggestions for Agreements

Many buyers neglect to review agreements, but doing so could be the most important step in acquiring new products and services from vendors. Experienced vendors may have hidden costs and unclear terminology written into the agreement, which could lead to wasted time and money.

There are usually three parts to the agreement: the master agreement, the license agreement, and the maintenance agreement. There may also be a development agreement, depending on whether you need programming or a custom design. Be sure that all parts of the agreement use specific and clearly defined terms.

The *master agreement* should include a number of terms, such as the goals of the company or program; interface guarantees; the capabilities required; all fees (including update and maintenance costs); frequency of contact between the two parties (daily or weekly updates on services rendered); proof-of-installation documentation; and access rights (for both parties). The *license agreement* should state the duration of the software license, the number of allowed users (for partners and alternative locations of the company or program), and permission to use or incorporate third-party software. The *maintenance agreement* should define all fees for maintenance and upgrades and set out the response guarantees for these services and for system malfunctions.

Each company or program should take into account the following criteria when negotiating the contract with the vendor (Fisher & Singh, 2000):

- The vendor is clear with respect to services required and the timeline in which these services will be delivered.
- The vendor guarantees to ensure proper functioning of the products or service.
- The agreement includes protection for unforeseen cost overrun.
- Prices are guaranteed for continued upgrades, support, and services.
- Legal requirements of third-party regulatory bodies, including HIPAA standards for privacy, security, and confidentiality of patient information, are met for the transmission of all sensitive information.

Vendor Options

As is true of all other services, companies, or vendors mentioned in this text, we have included these examples to acquaint you with capabilities and coverage; they are not intended to be endorsements.

- Confer.com offers software to optimize wellness and disease, case, and utilization management. It allows payers, providers, suppliers, and consumers to communicate seamlessly. Installation takes four months or longer, depending on the services requested. The company can consult, train, implement, and support a telemedicine or e-health program.

- Teraglobal.com has created a nationwide virtual private network using ATM technology.

- WilliamsComunication.com runs a fiber-optic network through which communications service providers and other businesses can obtain voice, data, Internet, and video services. It will install and maintain each product, and offers many types of security, videoconferencing, and information transportation systems.

- Webex.com offers teleconferencing and interactive multimedia services along with a virtual office that handles sales, marketing, and customer support services. The company's focus is on small businesses and requires only minimal computer hardware to use its services.

- Webcasting.com was originally created to host Internet projects for radio stations in the Dallas area, but this vendor soon expanded in response to a market demand for blending media and broadcasting. Some of the products and services currently offered are multimedia and corporate communications, audio- and videostreaming, and CD-ROM content.

- Videoscape.com allows customers to switch from the "one dimension" of traditional communications to videostreaming, data streaming, and Webcasting through the Internet. The company offers a twenty-four-hour subscription center, allowing the customer to purchase the desired service only when needed. It has a professional video production team that can help in all phases of the presentation production, from creating a presentation to editing the final version.

- Videogate.com has three main services. First, their VideoGateway provides a range of communications options, such as live video or Internet chat rooms. Second, the call request manager acts as a switchboard to globally connect any customer and representative through the desired medium. Third, the call center agent will connect the desired parties with the same information on both of their monitors, and allow interactivity for both parties.

Videoconferencing Room Requirements and Etiquette

VIDEOCONFERENCING ROOM REQUIREMENTS

Although equipment constitutes a significant portion of the start-up budget, you will also need to focus on the physical aspects of the site. The designing of a telehealth site involves many considerations that often require an outside consultant. The amount of attention you pay to room design can depend on the amount of time each business foresees using the room. Larger businesses, or businesses with employees in noncentralized locations, should devote more time to the preparation of this room. For many smaller businesses, placing portable equipment in any available room will do. Some businesses may find it more desirable to implement some type of portable or mobile system that would enable consultations to take place from multiple business sites; this approach reduces interruptions of work routines (Siden, 1998) and decreases access problems.

In clinic settings, a design that is consistent among videoconference rooms will help participants feel more comfortable and enable patients to feel as though they are in the same room with the clinician. This promotes a sense of closeness and privacy and removes the room as a variable in the health care exchange. A reasonable amount of money should be spent to ensure the comfort of patients and providers.

Room Location and Size

In a large-scale clinic, the location and physical attributes of the videoconference room are also important (assuming that voice and video are not yet available to every practitioner's desktop). A poorly chosen location for the video room can lead to scheduling problems and other frustrations. Consider the following factors when choosing a room.

The video room should be convenient to those who will be using it. It should allow unobstructed patient flow, especially in emergency consult situations. Bringing an unstable patient into a distant room can be awkward, if not dangerous. The videoconferencing room at both the remote and consulting sites must also be convenient for the medical practitioners, because if it is not, practitioners typically default to the desktop telephone for making many contacts that might be better served by videoconferencing (IOM, 1996). Telehealth technology allows the patient to be in a hospital bed or remote clinic or home while the practitioner remains in his or her own office.

The room should be in a central location in the facility and have extra room for program expansion. It should be in a location where it does not interfere with other clinical operations and is not exposed to excessive outside noise, such as adjoining stairwells, elevator shafts, emergency entrances, or—yes—flushing toilets in an adjoining restroom. Windows may also cause acoustical problems. Phone lines and fax machines should be easily accessible, and there must be a main source of power in the room. It is a good idea to have backups of each.

The room needs to be large enough for the technology being implemented and have room for additional equipment should it need to be brought in. It also must have adequate space for the personnel and patients using it.

Equipment Configuration

The arrangement of monitors, speakers, cameras, and microphones depends on the users' needs and on the physical layout of the room (Collins, 1996). Some telehealth clinicians using videoconferencing technology wish to work off the same documents and images, using digital whiteboarding. This feature may increase the sense of communication, as all participants can contribute to the interaction. One popular equipment configuration is to have the presentation camera mounted on the right wall so that it can focus on the presenter, the whiteboard, or a flip chart. It needs to be perpendicular to, and no more than twenty feet from, the whiteboard, which is used primarily for presentations. In most cases, the whiteboard should be positioned at an angle, to reduce glare and shadowing (Hodges, 1997).

Lighting

Proper lighting is crucial to telehealth applications. A high-quality camera cannot fully compensate for poor lighting, but excellent lighting can make a $100 video camera perform like a $10,000 broadcast-quality camera! If lighting is inadequate, the speaker's image may be blurred or darkened. Poor lighting can also accentuate light colors and create dark shadows under participant's eyes. Direct and indirect lighting must be designed to produce minimal shadows and ensure even illumination of people and objects in videoconferencing. The following are some tips:

• Each application requires different lighting. For example, lighting requirements for teleradiology will be different than for teledermatology. Experiment to find the optimal lighting for your specialty application.

• Position lighting behind the camera so that it shines directly on the subject.

• Avoid using a dark background. If the background creates too strong a contrast with the lighted images, the camera is unable to adjust its iris properly and may cause objects to appear out of focus.

• Glare from normal room lights can reduce the sharpness of the images displayed on the monitor. Experiment by turning room lights on and off to determine the best possible combination for your room.

• Avoid lighting that is too harsh or that is aimed directly at the eyes; participants may become uncomfortable or look distressed to the remote viewer, who will not necessarily know that a bright light is the cause.

Camera Specifications and Considerations

If your technology allows them, picture-in-picture (PIP) settings are recommended; this lets users see themselves and thereby realize when only half their face or body is on camera. If the transmitting site has a camera with far-end control, users are able to pan, tilt, and zoom the camera at the other end—all without any noise. Cameras with far-end control can zoom (change the focal length or width of view, move from close up to a longer view), focus, adjust exposure, pan (move left and right), and tilt (move up and down), but noisy camera movements can upset clients. Some cameras allow control from both local and remote locations. Having local camera control also enables users to switch among other video sources (in other words, documents, slides, or overhead projectors). Some videoconferencing arrangements allow a user to be viewed with two or more cameras simultaneously.

Motion Handling

A codec (from *coder-decoder*) is the core technology used for digital videoconferencing. Codecs convert analog audio and video signals to digital signals and compress them on the sending end. Codecs at the receiving end reverse this process. Frame rates determine how often images are refreshed, with faster refresh rates yielding more lifelike images. The standard frame rate (measured in frames per second, or fps) for television broadcasting is either 25 fps (PAL) or 30 fps (NTSC). This rate is fast enough to portray smooth, lifelike motion. The standard for an adequate frame rate for videoconferencing used to be approximately 15 fps. However, a number of projects (for example, Penn State University, the University of Kentucky, Kaiser Permanente, and the University of Kansas) are successfully using POTS-based solutions for some applications that transmit at a rate of 7 to 10 fps. At this speed, however, video quality can be marred by noticeable and potentially distracting pauses (Hawkins, 1997).

ISDN and LAN connections can handle much higher frame rates. ISDN- and LAN-based systems can support multipoint meetings with three or more parties, each appearing in their own video windows in a videoconferencing application (in "Hollywood Squares" configuration).

These systems also allow data sharing; for example, one person can launch an application, and both parties can work on a file via the videoconferencing connection. When more than two locations are involved in a videoconference, a multipoint control unit (MCU) is needed so that each member can participate in the conference simultaneously. MCUs are expensive. Most organizations will buy MCU services, otherwise known as videoconferencing bridge services, from a telecommunication service provider.

Audio

Successful telecommunication can occur only if the audio is coming through loud and clear. Audio is far more important than video in conveying information, yet too often it does not receive the priority attention it should. Poor video quality is much more tolerated by humans than poor audio quality. Too much background noise, room reverberation, or noise reflection can produce poor audio quality.

The quality of audio is dependent on the proper placement of the microphone and on room acoustics. Existing rooms can be modified with acoustical wall coverings and furniture that absorb sound. Hands-free devices, such as telephone headsets or speakerphones, are more natural than handsets and most readily enable face-to-face interactions.

With regard to audio input, there are three important considerations: (1) use of full-duplex versus half-duplex audio, (2) audio delays due to inadequate bandwidth, and (3) microphone characteristics and placement. We look at these considerations in the next paragraphs.

Full-duplex audio allows simultaneous transmission of audio communication from all users. It is more natural and is preferable to half-duplex audio, which allows only one side of the audio communication to be heard at any time. This results in clipped, rather unnatural audio exchanges. Communication through this form of audio transmission relies on taking turns. Walkie-talkies are a good example of half-duplex communications.

Audio delay is caused by bandwidth limitations. In our public telephone system, transmission delay is rarely more than 20 to 30 milliseconds (msec), whereas delay in an ISDN, a low- to medium-speed technology for digital telephony, is about 10 msec. Satellite links, often an expensive solution for two-way communication, add a 260 msec (quarter-second) delay due to the enormous distances a signal must travel.

In a video call, in contrast, the most important cause of delayed transmission is the video compression. All video compression techniques require processing time to perform their function. The more the compression, the more processing time it takes. Even though the compression and digitization of the audio channel only requires a few thousandths of a second, the typical delay in video compression is 200 to 400 msec (the exact length depending on the algorithm used and the amount of compression). Audio that precedes video by more than 100 msec will create the experience of watching a dubbed movie, in which lip motion and language are not synchronized. This can adversely affect the user's experience. Most manufacturers of video compression equipment assess the average delay incurred by video processing and attempt to offset it by artificially delaying the audio channel, thereby more closely synchronizing the image and the sound.

Microphone placement must take the size and dimensions of the room into account. Positioning microphones in various places around the room (ceiling, conference table, and wall) optimizes adequate audio pickup. In a tele-education environment, the "three-to-one" rule is often applied: the distance between microphones should be at least three times the distance from each microphone to the nearest person. Thus, if microphones are located one foot in front of each participant, they should be at least three feet apart from each other. Microphones placed too close to one another or too far away from the speaker may cause the screeching and yowling of feedback (Collins, 1996). Multiple microphones create a stereo effect that localizes each individual speaker around a conference table. The directionality of the microphone (omnidirectional versus unidirectional) is also important for ensuring that the speaker's voice energy is captured while also minimizing unwanted energy or noise.

Other microphone options that may have an effect on videoconferenced consultations include the use of specialized noise-canceling microphones, directional sound, lavaliere microphones, and multidirectional microphones (Collins, 1996).

VIDEOCONFERENCING ETIQUETTE

Improper etiquette while conducting a videoconference can lead to distraction, confusion, and annoyance. The points we discuss here are meant to ensure that the focus of the conference is on the speaker.

Distractions. Pay close attention to mannerisms of the face, hands, and torso. These can be annoying in a face-to-face encounter, and they may be much more so within the constricted image frame of a video monitor. Also be aware that when the practitioner is writing or taking notes, the patient will only see the top of his or her head.

Physical appearance and clothing. Stripes, whites or blacks, high-contrast colors, or prints that are too "busy" can cause low image quality. Yellows and oranges tend to "bleed." Darker, solid colors are best suited to videoconferencing. Dangling earrings and other ornaments can be very distracting on a small monitor.

Movement. Avoid rapid movement. Movement appears differently on various types of technology. Transmission at higher compression and lower bandwidths yields a lot of motion artifacts, which can be serious distractions (Hodges, 1997).

Body language and position. The user can fill up the screen and look overwhelming to the viewer. Avoid this by checking the self-view feature of the videoconferencing system. The user can, however, make therapeutic use of the camera in this way, appearing bigger on the screen to make a point. Many cameras can also freeze frames and capture still shots, so inappropriate scratching or engaging in an odd-looking activity can be captured as a picture for later use—or misuse.

GLOSSARY

Access control   The prevention of unauthorized access to information through the use of policies or software that determine who can have access to what data contained on a computer *network* (both within and outside the organization).

American National Standards Institute (ANSI)   A private, nonprofit organization that administers and coordinates standardization in the U.S. private sector. ANSI seeks to enhance the competitiveness of U.S. businesses in the global market and promote the American way of life by organizing voluntary consensus standards, promoting U.S. business integrity, and facilitating conformity assessment systems.

Analog   Describing wave-shaped electrical signals that continuously change size and shape depending on the information being transmitted. Signal variations lead to differences in volume, voice, and pitch.

Asynchronous   Describing a communication system, such as e-mail, in which there is a lapse between the time a message is sent and the time it is received.

Asynchronous transfer mode (ATM)   A data transmission technology in which a start signal precedes each data *packet,* and one or more stop signals follow it. These individual *packets* of information are easily prioritized and routed, which enables the seamless integration of audio, video, and data. ATM also denotes the complete system of *protocols* and equipment associated with *packet*-based communication *networks.*

Audioconferencing   Two-way remote voice communication among multiple individuals.

Audit trail   A comprehensive or selective method of monitoring every operation an individual performs on information.

Authentication   A method of verifying the identity of the individual sending or receiving information by use of passwords, *biometrics,* keys, digital or *electronic signatures,* and other automated identifiers.

Backbone network   A high-speed, high-capacity transmission facility that interconnects lower-speed distribution channels from smaller branches of the computer or *telecommunication network.*

Bandwidth   The measure of a communication channel's range of frequencies that a signal occupies. Generally, higher bandwidth carries information faster than lower bandwidth. In an *analog* transmission, the speed of information transfer increases in terms of megahertz (cycles per second); in digital transmissions, speed is measured in megabits per second *(Mbps).*

Biometrics   The scientific measurement and analysis of human biological data using technology. A common application of biometrics is identity *authentication* performed by verifying retinal or iris scans, fingerprint patterns, DNA sequence characteristics, or voice patterns.

Bit   A binary digit, the basic unit of data used by computers for information storage, transmission, and entry. Represented as off or on by the digits 0 or 1 and grouped into strings of eight bits known as *bytes,* these units take the place of numbers, letters, and symbols in electronic media.

Bit depth   The number of colors or *pixels* of gray supported by a monitor or scanner. Also known as *bit resolution* or *pixel depth.*

Broadband   Describing *telecommunication* over a single medium that provides multiple channels of data for high-speed transmission. Also applied to the higher *bandwidth* that will support real-time, full-motion *audioconferencing* and *videoconferencing.*

Browser   Program that runs on a client's computer and communicates with *Internet* Web servers by connecting to Web sites and sending information to enable interaction.

Charge-coupled device (CCD) A device that converts light into electronic information via sensors that collect light as a buildup of electrical charge. The signal that results from this conversion can be translated into computer code to form an image. This device is commonly used in television cameras, digital still-image cameras, and image scanners.

Chat room An *Internet* site or virtual community that provides real-time communication via the exchange of text messages (as well as sound and video files) between participants.

Click stream data Information used by Web advertisers showing the number of Web page visits or clicks of the mouse by a consumer visiting a Web site.

Coaxial cable A single or dual transmission wire that accommodates high *bandwidth.* Cable is used to transmit *broadband* data, voice, and video.

Codec Coder-decoder. *Hardware* or software (or both) that converts an *analog* video signal to digital, then compresses it. At the receiving end, the signal is decompressed and converted back to *analog* output by a *compatible* codec.

Compatible Describing the ability of *hardware,* software, and data to work together without data loss, changes, or other manipulations. Standards-based specifications of procedures, equipment interfaces, and data formats are essential for minimizing incompatibility.

Compressed video Video images that have been compressed to reduce the amount of *bandwidth* needed to transmit information. They can then be sent over less expensive transmission media (land-based T-1 lines rather than via satellite, *POTS* lines rather than ISDN, and so on).

Compression See *data compression.*

Computed radiography (CR) A system of creating digital radiographic images that uses a storage phosphor plate in a cassette. A laser beam scans the plate after it is exposed, producing a *digital image.*

Confidentiality   In the computer world, limiting the disclosure of privileged information by using authorization *protocols* to protect that information against theft or improper use. Confidentiality of patient records and communications is both a legal and an ethical requirement for health care professionals.

CPRI   Computer-Based Patient Record Institute, Inc., an independent institute that develops and recommends standards for computerized patient records.

Cryptopgraphy   Keeping data secret through the use of mathematical or logical functions that transform intelligible data into unintelligible data and back again.

Data compression   A technique designed to remove all extraneous characters and reduce data volume, thereby reducing image processing demands, transmission times, *bandwidth* requirements, and storage space requirements. Some compression techniques result in the loss of some information, which may or may not be clinically important, depending on the specific telehealth application.

Dedicated   Describing a permanent telephone or data line that is reserved exclusively for one specific purpose. Dedicated lines are usually digital and are also referred to as *leased* or *private lines.*

DICOM   Digital Imaging and Communications in Medicine. A set of protocols describing how radiological images are formatted and transferred from *point-to-point* digital medical imaging devices. DICOM was developed by the American College of Radiology and the National Electronic Manufacturers Association (ACR/NEMA).

Digital image   An image formed by independent *pixels,* each of which is distinguished by a digitally represented *luminance* level.

Digitization   The conversion of *analog* information into digital information. Digital signals transmit audio, video, and data coded as *bits.* Digital technology facilitates *data compression,* and digital signals are less susceptible to interference than *analog* technology.

Downlink   The transmission of data from a *satellite* to a receiver on the ground.

Duplex   Allowing *telecommunication* in opposite directions. Full-duplex communication channels can transmit data, audio, or video simultaneously; half-duplex channels can transmit in only one direction at a time.

Electronic signature   The attachment of specific codes to an electronic document for purposes of *authentication.* The *authentication* process may make use of such technologies as passwords, *cryptography,* and *biometrics.*

Encryption   A system of encoding data whereby the information can be transmitted, retrieved, and decoded only by the intended recipient, who holds the "key" to interpreting the message.

Fiber optics   Technology employing an insulated cable with a glass core; it relies on light pulses rather than electricity to transmit audio, video, and data signals at very high speeds (90 to 150 *Mbps*) with low error rates.

Firewall   Computer *hardware* and software designed to prevent internal and external unauthorized access between computer *networks.*

Frame rate   The number of frames per second (fps) displayed on a video monitor. Full-motion video is set at 25 to 30 fps. A frame rate of 15 fps or less is noticeably jerky and may be inadequate for some types of telehealth applications.

Geostationary   Describing the orbit of a *satellite* whose location relative to the earth's surface is constant, so that the *satellite* seems to hover over one spot.

Hardware   All physical equipment related to information technology, including the computers, *peripheral* devices (printers, disks, scanners, and so on), cables, switches, and other components of the *telecommunication* infrastructure.

Hub A single point of connection between workstations and other devices, enabling cost-effective *telecommunication* connections with remote sites.

Information technology (IT) Using various technologies for the storage, manipulation, networking, and communication of information in audio, data, and video formats.

Informed consent A careful explanation by the practitioner to the patient, usually in writing, that details proposed diagnostic or therapeutic procedures, along with their potential risks and benefits.

Intelligent agent A program that gathers information or performs some other service at a fixed interval without one's immediate presence. Typically, an agent program, using parameters one has provided, searches all or some part of the *Internet*, then gathers and presents the desired information.

Internet A collection of interconnected *networks* that speak the same computer language. The Internet now links thousands of independent *networks* in a global communication system.

Intranet A private *network* of interlinked computers used by the members of an organization or group. Many *security* systems allow sensitive information to be shared among intranet users.

Joint Commission on Accreditation of Healthcare Organizations (JCAHO) An independent nonprofit organization providing accreditation and related services that support performance improvement in health care organizations.

Local area network (LAN) A *network* of computers, printers, servers, and other equipment, typically all located within an enterprise, that can support audio, video, and data exchange. Differentiated from *metropolitan area networks (MANs)* and *wide area networks (WANs)* by the size of the area serviced and to some extent by the *protocols* used; the LAN is the smallest.

Low earth orbit (LEO)   Describing *satellite* technology aimed to serve two-way high-speed networking, teleconferencing, telehealth, and other interactive applications.

Master patient index   An index of patients, members of health care plans, physicians, health care practitioners, payers, employers, employees, and other individuals, along with patient demographic information—such as name, address, telephone number, date of birth, and visit dates—stored in a computerized database.

Mbps   Megabits (millions of *bits*) per second. A measure of *bandwidth* on a data transmission medium such as *twisted pair* copper cable, *coaxial cable,* or optical fiber. A typical uncompressed video signal requires at least 45 *Mbps* to facilitate transmission.

Microwave link   An antenna transmitting high-frequency radio signals (exceeding 800 megahertz) for audio, video, and data transmission. Microwave links require line-of-sight connection between transmission antennas.

Modem   Modulator-demodulator. A device that enables the transmission of digital data (by transforming it to and from *analog* form) over standard *analog* telephone lines and cable video lines.

Multimedia   Describing the transmission and manipulation of many types of information, including words, pictures, videos, music, numbers, and handwriting. In health care, integrated multimedia patient records can contain audio and video clips, still images, and other material.

Multiplexing   The aggregation of individual digital transmission lines (minimum of two, maximum of eleven) into one higher-speed line by means of a *hardware* device known as a *multiplexer*. Multiplexing allows transmission of multiple sources of audio, video, or data information in a single high-capacity communication channel.

National Committee for Quality Assurance (NCQA)   A private, nonprofit organization dedicated to assessing and reporting on the quality of managed care plans.

Network   Interconnected communication equipment used for data and information exchange. Networks can be classified by size (*LAN, MAN, WAN*) or by type of information carried (TCP/IP), who uses them (private or public), or how they are connected (*switched* or *dedicated,* using *fiber optics* or *coaxial cable*).

Newsgroups   Discussion groups on the *Internet* that allow users to submit and read other participants' submissions on a particular subject of mutual interest. Also referred to as the *Usenet.*

Nonrepudiation   Proof that only the signer could have created an *electronic signature.*

Packet   A basic message unit for communication in packet-switched *networks.* A single file may be broken up into packets for transmission, with each packet finding its own path to the destination, where the packets are reassembled. Most information transmitted over the *Internet* is in the form of packets.

Peripheral   Any externally connected device attached to a *videoconferencing* or *telemonitoring* system to augment its communication or medical capabilities. Examples include electronic stethoscopes, otoscopes, ophthalmoscopes, dermascopes, graphic stands, and scanners.

Pixel   The smallest and most fundamental picture element of a *digital image.* The greater the number of pixels in an image, the higher its *resolution.*

Point-to-point   Describing the transfer of data from one computer to another.

Portal   A Web site that is intended to be the first one people see when using the Web. A portal typically has a catalogue of Web sites, a search engine, or both, and may also offer e-mail and other services to entice people to use that site as their main "point of entry" to the Web.

POTS   Plain old telephone service. The *analog* public switched telephone *network* used throughout the world, capable of voice and data transmission at up to 56 Kbps.

Protocol   A system of guidelines and procedures, applying to both *hardware* and software, that controls communication between computer devices. Protocols are primarily concerned with three aspects of the communication process: how data are symbolized and coded, how data are transmitted, and how errors and failures are recognized and corrected.

Real-time transmission   The simultaneous capture, processing, and presentation of audio, video, and data at the time data are originated, without more than a fraction of a second delay when the *frame rate* is at least 30 fps.

Resolution   The level of detail that can be captured or displayed; in computer displays it refers to the spacing of *pixels* in the image and is measured in *pixels per inch* (ppi) or *dots per inch* (dpi). For example, if an image has a resolution of 72 ppi, it contains 5,184 *pixels* per square inch (72 *pixels* wide by 72 *pixels* high). For video displays (interactive video or *teleradiology*), resolution is measured in *pixels* by *pixels* (or lines) by *bit depth*.

Satellite   An instrument in orbit around the earth used to amplify, receive, or transmit electromagnetic signals over a wide geographical area, or *footprint*.

Security   Methods to control access and to protect information from accidental or intentional disclosure to unauthorized persons and from alteration, destruction, or loss.

Smart card   A plastic device, the size of a credit card, with embedded memory. Smart cards are used, especially in Europe, for people to carry their own medical records, images, and other information.

Store-and-forward   Describing an *asynchronous* connection that permits audio clips, video clips, still images, or data to be held now and transmitted or received at a later time. Store-and-forward technology can be used to create a *multimedia* computerized medical record.

Switched network   A *telecommunication* system in which every user has a unique address such that direct connections between any two users can be established.

Telecommunication   Transmitting or receiving information with the use of wire, radio, *satellite, fiber-optic,* or other electromagnetic or optical media for voice, data, and video communications.

Teleconferencing   Interactive electronic communication between multiple users at remote sites that allows the simultaneous exchange of voice, video, and data.

Teleconsultation   A clinical interaction between a clinician and patient, using *telecommunication* technology.

Telediagnosis   The detection or diagnosis of a disease by evaluating data transmitted electronically or by using *peripheral* instruments monitoring a remote patient.

Telementoring   An experienced clinician acting as a preceptor for a remote inexperienced clinician by observation via interactive *telecommunication* technology.

Telemetry   The automatic collection and transmission of data via wired or wireless media from stations based in remote locations (for example, patients' homes) to central receiving stations (such as clinics or hospitals) for recording and analysis.

Telemonitoring   The process of using audio, video, and other electronic *peripheral* devices to monitor the health status of a patient at a distance.

Telepresence   Generally, the quality of a *videoconference* that gives participants the feeling that they are actually in the same room together. This is affected by the extent to which nonverbal cues, such as facial expressions, posture, dress, and physical distance, are transmitted. An especially important part of telepresence is eye contact. More specifically, telepresence may refer to the close approximation of on-site presence afforded in, for example, telesurgery by the use of haptic feedback (force feedback) devices.

Teleradiology   A system that transmits radiographic images between enterprises.

Tunneling   A technique used to transmit data securely over a private *network*. The "tunnel" is the actual path over which the message travels. The *Point-to-Point* Tunneling *Protocol* (PPTP) has been proposed to provide rules that will allow the *Internet* to be used by companies as a "virtual private *network*."

Turnkey   Describing a complete product or system in which all of the services and components have been provided by a single vendor or contractor.

Twisted pair   A pair of copper wires that have been twisted to cancel out electronic interference. May be unshielded (standard phone wire) or shielded (enclosed in a shield that functions as a ground). Twisted pair wires form the residential portion of the hard-wired telephone system around the world.

Uplink   The path from a transmitting earth station to a *satellite*.

Videoconferencing   Two-way transmission of video images among multiple locations in real time to bring people at physically remote locations together for meetings and *teleconsultations*.

Virtual reality   A computer-based technology for simulating visual, auditory, and other sensory aspects of complex environments to create an illusion of being in a three-dimensional world. The world is designed by the computer; it is viewed through a special headset that responds to a person's head movements while a glove responds to the person's hand movements. For example, while in a virtual room, raising one's gloved hand will cause a virtual object seen through the headset to move upward.

Voice recognition   The ability of a computer to interpret auditory information in the form of spoken words. Also serves as a method for *authentication* with a wide variety of applications.

Whiteboarding Exchanging information on a *whiteboard,* a kind of electronic shared onscreen blackboard on which users can write or draw. Whiteboards are often supported by *broadband videoconferencing* or computer technology.

Wide area network (WAN) A data communication *network* that links distant *networks* and their computers to provide connectivity between separate *networks* located in different geographical areas.

BEST CONSULTING AND EVALUATION WEB SITES

Global Telehealth
    <http://www.globaltelehealth.com.au/>
International Telemedicine Center
    <http://int-telemedicine.com>
Feedback Research Services
    <http://www.feed-back.com>

BEST FEDERAL AGENCY AND GOVERNMENT PROGRAM WEB SITES (INCLUDING FUNDING)

Health Resources and Services Administration
    <http://www.hrsa.dhhs.gov>
Federal Telemedicine Gateway
    <http://www.tmgateway.org>
Health Care Financing Administration (HCFA)
    <http://www.hcfa.gov>
NASA Telemedicine Home Page
    <http://www.hq.nasa.gov/office/olmsa/aeromed/telemed/>
Office for the Advancement of Telehealth (OAT)
    <http://telehealth.hrsa.gov>
National Library of Medicine Telemedicine Initiative
    <http://www.nlm.nih.gov/nlmhome.html>
Veterans Administration Telemedicine Projects
    <http://www.va.gov/mediauto/telemed/nat.htm>

BEST GENERAL TELEMEDICINE RESEARCH WEB SITES

PubMed
    <http://www.ncbi.nlm.nih.gov/PubMed/>

Telemedicine Information Exchange
  <http://tie.telemed.org>
Galaxy's Professional Guide to Telemedicine
  <http://galaxy.einet.net/galaxy/Medicine/Medical-Informatics/
  Telemedicine.html>
MedWebPlus Telemedicine
  <http://www.medwebplus.com/subject/Telemedicine.html>

BEST LEGAL INFORMATION WEB SITES

Arent Fox
  <http://www.arentfox.com>
Center for Telemedicine Law
  <http://www.ctl.org>
Gray Cary Ware & Freidenrich
  <http://www.graycary.com>
Legamed
  <http://www.legamed.com>
National Partnership Guide to the HIPAA
  <http://www.nationalpartnership.org/healthcare/hipaa/guide.htm>
Joint Commission on Accreditation of Health Care Organizations (JCAHO)
  <http://www.jcaho.org>
National Committee for Quality Assurance (NCQA)
  <http://www.ncqa.org>
National Conference of State Legislatures
  <http://www.ncsl.org>
Thomas (federal bill tracking)
  <http://thomas.loc.gov>

BEST LISTSERVS FOR PROFESSIONAL DISCUSSIONS

E-Health Discussion List
  <http://telehealth.net/subscribe/ehealthsub.html>
  <http://telehealth.net/subscribe/subscribe_list.html>

Telemedicine Today Online Discussion
    <http://www.telemedtoday.com/discussionweb/disc2_toc.htm>
For other listservs, go to
    <http://tie.telemed.org/links/listserv.asp>

BEST PATIENT RECORD WEB SITES

Computerized Patient Records Institute (CPRI)
    <http://www.cpri.org>
Medical Records Institute
    <http://www.medrecinst.com>
PCASSO (Patient Centered Access to Secure Systems Online)
    <http://medicine.ucsd.edu/pcasso>

BEST APPLICATION SERVICE PROVIDER WEB SITES

Billing
    <http://www.claimsnet.com>
Scheduling
    <http://www.healinx.com>
Back-office duties
    <http://www.cybear.com>
Lab results
    <http://www.compulab.com>
Marketing
    <http://www.caredata.com>
Differential diagnosis
    <http://www.treeage.com>
Medical records
    <http://www.personalmd.com>
Evaluation and outcomes
    <http://www.elixis.com>
Virtual offices for physicians
    <http://www.webmd.com>

BEST CORRECTIONAL TELEMEDICINE WEB SITE

1999 Research Report Evaluating a Prison Telemedicine Network
  <http://www.ncjrs.org/telemedicine/toc.html>

BEST HOME CARE WEB SITES

American Medical Association's revised Guidelines for the Medical Management of the Home Care Patient
  <http://www.ama-assn.org/ama/pub/article/2036-2466.html>
American Telemedicine Association's Telehome Care Guidelines
  <http://www.atmeda.org/news/guidelines.html>
Home Health Care Extranet
  <http://www.telemedical.com/Telemedical/home.html>
HomeCare On-Line
  <http://www.nahc.org/home.html>

BEST MILITARY TELEMEDICINE WEB SITES

Pacific Regional Program Office
  <http://akamai.tamc.amedd.army.mil/>
Center for Total Access
  <http://www.cta.ha.osd.mil/>
Department of Defense Telemedicine Home Page
  <http://www.matmo.org>
Directorate of Telemedicine at the Walter Reed Army Medical Center
  <http://www.wramc.amedd.army.mil/departments/tmed/>

BEST NURSING WEB SITES

Telehealth Issues for Nursing
  <http://www.ana.org/readroom/tele2.htm>
Worldwide Nurse
  <http://www.wwnurse.com>

BEST PATHOLOGY WEB SITES

AFIP Department of Telepathology
    <http://www.afip.org/telepathology/>
TelePathology Consultants, P.C.
    <http://www.telepathology.com>

BEST PSYCHIATRY AND PSYCHOLOGY WEB SITE

TelehealthNet
    <http://telehealth.net>

BEST RADIOLOGY WEB SITES

CompuRAD Resource Center
    <http://www.compurad.com/index.asp?Sec=ref>
PACS and Networking News
    <http://www.pacsnews.com>
Telemedicine PACS Resource Page
    <http://www.dejarnette.com/users/efinegan/pacspage.htm>

BEST RELATED PROFESSIONAL ASSOCIATION WEB SITES

American Health Information Management Association (AHIMA)
    <http://www.ahima.org>
American Medical Informatics Association (AMIA)
    <http://www.amia.org>
American Psychiatric Association Telepsychiatry Committee
    <http://www.psych.org/pract_of_psych/telepsych.html>
American Telemedicine Association
    <http://www.atmeda.org>
Association of Telehealth Service Providers (ATSP)
    <http://www.atsp.org>
Canadian Society for Telehealth (CST)
    <http://www.ucalgary.ca/md/CST>

Center for Healthcare Information Management (CHIM)
    <http://www.chim.org>
College of Healthcare Information Management Executives
    <http://www.cio-chime.org/default.html>
Finnish Society of Telemedicine
    <http://www.fimnet.fi/telemedicine/engindex.htm>
Healthcare Information Management Systems Society (HIMSS)
    <http://www.himss.org>
International Society for Telemedicine (ISfT)
    <http://www.isft.org>
Internet Healthcare Coalition
    <http://www.ihc.net>
Joint Healthcare Information Technology Alliance
    <http://www.jhita.org>

BEST E-HEALTH, TELEHEALTH, AND TELEMEDICINE PUBLICATIONS

E-HealthCare Connections
    <http://www.ehealthcareconnections.com>
Journal of Telemedicine and Telecare
    <http://www.coh.uq.edu.au/>
MD Computing
    <http://www.mdcomputing.com>
Telehealth Magazine
    <http://telemedmag.com>
TelehealthNews
    <http://telehealth.net/subscribe/subscribe_telenews.html>
Telemedicine and Virtual Reality
    <http://search.medscape.com/LWW/TVR/public/TVR-journal.html>
Telemedicine Journal
    <http://www.liebertpub.com/tmj/default.htm>
Telemedicine Today Magazine
    <http://www.telemedtoday.com>

BEST SECURITY WEB SITES

Department of Health and Human Services
   <http://aspe.os.dhhs.gov/admnsimp/nprm/seclist.htm>
Electronic Privacy Information Center (EPIC)
   <http://www.epic.org>
International Computer Security Association (ICSA)
   <http://www.icsa.net>
MIS Training Institute
   <http://www.misti.com>
National Council for Prescription Drug Programs
   <http://www.ncpdp.org>
RSA Data Security
   <http://www.rsa.com>
Tunitas Group
   <http://www.tunitas.com>
Washington Publishing Company
   <http://www.wpc-edi.com>

BEST TECHNOLOGY-RELATED WEB SITES

Internet2
   <http://www.internet2.edu/home.html>
Webopedia
   <http://www.pcwebopedia.com>
Tech Encyclopedia
   <http://www.techweb.com/encyclopedia>
Videoconference Resource Center
   <http://www.videoconference.com/about.htm>
Videoconferencing FAQ
   <http://www.bitscout.com/faqtoc.htm>

REFERENCES

Abdel-Malek, A. (1996). Telemammography feasibility. *Telemedicine Today, 4*(6), 36–37.

Akay, M. (1996). VRT revolution. *Journal of the Institute of Electrical and Electronics Engineers, 15*(2), 31–33.

Allen, A. (1993). Patient-physician consultations via interactive video in 1993. *Telemedicine Newsletter* [now *Telemedicine Today*], *1*(4), 1.

Allen A. (1995a). Legal barriers to cross-state telemedicine? *Telemedicine Today, 3*(2), 7.

Allen, A. (1995b). The role of the consultant in telemedicine. *Journal of the Healthcare Information and Management Systems Society, 9,* 13–16.

Allen, A. (1998). A review of cost effectiveness research. *Telemedicine Today, 6*(5), 10–12, 14–15.

Allen, A., Bowersox, J., & Jones, G. G. (1997). Telesurgery: Telepresence, telementoring, telerobotics. *Telemedicine Today, 5*(3), 19–25.

Allen, A., Doolittle, G. C., Boysen, C. D., Komoroski, K., Wolf, M., Collins, B., & Patterson, J. D. (1999). An analysis of the suitability of home health care visits for telemedicine. *Journal of Telemedicine and Telecare, 5,* 90–96.

Allen, A., & Grigsby, B. (1998). Fifth annual program survey–part 2. Consultation activity in thirty-five specialties. *Telemedicine Today, 6*(5), 18–19.

Allen, A., & Perednia, D. A. (1996). Telemedicine and the healthcare executive. In *Telemedicine Today Buyer's Guide and Directory* [special issue], 4–34.

Allen, A., & Wheeler, T. (1998a). Annual survey: Teleradiology service providers. *Telemedicine Today, 6*(6), 33–34.

Allen, A., & Wheeler, T. (1998b). Fifth annual program survey–part 1: The leaders: U.S. programs doing more than 500 interactive consults in 1997. *Telemedicine Today, 6*(3), 36–37.

Alvarez, D. (1998). Tattling on teleradiology. *Telemedicine Today, 6*(6), 21–26.

Ambre, J., Guard, R., Perveiler, F., Renner, J., & Rippen, H. (1997). *Criteria for assessing the quality of health information on the Internet.* Retrieved May 16, 2000, from the World Wide Web: http://hitiweb.mitretek.org/docs/criteria.html

American College of Radiology. (1999). *ACR standards for teleradiology.* Retrieved May 5, 2000, from the World Wide Web: http://www.acr.org/

American Counseling Association. (1999, October). *Ethical standards for Internet online counseling.* Retrieved May 16, 2000, from the World Wide Web: http://www.counseling.org/gc/cybertx.htm

American Medical Association. (1990). *Legal implications of practice parameters.* Chicago: Author.

American Medical Association. (1999, July 30). *AMA testimony on the risks and benefits of on-line pharmacies.* Retrieved May 5, 2000, from the World Wide Web: http://www.ama-assn.org/ama/basic/article/

American Psychiatric Association. (1998). *Position statement on the ethical use of telemedicine.* Retrieved May 5, 2000, from the World Wide Web: http://www.psych.org/

American Psychological Association. (1992). Ethical principles of psychologists and code of conduct. *American Psychologist, 47,* 1597–1611.

American Psychological Association. (1997, November 5). *Services by telephone, teleconferencing, and Internet: A statement by the Ethics Committee of the American Psychological Association.* Retrieved September 10, 2000, from the World Wide Web: http://www.apa.org/ethics/stmnt01.html

American Psychological Association. (1998). Ethics Committee issues statement on services by telephone, teleconferencing and Internet. *APA Monitor, 29*(1), 38.

American Telemedicine Association. (1999). *American Telemedicine Association issues advisory on use of medical Web sites.* Retrieved May 5, 2000, from the World Wide Web: http://www.atmeda.org/news/

Anderson, A. H., Newlands, A., & Mullin, J. (1996). Impact of video-mediated communication on simulated service encounters. *Interactive Computing, 8,* 193–206.

Aneshensel, C. S., Frerichs, R. R., Clark, V. A., & Yokopenic, P. A. (1982). Measuring depression in the community: A comparison of telephone and personal interviews. *Public Opinion Quarterly, 46,* 110–121.

Baer, L., Brown-Beasley, M. W., Sorce, J., & Henriques, A. I. (1992). Computer-assisted telephone administration of a structured interview for obsessive-compulsive disorder. *American Journal of Psychiatry, 150,* 1737–1738.

Baer, L., Cukor, P., Jenike, M. A., Leahy, L., O'Laughlen, J., & Coyle, J. T. (1995). Pilot studies of telemedicine for patients with obsessive-compulsive disorder. *American Journal of Psychiatry, 152,* 1383–1385.

Baer, L., Elford, D. R., & Cukor, P. (1997). Telepsychiatry at forty: What have we learned? *Harvard Review of Psychiatry, 5*(1), 7–17.

Baker, D. B., & Cooper, T. (1995). *Information system security issues for health care.* Manuscript in preparation, Science Applications International Corp. and Kaiser Permanente.

Balas, E. A., Jaffrey, F., Kuperman, G. J., Boren, S. A., Brown, G. D., Pinciroli, F., & Mitchell, J. A. (1997). Electronic communication with patients: Evaluation of distance medicine technology. *Journal of the American Medical Association, 278,* 152–159.

Baldwin, G. (1999). The Internet can make strategic I.T. planning precarious. *Health Data Magazine, 7*(12), 42–48.

Ball, C., & McLaren, P. (1997). The tele-assessment of cognitive state: A review. *Journal of Telemedicine and Telecare, 3,* 126–131.

Barak, A. (1999). Psychological applications on the Internet: A discipline on the threshold of a new millennium. *Applied and Preventive Psychology, 8,* 231–245.

Bard, M. (2000, January). *The future of eHealth.* Retrieved September 8, 2000, from the World Wide Web: http://www.cyberdialogue.com

Bashshur, R. L. (2000). Telemedicine nomenclature: What does it mean? *Telemedicine Journal, 6,* 1–3.

Bashshur, R. L., & Lovett, J. (1997). Assessment of telemedicine: Results of the initial experience. *Aviation Space and Environmental Medicine, 48,* 65–70.

Bashshur, R. L., Scott, J., & Silva, J. (Eds.). (1994). *Report on a working conference on telemedicine policy for the NII.* Arlington, VA: Center for Public Service Communications.

Bates, D., Leape, L., Cullen, D., Laird, N., Petersen, L., Teich, J., Furdick, E., Hickey, M., Kleefield, S., Shea, B., Vander, M., & Seger, D. (1998). Effect of computerized physician order entry and a team intervention on prevention of serious medication errors. *Journal of the American Medical Association, 280,* 1311–1316.

Bergman, R. (1993). Computers make "house calls" to patients. *Hospitals, 67*(10), 52.

Biomedical sensors and telemetry for remote monitoring of patients. (1999). Retrieved May 5, 2000, from the World Wide Web: http://www.nttc.edu/telmed/bmfact.html

Blakeslee, B. S., & Satava, R. M. (1998). Military initiatives in telemedicine. In S. F. Viegas & K. Dunn (Eds.), *Telemedicine: Practicing in the information age* (pp. 69–76). Philadelphia: Lippincott-Raven.

Borowitz, S. M., & Wyatt, J. C. (1998). The origin, content, and workload of e-mail consultations. *Journal of the American Medical Association, 280,* 1321–1324.

Borzo, G. (1999, April 5). Who's record is it anyway? *American Medical News.* Retrieved May 5, 2000, from the World Wide Web: http://www.ama-assn.org/sci-pubs/amnews/

Bowersox, J., Cordts, P., & La Porta, A. J. (1998). Use of an intuitive telemanipulator system for remote trauma surgery: An experimental study. *Journal of the American College of Surgeons, 186,* 615–621.

Braden, J. (1999). *The future of HIM: An operational view.* Retrieved May 5, 2000, from the World Wide Web: http://www.ahima.org/publications/

Brandt, M. (1996). Information security: An overview. *Journal of the American Health Information Management Association, 67*(6). Retrieved May 5, 2000, from the World Wide Web: http://www.ahima.org/publications/

Brandt, M., & Carpenter, J. (1999, January). *Patient photography, videotaping, and other imaging (Updated).* American Health Information Management Association. Retrieved May 5, 2000, from the World Wide Web: http://www.ahima.org/publications/

Brecht, R. M., Gray, C. L., Peterson, C., & Youngblood, B. (1996). The University of Texas Medical Branch–Texas development of criminal justice telemedicine project: Findings from the first year of operation. *Telemedicine Journal, 2,* 25–35.

Brown, N. (1996). Twenty selected teleradiology references. *Telemedicine Today, 4*(6), 16–30.

Brown, S. G. (1910, May 5). A telephone relay. *Journal of the Institution of Electrical Engineers,* pp. 590–619.

Bruckman, A. (1996). Finding one's own space in cyberspace. *Technology Review, 99*(1), 48–54.

Bruderman, I., & Abboud, S. (1997). Telespirometry: Novel system for home monitoring of asthmatic patients. *Telemedicine Journal, 3,* 127–133.

Brunicardi, B. O. (1998). Financial analysis of savings from telemedicine in Ohio's prison system. *Telemedicine Journal, 4,* 49–54.

Burdick, A. E., Mahmud, K., & Jenkins, D. P. (1996). Telemedicine: Caring for patients across boundaries. *Ostomy/Wound Management, 42*(9), 26–37.

Cairncross, F. (1997). *The death of distance.* Boston: Harvard Business School Press.

California Healthcare Foundation. (1999, January 28). *Americans worry about the privacy of their computerized medical records.* Retrieved May 5, 2000, from the World Wide Web: http://www.chcf.org/press/

California Healthline. (1999, April 21). *Medical privacy: Agreement, but a long way to go.* Retrieved May 5, 2000, from the World Wide Web: http://www.chcf.org/press/

California Telehealth/Telemedicine Coordination Project. (1997, January). *Telehealth and Telemedicine: Taking distance out of caring.* Sacramento: Author.

Caramella, D., Lencioni, T., Mazzeo, S., & Bartolozzi, C. (1994). Transmission of radiological images using broadband communications. *European Radiology, 4,* 377–381.

Carrington, C. (1999a). For doctor-to-patient e-mail, does convenience trump privacy? *Telehealth Magazine, 5*(1), 41–44.

Carrington, C. (1999b). Internet2 promises healthcare benefits in not-too-distant future. *Telehealth Magazine, 5*(3), 13–14.

Carroll, E. T., Wright, S., & Zakoworotny, C. (1998). Securely implementing remote access within health information management. *Journal of the American Health Information Management Association, 69*(3), 46–49.

Center for Devices and Radiological Health. (1996). *Telemedicine-related activities.* Washington, DC: Food and Drug Administration.

Center for Telemedicine Law. (1997). Telemedicine and interstate licensure: Findings and recommendations of the CTL licensure task force. *North Dakota Law Review, 73*(1), 109–130.

Cepelewicz, B. (1998, October 8). *Telemedicine and strategies to minimize risks of liability.* Paper presented at the Telemedicine National Conference on Legal and Policy Developments, Washington, DC.

Cheriff, A. D., Schulam, P. G., Docimo, S. G., Moore, R. G., & Kavoussi, L. R. (1996). Telesurgical consultation. *Journal of Urology, 156,* 1391–1393.

Chin, T. (1999, November 8). Health sites to develop ethics guidelines. *American Medical News.* Retrieved May 5, 2000, from the World Wide Web: http://www.ama-assn.org/sci-pubs/amnews/

Civello, C. (1999). Cyberspace, trusted insiders, and organizational threat. *Psychologist-Manager Journal, 3,* 149–166.

Collins, J. (1996). Lighting design and layout of a telemedicine conference room. *Telemedicine Today, 4*(5), 26–28.

Computer-Based Patient Record Institute. (1999). *CPRI toolkit: Managing information security in health care.* Bethesda, MD: Author.

Computer Science and Telecommunications Board, National Research Council. (1996). *Cryptography's role in securing the information society.* Washington, DC: National Academy Press.

Cook, L. T., Insana, M. F., McFadden, M. A., Hall, T. J., & Cox, G. C. (1994). Assessment of low-contrast detectability for compressed digital chest images (Document No. 2166). *Proceedings of the Society of Photo-Optical Instrumentation Engineers.* Retrieved September 8, 2000, from the World Wide Web: http://www.spie.org/web/abstracts/abstracts_home.html

Cook, T. D., & Campbell, D. T. (1979). *Quasi-experimentation: Designs and analysis for field studies.* Skokie, IL: Rand McNally.

Corporate Technology Group. (2000). *Administrative procedures.* Retrieved May 11, 2000, from the World Wide Web: http://www.hipaasource.com/

Costa Rican Foundation for Sustainable Development. (1999). *Unwiring the world.* Retrieved May 5, 2000, from the World Wide Web: http://www.media.mit.edu/unwired/

Coy, P. (2000, January 11). Company closeup: Harris Interactive: A high opinion of online polling. *Business Week e.biz.* Retrieved September 9, 2000, from the World Wide Web: http://businessweek.com/ebiz/

Croweroft, J. (1997). Supporting videoconferencing on the Internet. In K. E. Finn, A. J. Sellen, & S. B. Wilbur (Eds.), *Video-mediated communication: Computers, cognition, and work* (pp. 519–540). Mahwah, NJ: Erlbaum.

Crowther, J. B., & Poropatich, R. (1995). Telemedicine in the U.S. Army: Case reports from Somalia and Croatia. *Telemedicine Journal, 1,* 73–80.

Cukor, P., Baer, L., Willis, S., Leahy, L., O'Laughlen, J., Murphy, M., Withers, M., & Martin, E. (1998). Use of videophones and low-cost standard telephone lines to provide a social presence in telepsychiatry. *Telemedicine Journal, 4,* 313–321.

Cunningham, N., Marshall, C., & Glazer, E. (1978). Telemedicine in pediatric primary care. *Journal of the American Medical Association, 240,* 2749–2751.

Curtis, C., & Fenton, S. (1999). *Health information managers and clinical data repositories: A natural fit.* Retrieved May 5, 2000, from the World Wide Web: http://www.ahima.org/publications/

Dakins, D. (1999, June). Increased investment and incremental expansion fuels optimism. *Telehealth Magazine, 5*(3), 28–31.

Dakins, D., & Jones, E. (1996). Cream of the crop: Ten outstanding telemedicine programs. *Telemedicine and Telehealth Networks, 2*(11), 24–41.

Day, S. X., & Schneider, P. L. (2000). *Psychotherapy using distance technology: Story and science.* Manuscript submitted for publication.

Deleon, P. H., Folen, R. A., Jennings, F. L., & Willis, D. J. (1991). The case for prescription privileges: A logical evolution of professional practice [Special issue: Child psychopharmacology]. *Journal of Clinical Child Psychology, 20,* 254–267.

Deleon, P. H., Vanden Bos, G. R., Sammons, M. T., & Frank, R. G. (1998). Changing healthcare environment in the United States: Steadily evolving into the twenty-first century. In A. S. Bellack, M. Hersen, & A. N. Wiens (Eds.), *Comprehensive clinical psychology: Vol. 2. Professional issues* (pp. 393–401). New York: Elsevier.

Deleon, P. H., & Wiggins, J. G. (1996). Prescription privileges for psychologists. *American Psychologist, 51,* 225–229.

Della Mea, V. (1999). Internet electronic mail: A tool for low-cost telemedicine. *Journal of Telemedicine and Telecare, 5,* 84–89.

De Nelsky, S. J., Haspel, M. B., & Lam, E. (1999). *E-health II: Beyond the business plan.* Boston: Crèdit Suisse/First Boston Equity Research.

Department of Health and Human Services. (1997a). *Confidentiality of individually-identifiable health information.* Retrieved May 5, 2000, from the World Wide Web: http://aspe.hhs.gov/admnsimp/

Department of Health and Human Services. (1997b). *Exploratory evaluation of rural applications of telemedicine.* Retrieved May 5, 2000, from the World Wide Web: http://www.ntia.doc.gov

Department of Health and Human Services. (1998, August 12). *Security and electronic signature standards.* Retrieved May 5, 2000, from the World Wide Web: http://aspe.os.dhhs.gov/admnsimp/

Department of Health and Human Services. (1999a). *Frequently asked questions about the National Provider Identifier.* Retrieved May 5, 2000, from the World Wide Web: http://aspe.os.dhhs.gov/admnsimp/

Department of Health and Human Services. (1999b). *Frequently asked questions about the National Standard Employer Identifier (EIN).* Retrieved May 5, 2000, from the World Wide Web: http://aspe.os.dhhs.gov/admnsimp/

Dertouzos, M. (1997). *What will be: How the new world of information will change our lives.* New York: HarperCollins.

Dick, R., Steen, E., & Detmer, D. (Eds.). (1998). *Computer based patient record: An essential technology for health care.* Washington, DC: National Institute of Medicine/National Academy Press.

Dishman, E., & Sherry, J. (1999). *Changing practices: Computing technology in the shifting landscape of American healthcare.* Santa Clara, CA: Intel Corp.

Dwyer, S. J., Stewart, B. K., Sayre, J. W., & Honeyman, J. C. (1992). Wide area network strategies for teleradiology systems. *Radiographics, 12,* 567–576.

Dyson, E. (1997). *Release 2.0: A design for living in the digital age.* New York: Broadway.

Eng, T., & Gustafson, D. (1999, April). Science panel on interactive communication and health. *Wired for health and well-being: The emergence of interactive health communication.* Washington, DC: U.S. Government Printing Office.

Ernst & Young LLP. (1997). *The role of the Internet in health care: Current state* [Brochure]. New York: Author.

Evans, R. L., Smith, K. M., Werkhoven, W. S., Fox, H. R., & Pritzl, D. O. (1986). Cognitive telephone group therapy with physically disabled elderly persons. *Geronotologist, 26,* 8–10.

Eysenbach, G., & Diepgen, T. (1998). Responses to unsolicited patient e-mail requests for medical advice on the World Wide Web. *Journal of the American Medical Association, 280,* 1333–1335.

Falconer, J. (1999). Telemedicine systems and telecommunications. In R. Wootton & J. Craig (Eds.), *Introduction to telemedicine* (pp. 17–36). London: Royal Society of Medicine.

Federal Trade Commission. (2000, May 15). *Federal Trade Commission Advisory Committee on online access and security.* Retrieved May 15, 2000, from the World Wide Web: http://www.ftc.gov/acoas/

Fenig, S., Levav, I., Kohn, R., & Yelin, N. (1993). Telephone vs. face-to-face interviewing in a community psychiatric survey. *American Journal of Public Health, 83,* 896–898.

Ferguson, E. W., Doarn, C. R., & Scott, J. C. (1995). Survey of global telemedicine. *Journal of Medical Systems, 19,* 35–46.

Ferguson, T. (1998). Digital doctoring: Opportunities and challenges in electronic patient-physician communication. *Journal of the American Medical Association, 280,* 1361–1362.

Fernandes, L., Brandt, M., Casey, D., Fletcher, D., Grant, K., Petrosky, C., Postal, S., Skeens, M., Wheatley, V., & Winter, T. (1997, July). Issue: Master patient (person) index (MPI): Recommended core data elements. *American Health Information Management Association practice brief.* Retrieved May 5, 2000, from the World Wide Web: http://www.ahima.org/publications/

Fiddleman, R., Hawthorn, E., & Jones, K. (1997, February). *Securing health information systems.* Paper presented at the conference of the Healthcare Information and Management Systems Society, San Diego, CA.

Fisher, R., & Singh, S. (2000, March). Checklist for a good contract for IT purchases. *Health Management Technology, 21*(3), 14–17.

Fisk, N. M., Bower, S., Sepulved, W., Garner, P., Cameron, K., Matthews, M., Ridley, D., Drysdale, K., & Wooton, R. (1995). Fetal telemedicine: Interactive transfer of realtime ultrasound and video via ISDN for remote consultation. *Journal of Telemedicine, 1*, 38–44.

Fitzmaurice, J. M. (1998, August 20). *Telehealth research and evaluation: Implications for decision makers.* Agency for Health Care Policy and Research. Retrieved May 5, 2000, from the World Wide Web: http://akamai.tamc.amedd.army.mil/PacMedTek/Presentations/Thursday/Fitzmaurice/index.htm

Fletcher, D. (1999). *Issue: Telemedical records.* American Health Information Management Association. Retrieved May 5, 2000, from the World Wide Web: http://www.ahima.org/publications/

Friedman, R. H., Kazis, L. E., Jette, A., Smith, M. B., Stollerman, J., Torgerson, J., & Carey, K. (1996). A telecommunications system for monitoring and counseling patients with hypertension: Impact on medication adherence and blood pressure control. *American Journal of Hypertension, 9*, 285–292.

Frisse, M., Kelly, E., & Mercalfe, E. (1994). An Internet primer: Resources and responsibilities. *Academic Medicine, 69*, 20–24.

Fuchs, M. (1979). Provider attitudes toward STARPAHC: A telemedicine project on the Papago Indian Reservation. *Medical Care, 17*, 59–66.

Garshnek, V. (1991). Applications of space communications technology to critical human needs: Rescue, disaster relief, and medical assistance. *Space Communications, 8*, 311–317.

Garshnek, V., & Burkle, F. (1999a). Application of telemedicine and telecommunications to disaster medicine: Historical and future perspectives. *Journal of the American Medical Informatics Association, 6*(1), 26–37.

Garshnek, V., & Burkle, F. (1999b). Telecommunications systems in support of disaster medicine: Applications of basic information pathways. *Annals of Emergency Medicine, 34*, 213–218.

Garshnek, V., & Hassell, L. (1997). The telemedicine frontier: Going the extra mile. *Space Policy, 13*(1), 37–46.

Garshnek, V., & Hassell, L. (1999). Evaluating telemedicine in a changing technological era. *Journal of Healthcare Information Management, 13*(4), 39–47.

Gershon-Cohen, J., & Cooley, A. G. (1950). Telediagnosis. *Radiology, 55*, 582–587.

Gibson, S. (2000, April). *Telepsychiatry in northern Arizona.* Paper presented at a symposium organized by the American Telemedicine Association, Phoenix, AZ.

Gilbert, F. (1999). HIPAA and the electronic record. In L. L. Brown, F. J. Cavanaugh, W. Rishel, P. Spitzer, & J. P. Tomes (Eds.), *Comprehensive guide to electronic health records* (pp. 351–363). Washington, DC: Faulkner & Gray.

Gillespie, G. (1999, December). Today's interactivity offers glimpse of tomorrow's Web sites. *Health Data Management, 7*(12), 50–56.

Glueckauf, R. L., Fritz, S., Sherod, T., Dages, P., Carney, P., & Maria, B. (in press). Home-based family videocounseling for rural teenagers with epilepsy: Phase I findings. *Rehabilitation Psychology.*

Glueckauf, R. L., Hufford, B. J., Whitton, J. D., Baxter, J., Schneider, P., Kain, J., & Vogelgesang, S. (1999). Tele-health: Emerging technology in rehabilitation and health care. In M. G. Eisenberg, R. L. Glueckauf, & H. H. Zaretsky (Eds.), *Medical aspects of disability: A handbook for the rehabilitation professional* (2nd ed., pp. 625–639). New York: Springer.

Glueckauf, R. L., Whitton, J. D., Baxter, J., Kain, J., Vogelgesang, S., Hudson, M., & Wright, D. (1998). Videocounseling for families of rural teens with epilepsy: Project update. *TelehealthNews, 2*(2), 1–3 [On-line magazine]. Retrieved September 5, 2000, from the World Wide Web: http://tele-health.net/subscribe/newslettr_3.html

Glueckauf, R. L., Whitton, J. D., & Nickelson, D. W. (in press). Tele-health: The new frontier in rehabilitation and healthcare. In M. J. Scherer (Ed.), *Assistive technology and rehabilitation psychology: Shaping an alliance.* Washington, DC: American Psychological Association.

Goldberg, A. I. (1997). Tele-home healthcare on call: Trends leading to the return of the housecall. *Telemedicine Today, 5*(4), 14–15.

Goldman, J., Hudson, Z., & Smith, R. M. (2000). *Report on the privacy policies and practices of health Web sites.* Retrieved May 5, 2000, from the World Wide Web: http://tie.telemed.org/

Goldstein, D. (2000). *E-healthcare: Harness the power of Internet e-commerce and e-care.* Gaithersberg, MD: Aspen.

Gould, R. L. (1996). The use of computers in therapy. In T. Trabin & M. Freeman (Eds.), *The computerization of behavioral healthcare: How to enhance clinical practice, management, and communications* (pp. 39–62). San Francisco: Jossey-Bass.

Graber, M. A., Roller, C. M., & Kaeble, B. (1999). Readability levels of patient education material on the World Wide Web. *Journal of Family Practice, 48*(1), 58–61.

Graham, C., Franses, A., Kenwright, M., & Marks, I. (2000). Psychotherapy by computer: A postal survey of responders to teletext article. *Psychiatric Bulletin, 24,* 331–332.

Granade, P. F. (1998, May 4). *Electronic medical records.* Paper presented at the Health Information and Technology Program conference of the American Health Lawyers Association, Chicago.

Graphics, Visualization and Usability Center (GVU). (1998). *GVU's tenth WWW user survey.* Georgia Tech Research Corp. Retrieved May 5, 2000, from the World Wide Web: http://www.cc.gatech.edu/gvu/

Greenberg, C. (1999). Technological innovations and advancements for psychologists working with organizations. *Psychologist-Manager Journal, 3,* 181–190.

Greene, J. (1997). Sign on and say "ah-h-h-h-h." *Hospitals and Health Networks, 71*(8), 45–46.

Grigsby, B., & Allen, A. (1997). Fourth annual program review. *Telemedicine Today, 5*(4), 30–38.

Grigsby, B., & Brown, N. (2000). *The 1999 ATSP report on U.S. telemedicine activity.* Portland, OR: Association of TeleHealth Service Providers.

Groves, R. M. (1989). *Survey errors and survey costs.* New York: Wiley.

Gustafson, D. H., Hawkins, R. P., Boberg, E. W., Bricker, E., Pingree, S., & Chan, C. L. (1994). *The use and impact of a computer-based support system for people living with AIDS and HIV infection.* Unpublished manuscript, University of Wisconsin at Madison.

Gustafson, D. H., Hawkins, R. P., Boberg, E. W., Pingree, S., Serlin, R., Graziano, F., & Chan, C. L. (1999). Impact of a patient-centered, computer-based health information/support system. *American Journal of Preventive Medicine, 16*(1), 1–9.

Gustafson, D. H., Wise, M., McTavish, F., Taylor, J. O., Wolberg, W., Stewart, J., Smalley, R. V., & Bosworth, K. (1993). Development and pilot evaluation of a computer-based support system for women with breast cancer. *Journal of Psychosocial Oncology, 11*(4), 69–93.

Haas, L. J., Benedict, J. G., & Kobos, J. C. (1996). Psychotherapy by telephone: Risks and benefits for psychologists and consumers. *Professional Psychology: Research and Process, 27,* 154–160.

Habash, T. (1999). The impact of audio- or video-conferencing and group decision tools on group perception and satisfaction in distributed meetings. *Psychologist-Manager Journal, 3,* 211–230.

Hagel, J., III, & Armstrong, A. (1997). *Net.gain: Expanding markets through virtual communities.* Boston: Harvard Business School Press.

Harris, G. (1999). Beyond a shadow of a doubt: Time for "gold-standard" acceptance of CCD radiographic digitizers/scanners? *Telemedicine Today, 7*(2), 27–33.

Harris, G. (2000). The final report: Kaiser Permanente tele-home health research project. *Telemedicine Today, 8*(2), 34–36.

Harris Poll. (1999, February 17). *Poll: Most net users want health info.* Retrieved May 8, 2000, from the World Wide Web: http://www.elibrary.com/

Haugh, R. (1999, December 1). The new consumer. *Hospitals and Health Networks.* Retrieved May 10, 2000, from the World Wide Web: http://www.hhn-mag.com/

Hawkins, R. (1997). *Effective implementation of videoconferencing systems for telemedicine applications.* Unpublished manuscript.

Health Care Financing Administration. (1998a). *HCFA Privacy Act: Internet security policy.* Retrieved May 5, 2000, from the World Wide Web: http://www.hcfa.gov/security/

Health Care Financing Administration. (1998b, November 2). Payment for tele-consultations in rural health professional shortage areas, 58879–58886. Extracted from the *Federal Register, 63*(211). Retrieved May 25, 2000, from the World Wide Web: http://www.arentfox.com

Health Care Financing Administration. (1999). *States where Medicaid reimbursement of services utilizing telemedicine is available.* Retrieved May 5, 2000, from the World Wide Web: http://www.hcfa.gov/medicaid/telelist.htm

Hipkins, J. H. (1997). Telemedicine in correctional systems. In R. L. Bashshur, J. H. Sanders, & G. W. Shannon (Eds.), *Telemedicine: Theory and practice* (pp. 375–389). Springfield, IL: Thomas.

Hodges, J. (1997). *Videoconference design guide.* Kansas City, MO: Author.

Hollenbeck, A. (1999). Using the Internet and World Wide Web (WWW): Amazing sites/amazing insights. *Psychologist-Manager Journal, 3*(2), 167–179.

Holt, M. (1997, December). Blueprint for healthcare's future found in collaborative telecommunities. *Telemedicine and Telehealth Networks.* Retrieved May 5, 2000, from the World Wide Web: http://www.telehealthmag.com/

House, A. M., & Roberts, J. M. (1977, August 20). Telemedicine in Canada. *Journal of the Canadian Medical Association, 117,* 386–388.

Hubbs, R. P., Rindfleisch, T. C., Godin, P., & Melmon, K. L. (1998). Medical information on the Internet. *Journal of the American Medical Association, 280,* 1363.

Hufford, B. J., Glueckauf, R. L., & Webb, P. M. (1999). Home-based videoconferencing for adolescents with epilepsy and their families. *Rehabilitation Psychology, 44,* 176–193.

Huling, T. (2000, May). Prisoners of the census. *Mojo Wire.* Retrieved August 28, 2000, from the World Wide Web: www.motherjones.com/reality_check/census.html

Impicciatore, P., Pandolfini, C., Casella, N., & Bonati, M. (1997). Reliability of health information for the public on the World Wide Web: Systematic survey of advice on managing fever in children at home. *British Medical Journal, 314,* 1875–1881.

Institute for the Future. (2000, January). *Health and Healthcare 2010: The Forecast, the Challenge.* San Francisco: Jossey-Bass.

Institute of Medicine. (1994). *Health data in the information age: Use, disclosure and privacy.* Washington, DC: National Academy Press.

Institute of Medicine. (1996). *Telemedicine: A guide to assessing telecommunications in health care* (M. J. Field, Ed.). Washington, DC: National Academy Press.

Intel Corp. (2000). *Online survey shows details of health content retrievers.* Retrieved May 5, 2000, from the World Wide Web: http://www.intel.com/intel/e-health/jdpower.htm

IntelliHealth. (2000). *Online health spending to soar.* Retrieved May 5, 2000, from the World Wide Web: http://ipn.intellihealth.com/

International Bar Association, Section on Legal Practice. (1999, June 2). Committee 2 (Medicine and the Law). *International Convention on Telemedicine and Telehealth* [Draft]. London: International Bar Association.

Internet Healthcare Coalition. (2000). *The draft code of ethics.* Retrieved May 5, 2000, from the World Wide Web: http://www.ihealthcoalition.org/community/join.html

Internet tools for telemedicine and medical education. (1999). Retrieved May 5, 2000, from the World Wide Web: http://www.nttc.edu/telmed/itfact.html

Jerant, A. F., Schlachta, L., Epperly, T. D., & Barnes-Camp, J. (1998). Back to the future: The telemedicine house call. *Family Practice Management, 5*(1), 20–29.

Jerome, L. (1997). E-mail therapy. *Journal of the American Academy of Child and Adolescent Psychiatry, 36,* 868.

Joint Commission on Accreditation of Healthcare Organizations. (1998). *Comprehensive accreditation manual for hospitals.* Oakbrook Terrace, IL: Author.

Joint Commission on Accreditation of Healthcare Organizations and the National Committee for Quality Assurance. (1998). *Protecting personal health information: A framework for meeting the challenges in a managed care environment.* Retrieved May 5, 2000, from the World Wide Web: http://www.jcaho.org

Joint Working Group on Telemedicine. (1998, January 6). *Report of the Interdisciplinary Tele-Health Standards Working Group.* Retrieved September 7, 2000, from the World Wide Web: http://www.arentfox.com/telemed/reports/telehlth.html

Jones, E. (1996, October). News uplink: Number crunching in Bosnia: Consults fall short. *Telemedicine Magazine.* Retrieved May 17, 2000, from the World Wide Web: http://www.telemedmag.com/

Jones, E. (1997, June). Global markets offer opportunity at a price. *Telemedicine and Telehealth Networks, 3*(3). Retrieved May 5, 2000, from the World Wide Web: http://www.telemedmag.com/

Jones, S. (1995). *CyberSociety: Computer-mediated communication and community.* Thousand Oaks, CA: Sage.

Jutras, A. J. (1959). Teleroentgen diagnosis made by means of videotape recording. *American Journal of Roentgentology, 82,* 1099–1102.

Jutras, A. J., & Duckett, G. (1957). Le radiodiagnostic ‡ distance: Tèlèfluoroscopie et cinèfluorographie [Remote x-ray diagnosis: Telefluoroscopy and kinescoping]. *Bulletin de l'Association des Medecins de Langue FranÂaise du Canada, 86,* 3–7.

Kane, B., & Sands, D. (1998). Guidelines for the clinical use of electronic mail with patients. *Journal of the American Medical Informatics Association, 5*(1), 104–111.

Karson, T. (2000, April). Visual integration: A new technology for the thinking physician. *MD Computing, 17*(2), 38–40.

Kassirer, J. (1995). The next transformation in the delivery of healthcare. *New England Journal of Medicine, 332,* 52–54.

Kerrigan, C. (1999). Trail blazer: Meeting the challenge of providing medical care to 750,000+ people: Maj. Gen. Nancy R. Adams, Commander, Tripler Army Medical Center. *Military Medical Technology, 3*(1), 16–18.

Kikuchi, H. (1999). Application development approach based on space technology. *Telemedicine Journal, 5,* 395–399.

Kincade, K. (1999, June). Telerehab project recasts home care. *Telehealth Magazine, 5*(3), 40.

Klein, N. (1999, Winter). Telehealth becomes new battleground: Psychiatry talks; HCFA listens. *AAP Advance,* p. 4.

Kobak, K. A., Taylor, L. H., Dottl, S. L., Greist, J. H., Jefferson, J. W., Burroughs, D., Mantle, J. M., Katzelnick, D. J., Norton, R., Henk, H. J., & Serline, R. C. (1997). A computer-administered telephone interview to identify mental disorders. *Journal of the American Medical Association, 278,* 905–910.

Koocher, G., & Morray, E. (1999). *Regulation of tele-psychology: A survey of state attorneys general.* Unpublished manuscript.

Koss, S. (2000a). *Health Insurance Portability and Accountability Act: Security standards: Implications for the health care industry.* Retrieved September 11, 2000, from the World Wide Web: www.ibm.com/solutions/healthcare/

Koss, S. (2000b). *Transaction standards: Implications for the health care industry.* Retrieved September 11, 2000, from the World Wide Web: www.ibm.com/solutions/healthcare/

Krosnick, J. A. (1999). Survey research. *Annual Review of Psychology,* pp. 537–567.

Krueger, R. A. (1988). *Focus groups: A practical guide for applied research.* Thousand Oaks, CA: Sage.

Kundel, H. (1986). Visual perception and image display terminals. *Radiologic Clinics of North America, 24*(1), 69–78.

Lamberg, L. (1997). Computers in psychiatry. *Journal of the American Medical Association, 278,* 799–801.

La Porte, R. E., Akazawa, S., Hellmonds, P., Boostrom, E., Gamboa, C., Gooch, T., Hussain, F., Libman, I., Marler, E., Roko, K., Sauer, F., & Tajima, N. (1994). Global public health and the information superhighway. *British Medical Journal, 308,* 1651–1652.

Larsen, A. (1999, July 12). Global security survey: Virus attack. *InformationWeek,* pp. 42–56.

Lavoie, F., Borkman, T., & Gidron, B. (1994). *Self-help and mutual aid groups: International and multicultural perspectives.* Binghamton, NY: Haworth Press.

Lazoff, M. (1997, December). EMR (in)security. *Medical Computing Today.* Retrieved May 3, 1999, from the World Wide Web: http://www.medical computingtoday.com/

Lee, J. K., Renner, J. B., Saunders, B. F., Stamford, P. P., Bickford, T. R., Johnston, R. E., Hsaio, H. S., & Phillips, M. L. (1998). Effect of real-time teleradiology on the practice of the emergency department physician in a rural setting: Initial experience. *Academic Radiology, 5*(8), 533–538.

Lee, R., Conley, D., & Preikschat, A. (2000, January 31). eHealth 2000: Healthcare and the Internet in the new millennium. *Wit Capital.* Retrieved September 5, 2000, from the World Wide Web: http://www.witcapital.com/

Lenoff, F. (Ed.). (2000). *State medical licensure requirements and statistics, 2000–2001.* Chicago: American Medical Association.

Levens, S. (1996). Video equipment testing: There's more to it than meets the eye. *Telemedicine and Telehealth Networks, 2*(11), 17–19.

Liebson, E. (1997). Telepsychiatry: Thirty-five years' experience. *Medscape Mental Health, 2*(7), 1. Retrieved November 15, 1997, from the World Wide Web: http://www.medscape.com

Lindberg, D.A.B., & Humphreys, B. L. (1995). Computers in medicine. *Journal of the American Medical Association, 273,* 1667–1668.

Lindberg, D.A.B., & Humphreys, B. L. (1998). Medicine and health on the Internet: The good, the bad, and the ugly. *Journal of the American Medical Association, 280,* 1303–1304.

Llewellyn, C. H. (1995). The role of telemedicine in disaster medicine. *Journal of Medical Systems, 19,* 29–34.

Lombard, M., & Ditton, T. (1997). At the heart of it all: The concept of telepresence. *Journal of Computer-Mediated Communication, 3*(2). Retrieved May 12, 2000, from the World Wide Web: http://www.ascusc.org/jcmc/vol3/issue2/lombard.html

Magaletta, P. R., Bartizal, D. E., & Pratsinak, G. J. (1999). Correctional telehealth. *Journal of Mental Health in Corrections Consortium, 44*(4), 4–5.

Magaletta, P. R., Fagan, T. J., & Ax, R. K. (1998). Advancing psychology services through telehealth in the Federal Bureau of Prisons. *Professional Psychology: Research and Practice, 29,* 543–548.

Maheu, M. (1997). Will online services for consumer self-help improve behavioral healthcare? *Behavioral Healthcare Tomorrow, 6*(6), 32–38.

Maheu, M. (1998). *Managing professional listservs.* Retrieved May 30, 2000, from the World Wide Web: http://telehealth.net/

Maheu, M. (1999a). Netiquette. *Selfhelp Magazine.* Retrieved May 5, 2000, from the World Wide Web: http://www.selfhelpmagazine.com/ppc/netpsy/netiquette.html

Maheu, M. (1999b, March 18). *Risk management in the retooling of healthcare.* Paper presented at the Behavioral Informatics Tomorrow conference, San Jose, CA. Retrieved May 16, 2000, from the World Wide Web: http://telehealth.net/articles/riskman3.html

Maheu, M. M. (2000a, Fall). The California Model for Psychotherapy Online (CAMPO): Suggestions for the ethical practice of behavioral e-health [Special issue]. *CAPP Bulletin*, pp. 2–10.

Maheu, M. (2000b). Telehealth: The furthering of psychology as a profession. *Independent Practitioner, 20*(1), 41–46.

Maheu, M., Callan, J., & Nagy, T. (1998). Call to action: Ethical and legal issues for behavioral telehealth including online psychological services. In S. Bucky (Ed.), *Comprehensive textbook of ethics and law on the practice of psychology.* Unpublished manuscript.

Maheu, M., & Gordon, B. (in press). Psychotherapy on the Internet: Legal, ethical and practice issues. *Professional Psychology: Research and Practice.*

Mahone, D. F., Tarlow, B., & Sandaire, J. (1998). A computer-mediated intervention for Alzheimer's caregivers. *Computers in Nursing, 16,* 208–216.

Mair, F., & Whitten, P. (2000). A systematic review of telemedicine patient satisfaction studies: Research which yields more questions than answers. *British Medical Journal, 320,* 1517–1520.

Mark, R. G. (1974). Telemedicine system: The missing link between homes and hospitals? *Modern Nursing Home, 32,* 39–42.

Marotta, R. E. (Ed.). (1986). *The Digital dictionary.* Bedford, MA: Digital Equipment Corporation.

Maxmen, J. S. (1977). Telecommunications in psychiatry. *American Journal of Psychotherapy, 32,* 450–456.

Mazmanian, P., McCue, M., Parpart, C. F., Marks, T. K., Fisher, E., Hampton, C., Krick, S., & Kaplowitz, L. (1996). Evaluating telemedicine [Abstract]. *International Conference on AIDS, 11,* 172.

McCarthy, P., Kulakowski, D., & Kenfield, J. A. (1994). Clinical supervision practices of licensed psychologists. *Professional Psychology: Research and Practice, 25,* 177–181.

McCormack, J. (1999). The top ten ways the Internet is changing health care I.T. *Health Data Management, 7*(12), 34–41.

McCue, M., Hampton, C., Marks, T. K., Fisher, E., & Parpart, C. F. (1997). The case of Powhatan Correctional Center/Virginia Department of Corrections and Virginia Commonwealth University/Medical College of Virginia. *Telemedicine Journal, 3,* 11–17.

McDonald, C., Overhage, M., Dexter, P., Blevins, L., Meeks-Johnson, J., Suico, J., Tucker, M., & Schadow, G. (1998). Canopy computing: Using the Web in clinical practice. *Journal of the American Medical Association, 280,* 1325–1329.

McLendon, K. (2000). E-commerce and HIM: Ready or not, here it comes. *Journal of the American Health Information Management Association, 71*(1), 22–23.

McLeod, S. (1998). The quality of medical information on the Internet: A new public health concern. *Archives of Ophthalmology, 116*(12). Retrieved May 5, 2000, from the World Wide Web: http://archopht.ama-assn.org/

Mehta, R., & Sivadas, E. (1998). Comparing response rates and response content in mail versus electronic mail surveys. *Journal of the Market Research Society, 37,* 429–439.

Mekhjian, H., Warisse, J., Gailiun, M., & McCain, T. A. (1996). An Ohio telemedicine system for prison inmates: A case report. *Telemedicine Journal, 2,* 17–24.

Mekhjian, H., Warisse, J., Turner, J., Gailiun, M., & McCain, T. A. (1999). Patient satisfaction with telemedicine in a prison environment. *Journal of Telemedicine and Telecare, 5,* 55–61.

Menduno, M. (1999, March 1). Net profits. *Hospitals and Health Networks.* Retrieved May 9, 2000, from the World Wide Web: http://www.hhnmag.com/

Menduno, M. (2000, January). Docs.com. *Hospitals and Health Networks.* Retrieved September 5, 2000, from the World Wide Web: http://www.hhnmag.com/

Menolascino, F., & Osborne, R. (1970). Psychiatric television consultation for the mentally retarded. *American Journal of Psychiatry, 127,* 157–162.

Microsoft announces Windows DNA for healthcare during annual Microsoft healthcare users group conference. (1999). Retrieved May 16, 2000, from the World Wide Web: http://www.microsoft.com/Industry/health/

Miller, D. (1996). Internet security: What health information managers should know. *American Health Information Management Association.* Retrieved May 5, 2000, from the World Wide Web: http://www.ahima.org/publications/

Mitchell, J. G., & Robinson, P. J. (2000, June). A multipurpose telehealth network for mental health professionals in rural and remote areas. *Telemedicine Today, 8*(3), 4–5.

Mitka, M. (1998). Developing countries find telemedicine forges links to more care and research. *Journal of the American Medical Association, 280,* 1295–1296.

Mitofsky, W. J. (1999). Pollsters.com. *Public Perspective,10*(4), 24–26.

Mittman, R., & Cain, M. (1999). *The future of the Internet in health care: Five-year forecast.* Menlo Park, CA: Institute for the Future. Retrieved May 16, 2000, from the World Wide Web: http://www.chcf.org/

Montgomery, J. (1997, November). *Broadband satellite systems stand ready to bring multimegabit data rates worldwide. Sounds great. What's the catch?* Retrieved May 5, 2000, from the World Wide Web: http://www.byte.com/

Montgomery, T. S. (1998). Distance healthcare education. *Telemedicine Today, 6*(5), 40–43.

Murphy, J. M., O'Hare, N. J., Wheat, D., McCarthy, P. A., Dowling, A., Hayes, R., Bowmer, H., Wilson, G. F., & Molloy, M. P. (1999). Digitized mammograms: A preliminary clinical evaluation and the potential for telemammography. *Journal of Telemedicine and Telecare, 5,* 193–197.

Murphy, R.L.H., & Bird, K. T. (1974). Telediagnosis: A new community health resource. *American Journal of Public Health, 64,* 113–119.

Murray, B. (1998, March). Data smog: Newest culprit in brain drain. *APA Monitor.* Retrieved May 5, 2000, from the World Wide Web: http://www.apa.org/monitor/

NASA satellite aids in Mexico City rescue effort. (1985). *NASA News*. Retrieved May 16, 2000, from the World Wide Web: http://www.nasa.gov/newsinfo/

NASA's telemedicine future: Terrestrial benefits. (1997). *Aerospace Technology Innovation, 5*(3). Retrieved May 5, 2000, from the World Wide Web: http://nctn.hq.nasa.gov/innovation/

National Committee for Quality Assurance. (1999). *2000 MCO surveyor guidelines*. Washington, DC: Author.

National Council of State Boards of Nursing. (1998). *Nurse licensure compact*. Retrieved May 5, 2000, from the World Wide Web: http://www.ncsbn.org/

National Research Council. (1997). *For the record: Protecting health information*. Washington, DC: National Academy Press.

National Research Council. (1999). Reinventing security. In F. B. Schneider (Ed.), *Trust in cyberspace*. Washington, DC: National Academy Press.

National Telecommunications and Information Administration. (1997, January 31). *Telemedicine report to Congress*. Retrieved September 7, 2000, from the World Wide Web: http://www.ntia.doc.gov/reports/telemed/

Navein, J., Arose, D., & Pietermich, A. (1999). A business model for telemedicine [Abstract]. *Journal of Telemedicine and Telecare, 5*, 76–78.

Net payoff. (1998, June 20). Retrieved May 9, 2000, from the World Wide Web: http://www.hhnmag.com

Nettleman, M. D., Olchanski, V., & Perlin, J. B. (1998). E-mail medicine: Dawn of a new era in physician-patient communication. *Clinical Performance and Quality Health Care, 6*, 138–141.

Newman, M. G. (1999). The clinical use of palmtop computers in the treatment of generalized anxiety disorder. *Cognitive and Behavioral Practice, 6*, 222–234.

Newman, M. G., Consoli, A., & Taylor, C. B. (1997). Computers in the assessment and cognitive-behavioral treatment of clinical disorders: Anxiety as a case in point. *Behavior Therapy, 28*, 211–235.

Newman, M. G., Kenardy, J., Herman, S., & Taylor, C. B. (1997). Comparison of cognitive-behavioral treatment of panic disorder with computer-assisted brief cognitive behavioral treatment. *Journal of Consulting and Clinical Psychology, 65*, 178–183.

New technologies breathe new life into the hospital communications equipment market. (1998). *Telemedicine and Virtual Reality, 3*(4), 41.

Newton, H. (1998). *Newton's telecom dictionary*. New York: Flatiron.

Next Generation Internet Initiative. (1999). *NGI overview*. Retrieved May 5, 2000, from the World Wide Web: http://www.ngi.gov/white-house/

Nickelson, D. (1998). Telehealth and the evolving health care system: Strategic opportunities for professional psychology. *Professional Psychology: Research and Practice, 29*, 527–535.

Nicogossian, A. (1989). *Final project report: U.S.-U.S.S.R. telemedicine consultation spacebridge to Armenia and Ufa*. Moscow: Joint Working Group on Space Biology and Medicine.

Nitzkin, J., Zhu, N., & Marier, R. (1997). Reliability of telemedicine examination. *Telemedicine Journal, 3,* 141–158.

Nua Internet Surveys. (1999, June). *How many online.* Retrieved May 5, 2000, from the World Wide Web: http://www.nua.ie/surveys/

Oberkirch, A. (2000, April). *Telepsychiatry in the management of five fragile patients: Improve quality and lower costs.* Paper presented at a symposium organized by the American Telemedicine Association, Phoenix, AZ.

O'Carroll, P. W. (1997). Beyond Odwalla: Epidemic investigation in an on-line world. *Washington Public Health, 15,* 40–43.

O'Conaill, B., & Whittaker, S. (1997). Characterizing, predicting, and measuring video-mediated communication: A conversational approach. In K. E. Finn, A. J. Sellen, & S. B. Wilbur (Eds.), *Video-mediated communication* (pp. 107–131). Mahwah, NJ: Erlbaum.

Office for the Advancement of Telehealth. (1999a). *Letter to the FCC: Comments on wireless medical telemetry service.* Retrieved May , 2000, from the World Wide Web: http://telehealth.hrsa.gov/

Office for the Advancement of Telehealth. (1999b, November). *Telehealth update: Future technology trends.* Retrieved May 5, 2000, from the World Wide Web: http://telehealth.hrsa.gov/

Office of Technology Assessment. (1995, September). *Bringing health care online: The role of information technologies* (Document No. OTA-ITC-624). Washington, DC: U.S. Government Printing Office. Retrieved May 5, 2000, from the World Wide Web: http://www.wws.princeton.edu/

Ong, K., Chia, P., Ng, W. L., & Choo, M. (1995). A telemedicine system for high-quality transmission of paper electrocardiographic reports. *Journal of Telemedicine and Telecare, 1,* 27–33.

Ota, D., Loftin, B., Saito, T., Lea, R., & Keller, J. (1995). Virtual reality in surgical education. *Computers in Biology and Medicine, 25,* 127–137.

Pasternack, A. (1998, July 20). www.Milwaukee.ER. *Hospitals and Health Networks.* Retrieved May 9, 2000, from the World Wide Web: http://www.hhnmag.com/

Pasveer, K. A., & Ellard, J. H. (1998). The making of a personality inventory: Help from the WWW. *Behavior Research Methods, Instruments, and Computers, 30,* 309–313.

Penk, W. E., Van Ormer, E. A., Osgood-Hynes, D., Ahern, D., Cukor, P., Baer, L., & Boyd, C. (1999, August 22). *Assessing patients in residential rehabilitation with Interactive Voice Response (IVR) technology.* Symposium conducted at the 107th annual meeting of the American Psychological Association, Boston.

Perednia, D. A., & Allen, A. (1995). Telemedicine technology and clinical applications. *Journal of the American Medical Association, 273,* 483–488.

Phillips, C. M., Burke, W. A., Schechter, A., Stone, D., Balch, D., & Gustke, S. (1997). Reliability of dermatology teleconsultations with the use of telecon-

352

ferencing technology. *Journal of the American Academy of Dermatology, 37,* 398–402.

Physician Insurers Association of America. (1996). *Telemedicine: An overview of applications and barriers.* Rockville, MD: Author.

Physician Insurers Association of America. (1998). *Telemedicine: A medical liability white paper.* Rockville, MD: Author.

Plastic surgery gets virtual reality test. (1997). *Telemedicine and Virtual Reality, 2*(1), 1.

Poitras, L. (1999). Telemedicine in a pediatric health network in Quebec. *Journal of Telemedicine and Telecare, 5*(Suppl. 1), 125–126.

Princeton Survey Research Associates. (1999). *Ethics survey of consumer attitudes about health Web sites.* Retrieved May 5, 2000, from the World Wide Web: http://ehealth.chcf.org/

Prussog, A., Muhlbach, L., & Bocker, M. (1994). *Telepresence in videocommunications.* Paper presented at the 38th annual meeting of the Human Factors and Ergonomics Society, Santa Monica, CA.

Puskin, D. S., Brink, L. H., Mintzer, C. L., & Wasem, C. J. (1997). Joint federal initiative for creating a telemedicine evaluation framework [Letter]. *Telemedicine Journal, 1,* 395–399.

Puskin, D. S., Mintzer, C. L., & Wasem, C. J. (1997). Telemedicine: Building rural systems for today and tomorrow. In P. F. Brennan, S. J. Schneider, & E. Tornquist (Eds.), *Information networks for community health.* New York: Springer.

Puskin, D. S., Morris, T., Hassol, A., Gaumer, G., & Mintzer, C. L. (1997). Patient and provider acceptance of telemedicine. *New Medicine, 1,* 55–59.

Rabasca, L. (1999, February). HCFA rejects telehealth payment for psychologists. *APA Monitor,* p. 27.

Rabinowitz, E. (1997). Correctional health care: Facilities look to reduce costs and improve the quality of inmate care. *Health Care Business Digest, 2*(11), 32–36.

Rauber, C. (1999, November). Disease management can be good for what ails patients and insurers. *Modern Healthcare,* pp. 48–54.

Reaser, J. (1999). New technologies and old issues: Using technology to enhance the elixir of discovery. *Psychologist-Manager Journal, 3*(2), 205–208.

Reents, S. (1999a, July). *Impacts of the Internet on the doctor-patient relationship: The rise of the Internet health consumer.* Retrieved May 16, 2000, from the World Wide Web: http://www.cyberdialogue.com/

Reents, S. (1999b, August). *Industry brief: Seizing the Internet health opportunity.* Retrieved September 5, 2000, from the World Wide Web: http://www.cyberdialogue.com/

Reents, S. (1999c, June). *The online health consumer: Unmet needs and opportunities.* Retrieved September 5, 2000, from the World Wide Web: http://www.cyberdialogue.com/

Reichertz, P., & Halpern, N. (1997). FDA regulation of telemedicine devices. *Food and Drug Law Journal, 52,* 517–523.

Reid, J. (1996). *A telemedicine primer: Understanding the issues.* Billings, MT: Innovative Medical Communications.

Rheingold, H. (1993). *The virtual community: Homesteading on the electronic frontier.* Reading, MA: Addison-Wesley.

Rhode, P., Lewinsohn, P., & Seeley, J. (1997). Comparability of telephone and face-to-face interviews in assessing Axis I and II disorders. *American Journal of Psychiatry, 154,* 1593–1598.

Rhodes, H. (1997). E-mail security. *Journal of the American Health Information Management Association, 68*(6). Retrieved May 5, 2000, from the World Wide Web: http://www.ahima.org/publications/

Rhodes, H. (1998). Electronic signatures (Updated). *Journal of the American Health Information Management Association, 69*(9). Retrieved May 5, 2000, from the World Wide Web: http://www.ahima.org/publications/

Rice, R. (1995). The Internet as a healthcare communication tool. *Telemedicine Today, 3*(1), 6–7, 27.

Rogelberg, S. G., & Luong, A. (1998). Nonresponse to mailed surveys: A review and guide. *Current Directions in Psychological Science, 7*(2), 60–65.

Rolnick, S., Owens, B., Botta, R., Sathe, L., Hawkins, R., Cooper, L., Kelley, M., & Gustafson, D. H. (1999). Computerized information and support for patients with breast cancer or HIV infection. *Nursing Outlook, 47*(2), 78–83.

Ruggiero, C. (1998). A teleradiology primer. *Telemedicine Today, 6*(6), 36–42.

Ruskin, P. E., Reed, S., Kumar, R., Kling, M. A., Siegel E., Rosen, M., & Hauser, P. (1998). Reliability and acceptability of psychiatric diagnosis via telecommunication and audiovisual technology. *Psychiatric Services, 49,* 1086–1088.

Rusovick, R., & Warner, D. (1998). The globalization of interventional informatics through Internet-mediated distributed medical intelligence. *New Medicine, 2,* 155–161.

Russo, H. (1999). *TIIAP supports innovations in health care.* Washington, DC: Telecommunications and Information Infrastructure Assistance Program, National Telecommunications and Information Administration.

Ryboski, L. (1998, July). *National health policy forum: Protecting the confidentiality of health information.* Washington, DC: George Washington University.

Salem, D. A., Bogat, G. A., & Reid, C. (1997). Mutual help goes online. *Journal of Community Psychology, 25,* 189–207.

Sampson, J. P., Jr. (1995). *Computer-assisted testing in counseling and therapy.* Greensboro, NC: ERIC Clearinghouse on Counseling and Student Services (Document No. ED 391 983).

Sampson, J. P., Jr., Kolodinsky, R. W., & Greeno, B. (1997). Counseling on the information highway: Future possibilities and potential problems. *Journal of Counseling and Development, 75,* 203–211.

Sanders, J. H., & Bashshur, R. L. (1995). Perspective: Challenges to the implementation of telemedicine. *Telemedicine Journal, 1,* 115–123.

Satava, R. M. (1995a, June). Medical applications of virtual reality. *Journal of Medical Systems, 19,* 275–280.

Satava, R. M. (1995b). Virtual reality, telesurgery, and the new world order of medicine. *Journal of Image-Guided Surgery, 1,* 12–16.

Satava, R. M. (1997). Telemedicine of the future: A pragmatic speculation. In R. L. Bashshur, J. H. Sanders, & G. W. Shannon (Eds.), *Telemedicine: Theory and practice* (pp. 393–405). Springfield, IL: Thomas.

Satcher, D. (1999, December 13). *Mental health report.* Washington, DC: Assistant Secretary for Health and Surgeon General's Office of Public Health and Science. Retrieved September 4, 2000, from the World Wide Web: http://surgeongeneral.gov/library/speeches/mentalhe.htm

Savas, S. D., Parekh, M., & Fisher, L. (1999, November 11). Health-e opportunities in e-health? *Goldman Sachs Investment Research,* p. 3.

Schanz, S. J. (1999a). Comprehensive Telehealth Act of 1999 introduced in Congress. *Telemedlaw, 4*(2), 8–9.

Schanz, S. J. (1999b). International telemedicine: Treaty on horizon? *Telemedlaw, 4*(3), 5–12.

Schanz, S. J. (1999c). *1999 compendium of telemedicine laws: Selected statute excerpts and article citations relating to telemedicine.* Raleigh, NC: Legamed.

Schlachta, L. (1998). Disease management via telehealth: Technology tools for the year 2005. In R. Nelson, T. Gelish, & S. Mun (Eds.), *Proceedings, Pacific Medical Technology Symposium.* Los Alamitos, CA: Institute of Electrical and Electronics Engineers Computer Society.

Schwartz, N. (2000, May 29). Dr. Koop and the greed disease. *Fortune,* pp. 156–163.

Sellen, A. (1995). Remote conversations: The effects of mediating talk with technology. *Human-Computer Interaction, 10,* 401–444.

Sentencing Project. (1995). *Americans behind bars: U.S. and international use of incarceration.* Retrieved May 16, 2000, from the World Wide Web: http://www.sentencingproject.org/

Sezeur, A. (1998). Surgical applications of telemedicine. *Annales de Chirurgie, 52*(5), 403–411.

Shellens, T., Jones, G., & Lang, J. (1999). A checklist for the lawyer. *Journal for Telemedicine and Telecare, 5*(Suppl. 1), 125.

Shields, R. (1996). *Cultures of the Internet: Virtual spaces, real histories, living bodies.* Thousand Oaks, CA: Sage.

Siden, H. B. (1998). A qualitative approach to community and provider needs assessment in a telehealth project. *Telemedicine Journal, 4,* 225–235.

Silberg, W. M., Lundberg, G. D., & Musacchio, R. A. (1997). Assessing, controlling, and assuring the quality of medical information on the Internet: *Caveat lector et viewor*—let the reader and viewer beware. *Journal of the American Medical Association, 277,* 1244–1245.

Siwicki, B. (1996). Network meets rural needs. *Health Data Management, 4*(5), 31–34.

Sleek, S. (1997, August). Providing therapy from a distance. *APA Monitor,* pp. 1–8.

Smith, H. A. (1998). Telepsychiatry. *Psychiatric Services, 49,* 1494–1495.

Smith, H. A., & Allison, R. A. (1998). *Telemental health: Delivering mental health care at a distance: A summary report.* Rockville, MD: Office for the Advancement of Telemedicine.

Smith, H. A., & Allison, R. A. (2000, April). *After five years of telemental health, what have we learned?* Paper presented at a symposium organized by the American Telemedicine Association, Phoenix, AZ.

Smith, M. A., & Leigh, B. (1997). Virtual subjects: Using the Internet as an alternative source of subjects and research environment. *Behavior Research Methods, Instruments, and Computers, 29,* 496–505.

Smithwick, M. (1995). Network options for wide-area telesurgery. *Journal of Telemedicine and Telecare, 1,* 131–138.

Solovy, A., & Serb, C. (1999, February 1). Health care's 100 most wired. *Hospitals and Health Networks.* Retrieved May 9, 2000, from the World Wide Web: http://www.hhnmag.com/

Spielberg, A. (1998). On call and online: Sociohistorical, legal, and ethical implications of e-mail for the patient-physician relationship. *Journal of the American Medical Association, 280,* 1353–1359.

Squibb, N. J. (1999). Video transmission for telemedicine. *Journal for Telemedicine and Telecare, 5,* 1–11.

Stamm, B. H. (1998). Clinical applications of telehealth in mental health care. *Professional Psychology: Research and Practice, 29,* 536–542.

Stamm, B. H. (2000). Shifting gears: Integrating models of telehealth and telemedicine into current models of mental health care. In L. G. Lawrence (Ed.), *Innovations in clinical practice* (Vol. 17). Sarasota, FL: Professional Resource Press.

Stamm, B. H., & Friedman, M. J. (2000). Cultural diversity in the appraisal and expression of traumatic exposure. In A. Shalev, R. Yehuda, & A. McFarlane (Eds.), *International handbook of human response to trauma* (pp. 69–85). New York: Plenum Press.

Stamm, B. H., & Pearce, F. W. (1995). Creating virtual community: Telemedicine and self-care. In B. H. Stamm (Ed.), *Secondary traumatic stress: Self-care issues for clinicians, researchers, and educators* (pp. 179–207). Lutherville, MD: Sidran Press.

Stamm, B. H., & Perednia, D. A. (2000). Evaluating psychosocial aspects of telemedicine and telehealth systems. *Professional Psychology: Research and Practice, 31,* 184–189.

Stanton, J. M. (1998). An empirical assessment of data collection using the Internet. *Personnel Psychology, 51,* 709–725.

Stoloff, P. H., Garcia, F. E., Thomason, J. E., & Shia, D. S. (1998). A cost-effectiveness analysis of shipboard telemedicine. *Telemedicine Journal, 4,* 293–304.

Straker, N., Mostyn, P., & Marshall, C. (1972). The use of two-way TV in bringing mental health services to the inner city. *American Journal of Psychiatry, 133,* 1202–1218.

Suler, J. (1998). Keeping record: The e-mail archive. *Self-Help and Psychology Magazine.* Retrieved May 5, 2000, from the World Wide Web: http://www.selfhelpmagazine.com/articles/

Sullivan, P., & Lugg, D. J. (1995). *Telemedicine between Australia and Antarctica, 1911–1995.* Warrendale, PA: Society of Automotive Engineers.

Sund, T. (1997). Digital pictures seen with new eyes: What digital pictures do that traditional films don't. *Telemedicine Today Buyer's Guide* [Special issue], pp. 26–36.

Swartz, D. (1998). The webification of information systems and the emergence of the Internet as the WAN of choice. *Telemedicine Today, 7*(1), 34–35.

Swinson, R. P., Fergus, K. D., Cox, B. J., & Wickwire, K. (1995). Efficacy of telephone-administered behavioral therapy for panic disorder with agoraphobia. *Behavior Research and Therapy, 33,* 465–469.

Swoboda, W. J., Muhlberger, N., Weitkunat, R., & Schneeweib, S. (1997). Internet surveys by direct mailing. *Social Science Computer Review, 15,* 242–255.

Teledesic overview. (1999). Retrieved September 20, 1999, from the World Wide Web: http://www.teledesic.com/about/over.htm

Telemedicine Development Act of 1996. (1996). Calif. S. B. 1665. Retrieved September 5, 2000, from the World Wide Web: http://www.arentfox.com

Thompson, J. M. (1997, January-February). The Telemedicine Development Act of 1996. *Sonoma County Physician,* pp. 22–24.

Thompson, J. M., Ottensmeyer, M. P., & Sheridan, T. B. (1999). Human factors in telesurgery. *Telemedicine Journal, 5,* 129–137.

Thrall, T. (1999, May 1). Marketing nets out. *Hospitals and Health Networks.* Retrieved May 16, 2000, from the World Wide Web: http://www.hhnmag.com/

Tieman, J. (2000, April 10). HIMSS preview: A sea of dot-coms. *Modern Healthcare.* Retrieved May 5, 2000, from the World Wide Web: www.modernhealthcare.com/

Tracy, J., McClosky, T., Sprang, R., & Burgiss, S. (1999). *Medicare reimbursement for telehealth: An assessment of telehealth encounters, January 1, 1999, to June 30, 1999.* Unpublished manuscript.

Trafton, C. E. (1999, July 2). Statistical abstracts of the United States. In *Healthcare industry report: Healthcare plays on the Internet.* New York: Adams, Harkness & Hill.

Troester, A. I., Paolo, A. M., Glatt, S. L., Hubble, J. E., & Koller, W. C. (1995). "Interactive video conferencing" in the provision of neuropsychological services to rural areas. *Journal of Community Psychology, 23,* 85–88.

Trott, P., & Blignault, I. (1998). Cost evaluation of a telepsychiatry service in northern Queensland. *Journal of Telemedicine and Telecare, 4,* 66–68.

Tschida, M. (1999, December). *Ethics online: Healthcare sites form alliances to create voluntary standards.* Retrieved May 5, 2000, from the World Wide Web: http://www.healthwise.org/Hi-EthicsHome.htm

Tufo, H. M., & Speidel, J. J. (1971). Problems with medical records. *Medical Care, 9,* 509–517.

Turkle, S. (1995). *Life on the screen: Identity in the age of the Internet.* New York: Touchstone.

Turner, D. J. (1996). Solo surgery—with the aid of a robotic assistant. *Journal of Telemedicine and Telecare, 2,* 46–48.

U.S. Department of Justice. (1999, March). *Telemedicine can reduce correctional health care costs: An evaluation of a prison telemedicine network.* Washington, DC: Abt Associates. Retrieved May 5, 2000, from the World Wide Web: http://www.ncjrs.org/

U.S. General Accounting Office. (1991). *Medical ADP systems: Automated medical records hold promise to improve patient care.* Washington, DC: Author.

U.S. General Accounting Office. (1999, February 24). *Medical records/privacy: Access needed for health research, but oversight of privacy protections is limited* (Publication No. B-280657). Washington, DC: Author. Retrieved May 5, 2000, from the World Wide Web: http://frwebgate.access.gpo.gov/

Wachter, G., & Grigsby, B. (1997). External vs. internal funding: Does it matter who pays the bills? *Telemedicine Today, 5*(1), 30–32.

Wallace, B. (1996). Savings in focus. *Computerworld, 30*(22), 57.

Waller, A., & Alcantara, O. (1998). Ownership of health information in the information age. *Journal of American Health Information Management Association, 69*(3), 28–38.

Weber, J., Yang, C., & Capel, K. (1999, July 12). The global 1000. *Business Week Online.* Retrieved May 9, 2000, from the World Wide Web: http://www.businessweek.com/

Weil, M., & Rosen, L. (1997). *TechnoStress: Coping with technology @work @home @play.* New York: Wiley.

Wellman, B. (1997). An electronic group is virtually a social network. In S. Kiesler (Ed.), *Culture of the Internet* (pp. 179–205). Mahwah, NJ: Erlbaum.

Wellman, B., & Gulia, W. (1995). *Communities in cyberspace.* Berkeley: University of California Press.

Wheeler, T. (1998). Corrections-based telemedicine programs top most-active list. *Telemedicine Today, 6*(3), 38–44.

Whitfield, D. (1988). The first ten years of public-key cryptography. *Proceedings of the IEE, 76,* 560–577.

Whiting, R. (2000, March 6). Mind your business. *InformationWeek,* p. 24.

Whittaker, S., & O'Conaill, B. (1997). The role of vision in face-to-face and mediated communication. In K. E. Finn, A. J. Sellen, & S. B. Wilbur (Eds.), *Video-mediated communication* (pp. 23–49). Mahwah, NJ: Erlbaum.

Whitten, P., & Allen, A. (1995). Analysis of telemedicine from an organizational perspective. *Telemedicine Journal, 1,* 203–213.

Whitten, P., Collins, B., & Mair, F. (1998). Nurse and patient reactions to a developmental home telecare system. *Journal of Telemedicine and Telecare, 4,* 152–160.

Whitten, P., Cook, D. J., Shaw, P., Ermer, D., & Goodwin, J. (1998). Telekid care: Bringing health care into schools. *Telemedicine Journal, 4,* 335–343.

Whitten, P., Cook, D. J., Swirczynski, D., Kingsley, C., & Doolittle, G. (1999, December). *School-based telemedicine: An empirical analysis of teacher, nurse, and administrator perception.* Paper presented at TeleMed99, London.

Whitten, P., & Franken, E. A. (1995). Telemedicine for patient consultation: Factors affecting use by rural primary care physicians in Kansas. *Journal of Telemedicine and Telecare, 1,* 139–144.

Whitten, P., Sypher, B. D., & Patterson, J. (2000). Transcending the technology of telemedicine: A case study of telemedicine in North Carolina. *Health Communication, 12*(2), 109–135.

Whitten, P., Zaylor, C., & Kingsley, C. (1999). An empirical analysis of the busiest telepsychiatry programs [Abstract]. *Telemedicine Journal, 5,* 51.

Whitten, P., Zaylor, C., & Kingsley, C. (2000). An analysis of telepsychiatry programs from an organizational perspective. *Cyberpsychology and Behavior, 3*(6).

Willemain, T. R., & Mark, R. G. (1971). Models of remote health systems. *Biomedical Sciences Instrumentation, 8,* 9–17.

Winker, M., Flanagin, A., Chi-Lum, B., White, J., Andrews, K., Kennett, R., De Angelis, C., & Musacchio, R. (2000, March). *Guidelines for medical and health information sites on the Internet.* Chicago: American Medical Association. Retrieved May 11, 2000, from the World Wide Web: http://www.ama-assn.org/about/guidelines.htm

Wittson, C. L., Afflect, D. C., & Johnson, V. (1961). Two-way television in group therapy. *Mental Hospitals, 12,* 22–23.

Wootton, R., Loane, M., Mair, F., Montray, M., Harrison, S., Sivananthan, S., Allen, A., Doolittle, G., & McLernan, A. (1998). The potential for telemedicine in home nursing. *Journal of Telemedicine and Telecare, 4,* 214–218.

World Health Organization. (1997, December 23). *Telehealth and telemedicine will henceforth be part of the strategy for health for all.* Geneva: Author.

Retrieved September 2, 1999, from the World Wide Web: www.who.int/archives/
inf-pr-1997/en/pr97-98.html

Xiao, Y., Mackenzie, C., Orasanu, J., Spencer, R., Rahman, A., Gunawardane, V., &
the Lotas Group. (1999). Information acquisition from audio-video-data
sources. *Telemedicine Journal, 5,* 139–155.

Zarate, C. A., Jr., Weinstock, L., Cukor, P., Morabito, C., Leahy, L., Burns, C., &
Baer, L. (1997). Applicability of telemedicine for assessing patients with
schizophrenia: Acceptance and reliability. *Journal of Clinical Psychiatry, 58,*
22–25.

Zaylor, C. (1999, February). Psychiatric patients prefer care provided via telemedicine technologies. *Telehealth Magazine, 5*(1), 15–18.

Zaylor, C. (2000, April). *Telepsychiatry services to a rural jail.* Paper presented at a
symposium organized by the American Telemedicine Association, Phoenix,
AZ.

Zaylor, C., Whitten, P., & Kingsley, C. (1999, December). *Telemedicine services to a
county jail.* Paper presented at Telemed99, London.

Zincone, L. H., Jr., Doty, E., & Balch, D. C. (1997). Financial analysis of telemedicine in a prison system. *Telemedicine Journal, 3,* 247–255.

SUBJECT INDEX

A

Access: to health care, with telehealth, 14; to health care information on Internet, 19; to medical records, by patients, 135; to patient information, with computerized patient records (CPRs), 130–131

Access control, 158

Accountability, identifying, as business plan step, 243–244

Administration: Internet support for, 19–20; telecommunication technology applied to, 12; telehealth as reducing costs of, 19

Advertising, for e-health sites, 227

Agency for Health Care Policy and Research (AHCPR), telehealth evaluation requirements of, 268

Alternative medicine, Web sites on, 117, 126–127

American College of Radiology (ACR), 72, 73, 75, 165; data integrity guidelines of, 165–166; telehealth standards of, 187

American Counseling Association (ACA), 188

American Health Information Management Association, 22

American Medical Association (AMA), 36, 85; on confidentiality, 147; information on computerized patient

records (CPRs) from, 133; medical malpractice definition of, 192; prescription guidelines from, 202; on privacy on Internet, 147; on telehealth licensure, 177–178; telehealth standards of, 187–188

American Medical Informatics Association, 22

American National Standards Institute (ANSI), document image capture standards from, 166

American Psychiatric Association, 198

American Psychological Association, 82, 258; Telephone Therapy Task Force, 78

American Telemedicine Association (ATA), 35, 92

Analog, 56

Application service providers (ASPs), 124–125; Web sites on, 329

Association for Information and Image Management (AIIM), document image capture standards from, 166

Asymmetric DSL (ADSL), 55, 57–59

Asynchronous communication, 49–50, 51

Asynchronous transfer mode (ATM), 54, 57–59

Audioconferencing, 15

Audit trails, 161, 162

Authentication, 154, 159–160

B

Backbone networks, 54

Bandwidth, 7; as consideration in selecting transmission equipment, 52–53; and transmission time, 50

Behavioral health care, 76–90; cost-effectiveness of, 90; e-mail and chat rooms for, 80–82; ethical concerns in, 85–89; organizational considerations in, 89–90; services offered in, 76; telephone as technology for, 77–79, 82–83; utilization of, 76–77; videoconferencing technology for, 80, 82–85; virtual reality psychotherapy for, 291–292; Web site on, 331

Behaviorial health care, computer-assisted self-help programs for, 79

Biomedical Sensors, 288

Biosensors, 287–290

Bit depth, 63

Bits, 53

Branding, by e-health companies, 227–228

Broadband ISDN (B-ISDN), 54

Browser, 20

Business: forms of, for marketing e-health, 43–46; as interested in e-health, 31–32

Business plan: as element of evaluation plan, 265; steps in developing, 216–217

C

Cable modems, 55, 57–59

California Healthcare Foundation, 132, 152

California Healthline, 206

California Telehealth Initiative, 10

California Telehealth/Telemedicine Coordination Project, 91, 223

California Telemedicine Development Act of 1996, 179, 180

Caregivers, benefits of telehealth for, 16

Center for Clinical Computing and Sapient Health Network, 29

Center for Devices and Radiological Health (CDRH), 182, 183

Center for Telemedicine Law (CTL), 176

Charge-coupled device (CCD), 60

Chat rooms, 12, 80–82

Children's Memorial Hospital (Chicago) Telecardiology Project, 10

Children's Online Privacy Protection Act of 1999, 174

Click stream data, 36

Clinical Context Manager, 143

Clinical practice: basic, and risk management, 205; telecommunication technology applied to, 12; Web sites on, 117, 122–125. *See also* Professional practice; *specific areas of specialty*

Coaxial cable, 55

Codec, 60

College of Americn Pathologists (CAP), telehealth standards of, 188

Commission on Accreditation of Rehabilitation Facilities (CARF), security requirements of, 155

Compatibility, 66

Competence: multilingual and multicultural, 207; and risk management, 199–200

Compression. *See* Data compression

Computed radiography (CR), 63

Computer Science and Telecommunications Board, 160

Computer-assisted self-help programs, for behavioral health care, 79

Computer-Based Patient Record Institute (CPRI), 160, 161, 174

Computerized information systems, history of, in health care industry, 129–130

Computerized patient records (CPRs): benefits of, 130–132, 143–144; confidentiality of, 22, 132–133; data mining of, 136–138; device for personal storage of, 273–274; and e-health, 133; health information management (HIM) professionals' role with, 140–143; identifiers used with, 139–140; multiple provider use of,

138–140; ownership of, 133–135; privacy of, 147; reusing and reselling information from, 136; security of, 132, 155, 157, 206; software for managing, 143; Web sites on, 329. *See also* Personal medical records (PMRs)

Concepts, 257–258

Confidentiality, 20, 147–154; of computerized patient records (CPRs), 22, 132–133; data, 148; defined, 146, 147; of e-mail, 149–150, 213; factors influencing maintenance of, 148–149; laws on, 174; proposals for maintaining, of patient information on Internet, 153–154; and risk management, 208; with telecommunication technology, 22. *See also* Privacy

Consent agreements, 203–205

Constructs, 258

Consultants: as resource consideration in business plan, 236–237; Web sites on, 327. *See also* Teleconsultation

Consumer protection: with behavioral health care, 81; for privacy of information on e-health Web sites, 36–37, 147, 149–153; for quality and accuracy of health care information on Internet, 34–36

Consumers, transformation of patients into, 32–33

Continuing education: for risk management, 208; telehealth provision of, 15; via Internet, 118–120. *See also* Training

Cookies, and Web sites, 151

Copyright Act of 1976, 170–171; security requirements of, 155

Correctional facilities:
telehealth in, 100–105

advantages of, 100–102; cost-effectiveness of, 102–104; example of, 104–105; Web site on, 330

Cost-effectiveness: of behavioral health care, 90; of computerized patient record (CPR) systems, 131; of tele-

health administration, 19; of telehealth in correctional facilities, 102–104; of telehealth in military settings, 107–108; of telehealth in schools, 112; of telehealth technology use, 275; of telehealth for tribal communities, 109–110; of telehome care, 92–93; of teleradiology, 76. *See also* Costs

Costa Rican Foundation for Sustainable Development, 279

Costs: forecasting, for e-health and telehealth startups, 244–245, 248; incorrect media report of, of telemedicine services, 297–298; of telecommunication technology, as barrier to adoption, 25. *See also* Cost-effectiveness

Credentialing, telehealth, 183–185. *See also* Licensure

Cryptography, 159

Cyber Dialogue, Inc., 30

D

Data compression, 7, 64

Data confidentiality, 148

Data integrity, 165–167; American College of Radiology guidelines on, 165–166; defined, 146; document image capture standards for, 166

Data mining, 136–138

Dedicated connections, 52

Dedicated lines, 20

Department of Health and Human Services (DHHS). *See* U.S. Department of Health and Human Services (DHHS)

Dial-up services, 52

Digital image: in PACS, 72; in teleradiology, 74–75

Digital Imaging and Communications in Medicine (DICOM), 63, 75

Digital subscriber line (DSL), 55, 57–59

Digitization, 7

Disaster assistance, early telemedicine efforts for, 5–6

Disease management, telehome care programs for, 96–98

Documentation: as evaluation step, 266; as risk management technique, 205

Downlinks, 49, 55

Drugs. *See* medications

E

E-care, 42

E-health: business's interest in, 31–32; categories of Web sites for, 115–127; changes in health care environment facilitated by, 32–34; and computerized patient records (CPRs), 133; defined, 3–4, 27; distinction between telehealth, telemedicine and, 4, 28; five C's of services of, 4, 115; future benefits of, 282–284; future challenges for, 284–287; and Internet, 29–31, 281–282; marketing of, 42–46; privacy and confidentiality of information in, 149–154; research on, 269–272. *See also* E-health companies

E-health companies: business plan for, 216–217; challenges in starting, 233–235; forecasting costs for, 248; identifying funding sources for, 248–250; lessons from early, 232; personnel of, 229–232; retention of consumers by, 226–229

E-mail: as behavioral health care technology, 80–82; for patient support groups, 37; for practitioner contact with colleagues, 40–41; for practitioner-patient communication, 37–40; privacy and confidentiality of, 149–150, 213; risk management with, 211–213; security of, 39, 213; as training tool, 41

Education: patient, Web sites for, 117, 118; practitioner, Web sites for, 117, 118–120; telecommunication technology applied for, 12–13. *See also* Continuing education; Training

Efficiency, e-health as contributing to, 33–34

Electronic medical records. *See* computerized patient records (CPRs)

Electronic signatures, 154, 161

Employer Identification Numbers (EINs), 139, 140

Encryption, 64, 159–160

Equipment: general telemedicine, 63–65; medical, Web sites for, 121–122; for radiology, 62–63; as resource consideration in business plan, 235–236; for transmission, 52–59; for videoconferencing, 60–62

Ernst & Young LLP, 43

Error reduction, with computerized patient record (CPR) systems, 131

Ethics, 185–190; in behavioral health care, 85–89; e-health organization guidelines for, 188–190; key issues involving, 185–186; professional association standards for, 186–188; for working with research participants, 258

Evaluation: categories of, 264; creating plan for, 263–267; elements of plan for, 264–266; federal government requirements for, 267–268; principles for designing research for, 256–261; problems encountered in, 266; and program funding, 261–262; Web sites on, 327. *See also* Research

Extranets, 163–164

F

Federal government: evaluation requirements of, 267–268; telehealth funding by, 245–246; telehealth regulatory bodies of, 181–183; telemedicine funding by, 6–7, 8–10; Web sites of, 327

Federal Trade Commission (FTC), 155, 174

Federation of State Medical Boards (FSMB): telehealth licensing legislation developed by, 177; telehealth standards of, 188

Feedback, mechanisms for, in business plan, 53

Fees, and risk management, 207

Fetal health monitoring system (FHMS), 288

Fiber optics, 48

Firewalls, 154, 163–164

Focus groups, for needs assessment, 222–223

Frame rate, 60

Funding: for e-health startups, 248–250; for early telemedicine programs, 6–7, 8–10; internal or state-initiated, 11; and program evaluation research, 261–262; renewed, of telemedicine projects, 7, 8–9; for telehealth projects, 11, 245–248; Web sites on, 327

G

Georgetown University, Health Privacy Project, 152

Geostationary satellites, 6, 277, 278

Geosynchronous satellites, 56

Globalization, of health care delivery, 280

Goals, in business plan, 217–218, 250

Graphics, Visualization and Usability Center (GVU), 146

Guardian Angel, 273–274

H

Harris Poll, 44

Health Care Financing Administration (HCFA), 23, 142, 180, 181; evaluation requirements of, 267

Health care information: access to, on Internet, 19; quality and accuracy of, on Internet, 34–36; as transforming patient into consumer, 32–33; Web sites offering, 117, 118. *See also* Health information

Health care organizations: business opportunities for, with telehealth, 18; future benefits of e-health for, 284

Health care professionals. *See* Practitioners

Health information, defined, 135–136. *See also* Health care information

Health information management (HIM) professionals, role of, with computerized patient records (CPRs), 140–143

Health insurance, Web sites on, 117, 125–126

Health Insurance Portability and Accountability Act (HIPAA), 142, 171–174; compliance with, 173–174; and confi-

dentiality, 148–149, 174; on privacy, 173; security standards of, 155, 172; standard identifiers outlined in, 139–140; transaction standards of, 172; vendor accountability requirements of, 213, 214

Health Internet Ethics (Hi-Ethics), 189

Health on the Net (HON), 189–190

HealthSat satellites, 6

Home care. *See* Telehome care

Hub hospitals, 11–12

Hypotheses, 257

I

Identifiers: standard, 139–140; universal patient, 162–163

Information technology (IT), 141

Informed consent, 21

Institute for the Future, 30, 42

Institute of Medicine (IOM), 5, 13, 22, 24, 49, 148, 162, 176, 177, 184, 193, 195, 196, 245, 256, 261, 264–266, 267, 308

Integrated services digital network (ISDN), 53–54, 57–59

Intel Corp., 44

Intelligent agent software systems, 283

IntelliHealth, 32

Interactive televideoconferencing (ITV). *See* Videoconferencing

International Bar Association, Section on Legal Practice, 178

International settings, telehealth projects in, 10–11, 113–115

International Telecommunications Union (ITU), 280

Internet, 2; audio services through, 49; characteristics of, advantageous for e-health, 29–31; demographics of users of, 30; future of, and e-health, 281–282; growth of, 30–31; integrated e-health services using, 41–42; privacy and confidentiality of e-health information on, 149–154; solutions to health care problems offered by, 19–20; video transmission using, 62. *See also* E-mail; Web sites

Internet Healthcare Coalition (IHC), 188–189

Internet Tools, 10

Internet2, 281–282

Interstate Nurse Licensure Compact, 177, 188

Intranets, 146, 163

J

Joint Commission on Accreditation of Healthcare Organizations (JCAHO), 161, 174, 184; credentialing standards of, 184–185; security requirements of, 155, 161

Joint Working Group on Telemedicine (JWGT), 89; establishment of, 9; evaluation goals of, 267; telehealth regulation by, 181–182, 183

Jurisdiction: for licensure, 175; for malpractice, 197–198

K

Kennedy-Kassenbaum Act. *See* Health Insurance Portability and Accountability Act (HIPAA)

L

Legal information, Web sites for, 328

Legislation: on telehealth reimbursement, 179–181, 243, 295; on telehealth security and confidentiality issues, 169–174. *See also specific laws*

Licensure, telehealth, 175–179; by states, 21, 176; human factor in, 178–179; international approach to, 178; interstate, 175; national approach to, 177–178; and risk management, 200–201. *See also* Credentialing

Listservs, for professional discussions, 328–329

Local area networks (LANs), 20

Lotas Group, 24

Low earth orbit (LEO) satellites, 6, 56, 277

Luminance, 74–75

M

Malpractice, 192–198; and collegial relationships, 196–197; defined, 192; jurisdiction for, 197–198; and practitioner-patient relationship, 192–196; with telecommunication technology, 22–23

Malpractice insurance, and risk management, 201

Marketing: of e-health, 42–46; product, Web sites for, 116, 117

Massachusetts Institute of Technology (MIT), Guardian Angel technology of, 273–274

Master patient index, 131

Mbps (megabits per second), 54

Medicaid, reimbursement by, for telehealth services, 181

Medical equipment, Web sites on, 117, 121–122

Medical Information Protection Act (MIPA), 174

Medical records: ownership of, 134–135; personal (PMRs), 33; Web sites on, 329. *See also* Computerized patient records (CPRs)

Medical Records Confidentiality Act of 1995, 171

Medical Records Institute, 133

Medicare, reimbursement by, for telehealth services, 180, 295

Medications: risk management with, 202; Web sites on, 117, 120–121

Mental health care. *See* Behavioral health care

Mentoring, 197

Metasites, 116–118

Microsoft Announces, 286

Microwave links, 52, 56

Military settings, telehealth in, 105–109; advantages of, 105–107; cost-effectiveness of, 107–108; sample projects for, 108–109; Web sites on, 330

Minors, parental consent when working with, 208

Mission, organizational, and business plan, 217–218

Modems, 37; cable, 55, 57-59
Multiplexing, 54

N

"NASA Satellite," 6
"NASA's Telemedicine Future," 288, 289
National Aeronautics and Space Administration (NASA): biosensor development by, 288–289; telemedicine development by, 5–6
National Committee for Quality Assurance (NCQA), 174, 184, 202, 203, 205, 210
National Council of State Boards of Nursing, licensing standards of, 177, 188
National Electrical Manufacturers Association (NEMA), 75
National Provider Identifers (NPIs), 139–140
National Provider System, 140
National Research Council (NRC), 146, 147, 159, 160, 162, 165
National Standard Employer Identifiers. *See* Employer Identification Numbers (EINs)
National Telecommunications and Information Administration (NTIA), 89, 146, 187, 188
Needs assessment: as business plan step, 218–220; focus groups for, 222–223; information on, 225
Net payoff, 29
"New Technologies," 351
Newsgroups, 151
Next Generation Internet (NGI), 281–282
Nonrepudiation services, 161
Norwegian Telemedicine Project, 11
Nova Scotia Telehealth Initiative, 10
Nua Internet Surveys, 31, 146
Nursing, Web sites on, 330

O

Office for the Advancement of Telehealth (OAT), 30, 280, 283; on benefits of telehome care, 91–92; establishment of, 9–10
Office functions, Web sites on, 117, 123–125

Office of Rural Health Policy, 225, 245, 267
Office of Technology Assessment, 132, 139, 171, 209
Optum, 163–164
Organizational structure: designing, in business plan, 237–243; referral patterns component of, 241–242; reimbursement component of, 242–243; scheduling component of, 241; staffing component of, 239–241

P

Packets, 54
Parental consent, when working with minors, 208
Pathology, Web sites on, 331
Patient information: data mining of, 136–138; nonidentifiable, 136–138; reuse and resale of, 136; risk management when releasing, 205–206. *See also* Computerized patient records (CPRs); Medical records
Patients: acceptance of telecommunication technology by, 23–24; access to medical records by, 135; consent agreements by, 203–205; e-mail communication with, by practitioners, 37–40; e-mail support groups for, 37; future benefits of e-health for, 283; information and support for, with telehealth services, 15–17; as owners of medical records, 134–135; relationship between practitioners and, 192–196; risk management considerations related to, 203–207; transformed into consumers, 32–33; Web sites for education of, 117, 118
Peer review, and risk management, 202–203
Peripherals, 60
Personal medical records (PMRs), 33. *See also* Computerized patient records (CPRs)
Personal status monitor (PSM), 288
Personnel. *See* Staff
Physician Insurers Association of America, 23, 199

Picture archiving and communications system (PACS), 72, 262
Pixels, 60
Plain old telephone service (POTS). *See* Telephone
Planning. *See* Business plan
"Plastic Surgery," 292
Point-to-point data transfer, 29
Practitioners: acceptance of telecommunication technology by, 23–24; collegial relationships of, 40–41, 196–197; e-mail communication by, 37–41; future benefits of e-health for, 283–284; integrated Internet services for, 41–42; as owners of medical records, 134; relationship between patients and, 192–196; risk management considerations related to, 199–203; Web sites for education of, 117, 118–120
Prescriptions. *See* Medications
Princeton Survey Research Associates, 162
Prisoners. *See* Correctional facilities
Privacy, 146–147; defined, 146; of e-mail communication, 39; Health Insurance Portability and Accountability Act (HIPAA) on, 173; of information on e-health Web sites, 36–37, 147, 149–153. *See also* Confidentiality
Privacy Act of 1974, 142, 170; security requirements of, 155, 170
Product marketing, Web sites for, 116, 117
Professional associations: and ethical standards, 186–187; exemplary, 187–188; exemplary e-health, 188–190; Web sites of, 331–332
Professional practice: concerns about telecommunication technology in, 21–24; listservs for, 328–329. *See also* Clinical practice
Protocols, 29
Providers. *See* Practitioners
Psychiatry. *See* Behavioral health care
Psychology. *See* Behavioral health care
Public health, telehome care programs for, 95
Publications, Web sites of, 332

R

Radiology. *See* Teleradiology
Real-time transmission, 11
Referral patterns, as consideration in designing organizational structure, 242
Reimbursement: as area of concern for telehealth, 23; as consideration in designing organizational structure, 242–243; as future challenge for e-health, 286–287; telehealth, legislation on, 179–181, 243, 295
Remote medical instruments, 12
Research: approvals required before conducting, 206; on e-health, 269–272; general principles for designing, 256–261; major types of, 256–257; qualitative vs. quantitative approach to, 259, 261; steps in, 257–261; on telemedicine, 268–269; validity of, 260; Web sites on, 327–328. *See also* Evaluation
Resolution, 53, 75
Resources: annual report on, 253; consultants as, 236–237; equipment as, 235–236; identifying, as business plan step, 229–237; improved distribution of, with telehealth, 17; personnel as, 229–232; transmission channels as, 236
Risk management, 198–214; with e-mail, 211–213; organizational considerations for, 209; patient-related considerations for, 203–207; practitioner-related considerations for, 199–203; staff training for, 207–209; technological considerations for, 209–211; with vendors, 213–214
Ruiz v. Texas, 100

S

SatelLife/HealthNet program, 6
Satellites: downlinks from, 49, 55; early telemedicine efforts using, 5–6; as future wireless technology, 277–279; geostationary, 6, 277, 278; geosynchronous, 56; LEO, 6, 56, 277; as transmission technology, 56, 57–59; uplinks from, 55

Scheduling, in designing organizational structure, 241–242

Schools, telehealth in, 110–113; cost-effectiveness of, 112; sample programs for, 110–111, 112–113

Security, 20, 154–165; assessing needs for, 156–157; of computerized patient records (CPRs), 132, 155, 157, 206; defined, 146; of e-mail communication, 39, 213; Health Insurance Portability and Accountability Act (HIPAA) standards for, 155, 172; recommended approaches to, 157–165; and risk management, 206, 210–211; Web sites on, 333

Self-help programs, computer-assisted, 79

Senior care, telehome care programs for, 93–94

Sentencing Project, 100

Smart cards, 160, 290–291

Space Bridge to Russia, 6, 10

Staff: as consideration in designing organizational structure, 238–241; as resource consideration in business plan, 229–232. *See also* Training

Standards: of care, and risk management, 201–202, 208; ethical, 186–190; for images in teleradiology, 75; security, 172; transaction, 172; for videoconferencing, 280

STARPAHC (Space Technology Applied to Rural Papago Health Care), 5

State governments, telemedicine licensure by, 176–178

Store-and-forward (S&F) technologies, 8, 49–50

Strategic partners, selecting, 223–225. *See also* Vendors

Support: for patients and families, 15–16, 37; technical, from vendors, 68–70

Switched 56, 54, 57–59

Switched network, 54

Synchronous communication, 48–49, 51

T

T-1, 55–56, 57–59

Target audience, identifying, 229–232

Technical support, from vendors, 68–70

Technology: adopting new, 297; of future, 287–294; and risk management, 209–211; Web sites on, 333. *See also* Telecommunication technology

Telecommunication technology: asynchronous, 49–50, 51; benefits of, 13–20; as changing health care industry, 2; considerations in selecting vendor for, 65–70; cost-effectiveness of using, in health care, 275; effects of applications of, in health care system, 12–13; history of, in health care, 4–11; issues of concern in adopting, 21–25; for radiology, 62–63; for reception, 60–62; synchronous, 48–49, 51; for transmission, 52–59; wireless, 275–279

Teleconsultation, 21–22, 56

Teledermatology, 50

Teledesic Overview, 278

Telehealth: benefits of, 14–19; current activities for, 10–11; distinction between e-health, telemedicine and, 3, 4, 28; as evolving behavior, 297; legislation on security and confidentiality in, 169–174; reimbursement for, 179–181, 242–243, 295; typical model for, 11–12. *See also* Telehealth projects; Telemedicine

Telehealth Improvement and Modernization Act of 2000, 180, 243

Telehealth projects: business plan for, 216–217; challenges in starting, 220–222; in correctional facilities, 100–105; forecasting costs for, 244–245; funding of, 11, 245–248; in international settings, 10–11, 113–115; lessons from early, 218–220; in military settings, 105–109; in schools, 110–113; in tribal settings, 109–110

Telehome care: clinical applications of, 91–92; cost-effectiveness of, 92–93; defined, 90–91; sample programs for, 93–98; Web sites on, 330

Telemammography, 73–74

Telemedicine: defined, 2; distinction between e-health, telehealth and, 3, 4, 28; early examples of, 2–3; funding of programs for, 6–7, 8–10; general equipment for, 63–65; lessons from early programs for, 218–220; origin of, 4–7; positive experiences with, 298–302; renaissance of, 7–9; research on aspects of, 268–269; Web sites on, 327–328, 330. *See also* Telehealth

Telementoring, 13

Telemetry, 3

Telemonitoring: equipment for, 64; virtual reality (VR) technology for, 291

Telephone: as behavioral health care technology, 77–79, 82–83; as synchronous communication, 48–49; as transmission technology, 53, 57–59; videophones, 61

Telepresence, 83

Teleradiology, 11, 50, 72–76; clinical applications of, 72–74; cost-effectiveness of, 76; defined, 72; distinction between PACS and, 72; equipment for, 62–63; image resolution in, 74–75; standards for images in, 75; utilization of, 75; Web sites on, 331

Telesurgery, 292–294

Televillage, 17

Texas Department of Criminal Justice, telehealth project of, 104–105

Texas, Ruiz v., 100

Timeline, project, in business plan, 250–251

Training: as area of concern for telehealth, 23; e-mail as tool for, 41; for risk management, 207–209. *See also* Continuing education

Transmission channels, 52–59; considerations in selecting, 52–53; dedicated connections for, 52; dial-up services for, 52; overview of, 57–59; as resource consideration in business plan, 237; technologies used for, 53–59; terminology used with, 56

Tribal communities, telehealth in, 109–110; cost-effectiveness of, 109–110; sample programs for, 110

TRUSTe, 189

Tunneling, 20, 163

Turnkey, 61

Twisted pair, 55

U

Uniform Electronic Transactions Act (California), 161

Universal patient identifiers, 162–163

Uplinks, 55

U.S. Department of Health and Human Services (DHHS), 22, 136, 140, 155, 158, 161, 198; Joint Working Group on Telemedicine (JWGT) set up by, 9; Office for the Advancement of Telehealth (OAT), set up by, 9–10

U.S. Department of Justice, 101

U.S. Food and Drug Administration (FDA), telehealth regulation by, 35, 181–183

U.S. General Accounting Office (GAO), 131, 146

V

Variables, 258

Vendors: agreements with, 303–304; considerations in selecting, 65–66; risk management with, 213–214; sample, 304–305; technical support from, 68–70; tips on working with, 66–68. *See also* Strategic partners

Videoconferencing: adopted throughout organization, 296–297; as behavioral health care technology, 80, 82–85; equipment for, 60–62; etiquette for, 313; international standards for, 280; joint liability with, 196; patient-practitioner relationship with, 193–194; risk management with, 209; room requirements for, 307–313; as synchronous communication, 49; telemedicine programs using, 7–8; telepresence with, 83; Web sites on, 333

Videophones, 61
Videotapes: and malpractice, 195–196; risk management when storing, 206
Virtual communities, 228
Virtual private networks (VPNs), 158–159, 163, 164
Virtual reality (VR), 291–292
Voice recognition, 41 [bf]

W

Web sites: best, 327–333; and cookies, 151; e-health categories of, 115–127; privacy and confidentiality of information on e-health, 36–37, 147, 149–153; quality of health care information on, 34–36. *See also* Internet
Whiteboarding, 60, 85
Wide area network (WAN), 20, 29
Wireless technologies, 275–279; barriers to, 279; satellites as, 277–279; as transmission technologies, 56, 57–59
World Health Organization, 3
World Trade Organization (WTO), 280

NAME INDEX

Brown, N., 11, 73, 77
Brown, S. G., 5
Brown-Beasley, M. W., 78
Bruckman, A., 37, 194
Bruderman, I., 79
Brunicardi, B. O., 103
Burdick, A. E., 91, 106
Burgiss, S., 89
Burke, W. A., 23
Burkle, F., 6, 10, 106, 107
Burns, C., 87
Burroughs, D., 78

C

Cain, M., 281, 284, 287
Cairncross, F., 281
Callan, J., 88, 186, 192, 194
Cameron, K, 268
Campbell, D. T., 260
Capel, K., 31
Caramella, C., 269
Carey, K., 79
Carpenter, J., 196, 198, 206
Carrington, C., 282, 283
Carroll, E. T., 162, 198
Casella, N., 35
Casey, D., 130, 131, 141
Cepelewicz, B., 22, 136, 179, 180, 185, 198, 285
Chan, C. L., 80, 98
Cheriff, A. D., 292
Chi-Lum, B., 147
Chia, P., 268
Chin, T., 36
Choo, M., 268
Civello, C., 156, 157, 158
Clark, V. A., 78
Collins, B., 92, 93, 94
Collins, J., 308, 312, 313
Conley, D., 4, 45
Consoli, A., 79
Cook, D. J., 76, 112, 113
Cook, L. T., 269
Cook, T. D., 260
Cooley, A. G., 5
Cooper, L., 98

Cooper, T., 161
Cordts, P., 293
Cox, B. J., 78
Cox, G. C., 269
Cox, R., 17, 66, 221, 253, 295
Coy, P., 271
Coyle, J. T., 83
Croweroft, J., 85
Crowther, J. B., 107
Cukor, P., 78, 79, 82, 83, 87, 90, 194
Cullen, D., 131
Cunningham, N., 3
Curtis, C., 141

D

Dakins, D., 104, 105, 225, 286
Davis, G., 161
Davis, S., 252, 295
Day, S. X., 84
De Angelis, C., 147
De Leon, P. H., 9, 76, 176, 179
De Nelsky, S. J., 44
Della Mea, V., 38
Dertouzos, M., 13, 274, 284
Detmer, D., 131
Dexter, P., 42, 131
Dick, R., 131
Diepgen, T., 39, 283
Dishman, E., 45
Doarn, C. R., 6
Docimo, S. G., 292
Doolittle, G., 92, 93, 269
Dottl, S. L., 78
Doty, E., 102
Dowling, A., 74
Drysdale, K., 268
Duckett, G., 3, 73
Dwyer, S. J., 74
Dyson, E., 150

E

Ellard, J. H., 79
Eng, T., 114
Epperly, T. D., 97
Ermer, D., 76, 112, 113
Evans, R. L., 78
Eysenbach, G., 39, 283

F

Fagan, T. J., 102
Falconer, J., 50
Fenig, S., 78
Fenton, S., 141
Fergus, K. D., 78
Ferguson, E. W., 6
Ferguson, T., 194, 284
Fernandes, L., 130, 131, 141
Fiddleman, R., 155, 160
Fisher, E., 102, 103, 265
Fisher, L., 4
Fisk, N. M., 268
Fitzmaurice, J. M., 268
Flanagan, R., 224, 233, 240
Flanagin, A., 147
Fletcher, D., 130, 131, 141, 184
Folen, R. A., 76
Fox, H. R., 78
Frank, R. G., 9, 176, 179
Franken, E. A., 242, 264
Franses, A., 86
Frerichs, R. R., 78
Friedman, M. J., 220
Friedman, R. H., 79
Fuchs, M., 3, 5
Furdick, E., 131

G

Gailiun, M., 15, 18, 101, 103, 221, 247
Gamboa, C., 113, 114
Garcia, F. E., 107, 264
Garner, P., 268
Garnier, A., 234
Garshnek, V., 6, 10, 106, 107, 109
Gaumer, G., 23, 24, 239
Gershon-Cohen, J., 5
Gibson, S., 76
Gidron, B., 37
Gilbert, F., 149, 150, 171, 174
Gillespie, G., 121
Glatt, S. L., 87
Glazer, E., 3
Glueckauf, R. L., 52, 82, 84, 87
Godin, P., 34

Gold, M. H., 227, 233, 240
Goldberg, A. I., 92
Goldman, J., 152, 153
Goldstein, D., 142, 155, 227
Gooch, T., 113, 114
Goodwin, J., 76, 112, 113
Gordon, B., 38, 81, 88, 179, 186, 285
Gore, A., 295
Graber, M. A., 34
Graham, C., 86
Granade, P. F., 157
Grant, K., 130, 131, 141
Gray, C. L., 14, 104, 105
Graziano, F., 80, 98
Greenberg, C., 270
Greene, J., 122
Greeno, B., 285
Greist, J. H., 78
Grigsby, B., 11, 77, 245, 246
Groves, R. M., 271
Guard, R., 35
Gulia, W., 194
Gunawardane, V., 24
Gustafson, D. H., 80, 98, 114
Gustke, S., 23

H

Haas, L. J., 78, 82
Habash, T., 194
Hagel, J., III, 228
Hall, T. J., 269
Halpern, N., 182
Hampton, C., 102, 103, 265
Harris, G., 63, 94
Harrison, S., 93
Haspel, M. B., 44
Hassell, L., 6, 10, 109
Hassol, A., 23, 24, 239
Haugh, R., 227
Hauser, P., 23
Hawkins, R., 56, 80, 98, 310
Hawthorn, E., 155, 160
Hayes, R., 74
Hellmonds, P., 113, 114
Henk, H. J., 78
Henriques, A. I., 78

Herman, S., 79
Hickey, M., 131
Hipkins, J. H., 102
Hodges, J., 68, 70, 309, 313
Hollenbeck, A., 271
Holt, M., 275, 285, 287
Honeyman, J. C., 74
House, A. M., 7
Hsaio, H. S., 73
Hubble, J. E., 87
Hubbs, R. P., 34
Hudson, M., 84
Hudson, Z., 152, 153
Hufford, B. J., 84
Huling, T., 100
Humphreys, B. L., 130
Hussain, F., 113, 114

I

Ierdme, L., 109
Impicciatore, P., 35
Insana, M. F., 269

J

Jaffrey, F., 17
Jefferson, J. W., 78
Jenike, M. A., 83
Jenkins, D. P., 91, 106
Jennings, F. L., 76
Jerant, A. F., 97
Jerome, L., 80
Jette, A., 79
Johnson, V., 3, 5
Johnston, R. E., 73
Jones, E., 104, 105, 106, 225, 280
Jones, G., 195
Jones, G. G., 293
Jones, K., 155, 160
Jones, S., 37
Jutras, A. J., 3, 5, 73

K

Kaeble, B., 34
Kain, J., 84
Kane, B., 22, 38, 198, 199, 284

Kaplowitz, L., 103, 265
Karp, W. B., 16, 67, 112, 113, 221, 237, 251, 297
Karson, T., 143
Kassirer, J., 15
Katzelnick, D. J., 78
Kavoussi, L. R., 292
Kazis, L. E., 79
Keller, J., 291
Kelley, M., 98
Kenardy, J., 79
Kenfield, J. A., 76
Kennett, R., 147
Kenwright, M., 86
Kerrigan, C., 109
Kikuchi, H., 283
Kincade, K., 291
Kingsley, C., 76, 89, 230, 269
Kleefield, S., 131
Klein, N., 242
Kling, M. A., 23
Kobak, K. A., 78
Kobos, J. C., 78, 82
Kohn, R., 78
Koller, W. C., 87
Kolodinsky, R. W., 285
Komoroski, K., 92
Koocher, G., 183, 186
Kormylo, T., 112, 113
Koss, S., 172, 173
Krick, S., 103, 265
Kriese, G. E., 224
Krosnick, J. A., 271
Krueger, R. A., 223
Kulakowski, D., 76
Kumar, R., 23
Kundel, H., 74
Kuperman, G. J., 17
Kuraitis, V., 234

L

La Porta, A. J., 293
La Porte, R. E., 113, 114
Laird, N., 131
Lam, E., 44

Thrall, T., 119
Tieman, J., 44
Torgerson, J., 79
Trabin, T., 124
Tracy, J., 89
Trafton, C. E., 31, 32
Troester, A. I., 87
Trott, P., 90
Tschida, M., 189
Tsukahara, C., 234, 228
Tucker, M., 42, 131
Tufo, H. M., 131
Tullman, G., 234, 240
Turkle, S., 37, 194
Turner, D. J., 293

V

Van Ormer, E. A., 79
Vanden Bos, G. R., 9, 176, 179
Vander, M., 131
Vogelgesang, S., 84

W

Wachter, G., 245, 246
Wallace, B., 103
Waller, A., 131, 133, 134, 135, 136, 139, 285
Warisse, J., 101, 103
Warner, D., 285
Wasem, C. J., 17, 66, 265, 267
Webb, P. M., 84
Weber, J., 31
Weil, M., 24, 285
Weinstock, L., 87
Weiss, M., 224, 240
Weitkunat, R., 271
Wellman, B., 37, 194
Werkhoven, W. S., 78
Wheat, D., 74
Wheatley, V., 130, 131, 141
Wheeler, T., 50, 55, 75, 105
White, J., 147

Whitfield, D., 159
Whiting, R., 36
Whittaker, S., 83, 194
Whitten, P., 76, 89, 93, 94, 112, 113, 226, 230, 237, 242, 251, 262, 264, 269
Whitton, J. D., 52, 82, 84, 87
Wickwire, K., 78
Wiederhold, B., 291–292
Wiggins, J. G., 76
Willemain, T. R., 3
Willis, D. J., 76
Willis, S., 78, 82, 83, 90
Wilson, G. F., 74
Winker, M., 147
Winter, T., 130, 131, 141
Withers, M., 78, 82, 83, 90, 194
Wittson, C. L., 3, 5
Wolf, M., 92
Wooton, R., 268
Wootton, R., 93
Wright, D., 84
Wright, S., 162, 198
Wyant, J., 148
Wyatt, J. C., 38

X

Xiao, Y., 24

Y

Yang, C., 31
Yelin, N., 78
Yellowlees, P., 18, 68, 222, 238, 253, 301
Yokopenic, P. A., 78
Youngblood, B., 14, 104, 105

Z

Zakoworotny, C., 162, 198
Zarate, C. A., Jr., 87
Zaylor, C., 76, 89, 194, 230, 269
Zhu, N., 23
Zincone, L. H., Jr., 102